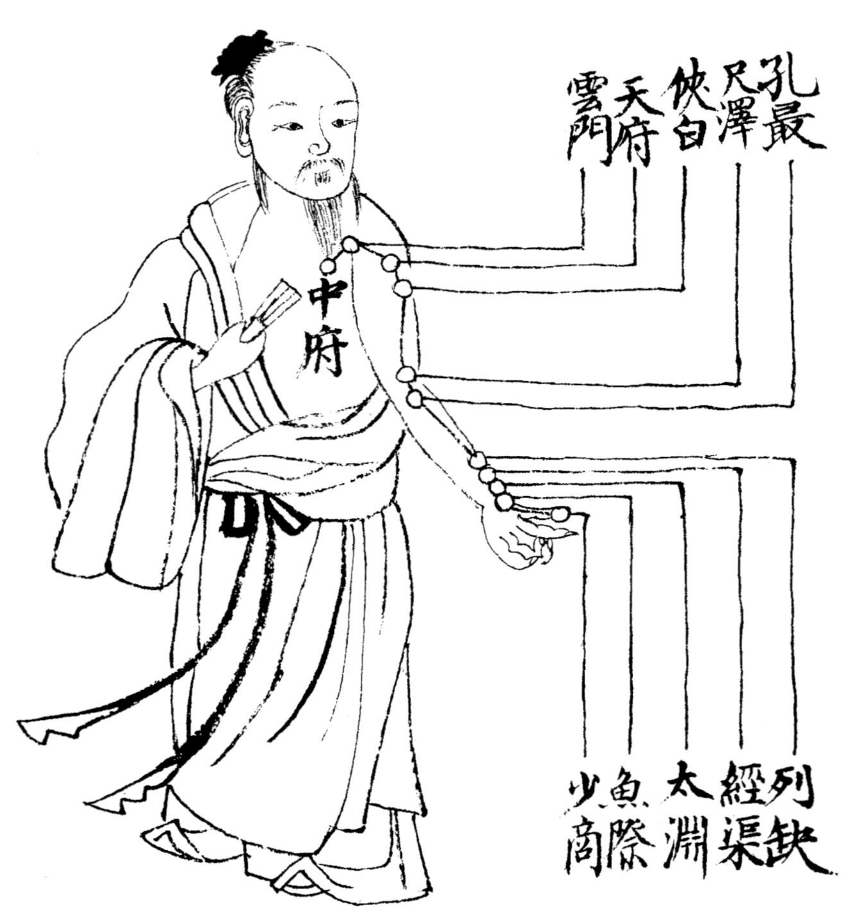

孔最
尺澤
俠白
天府
雲門
中府
列缺
經渠
太淵
魚際
少商

Paul U. Unschuld

# Medicine in China

## Historical Artifacts and Images

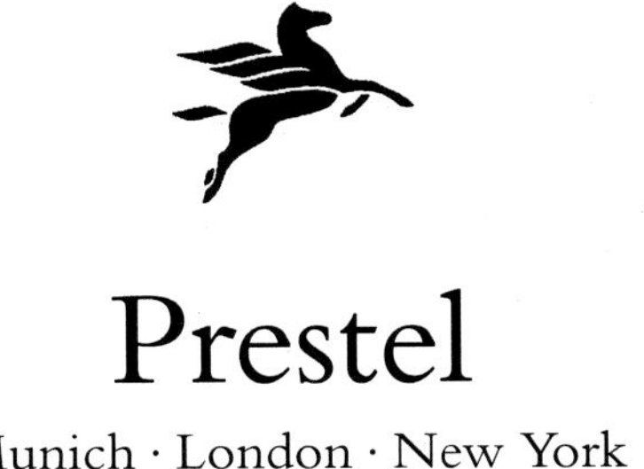

## Prestel

Munich · London · New York

Front cover: Pharmacy delivery containers (see plate 88)
Back cover: "The Foot Bright Yang Conduit of the Stomach"
Private medical handbook, undated manuscript (see plate 19)
Frontispiece: "The Hand Great Yang Conduit of the Lung"
Unpublished manuscript

Editorial direction by Daniela Küster, Munich
Translated from the German by Sabine Wilms, Texas
Copyedited by Courtenay Smith, Munich

© Prestel Verlag, Munich · London · New York, 2000

Library of Congress Catalog Card Number: 99-63867

Photo credits: The photos for the works illustrated come from
the picture archive of the Preussischer Kulturbesitz SMB, Berlin
(plates, pp.121-216); the Bodleian Library, Oxford (p.104 bottom);
H. Roger Viollet, Paris (p.114 right); Roger-Viollet (Boyer-Viol-
let), Paris (p.50 top); Roger-Viollet (Collection Viollet), Paris
(p.76); Roger-Viollet (Harlingue-Viollet), Paris (p.74 bottom);
and The Wellcome Centre for Medical Science, London (p.106)

Prestel Verlag
Mandlstrasse 26 · 80802 Munich
Tel. +49 (89) 381-7090, Fax +49 (89) 381-70935

175 Fifth Avenue · New York, NY 10010
Tel. +1 (646) 602-8616, Fax +1 (646) 602-8639

4 Bloomsbury Place · London WC1A 2QA
Tel. +44 (171) 323-5004, Fax +44 (171) 636-8004

Prestel books are available worldwide.
Please contact your nearest bookseller or one of the above Prestel
offices for details concerning your local distributor.

Typography by Dr. Hu Bo, Munich
Lithography by Gerber Satz, Munich
Printed and bound by Schoder Druck, Gersthofen

Printed in Germany on acid-free paper

ISBN 3-7913-2149-8

# Contents


THE HISTORY OF MEDICINE IN CHINA: AN OVERVIEW
Preliminary remarks    7
Theoretical Foundations of Traditional Chinese Medicine and its Cultural Environment    9
"Western" Medicine in China    16

THE LITERATURE OF TRADITIONAL CHINESE MEDICINE AND PHARMACEUTICS
The Mawangdui Texts as the Starting Point for Medical Literature in China    19
Pharmaceutical Literature    23
Formulary Literature    24
Literature of Medical Theory    30

THE CHINESE PHARMACY
Drug Use and Chinese Pharmacology    42
Pharmacies: Historical Testimonies    48
Equipment and Containers    50
Dates and Names of Chinese Pharmacies    51
Mass-Produced Drugs and Marketing    54

THE CHINESE PHYSICIAN, HIS PATIENTS AND HIS INSTRUMENTS
Medical Training and Social Standing of Physicians in China before the Twentieth Century    62
Medical Officials and Palace Physicians    63
Medical Scholars and Scholar Physicians    64
Criticism of Physicians and Ethical Maxims    68
Itinerant Doctors    73
The Instruments of Traditional Chinese Medicine    82

MEDICINE, HEALING, AND POPULAR RELIGION
The Tang Period Physician Sun Simiao: From Healer to Medicine God    88
Other Metaphysical Helpers and Acts of Assistance    95

CHINESE MEDICINE IN ART AND LITERATURE
Medicine and Art in Europe and China    97
Examples of Medicine and Art in China    99
Illustrations in Medical Literature    101
Medicine as a Topic in Literature, Drama, and Film    107
Chinese Medicine through European Eyes    110

PLATES
Literature    120
Teaching  Charts for Acupuncture    135
Advertising    142
Processing and Storage of Medicinal Drugs in Pharmacies    150
The Delivery Containers of Pharmacies    162
Therapeutic Instruments    191
Magic, Religion, and Art    199

CHRONOLOGICAL CHART    217

INDEX    218

Dedicated to Irml Mensdorff-Pouilly who opened my eyes to the beauty of Chinese artifacts three decades ago.

# THE HISTORY OF
# MEDICINE IN CHINA:
# AN OVERVIEW

## PRELIMINARY REMARKS

The theoretical content and clinical application of Chinese medicine have attracted attention in Europe since the seventeenth century.[1] In 1682, the German physician Andreas Cleyer published the first translation (into Latin) of a medical text from China as well as his own findings, which he had gained during his service for the Dutch East India Company in Batavia.[2] Although the interest in Chinese medicine, and especially in the therapeutic technique of needling (so-called acupuncture), never subsided completely over the course of the following three centuries, a systematic investigation of the history, the theoretical foundations, and, particularly, the practical applicability of Chinese medicine has only begun in the recent past.

One difficulty lies in the definition of the term "Chinese medicine", which can carry very different meanings and therefore be misunderstood.

First, "Chinese medicine" is referred to as the historical reality of a multi-layered, dynamic medical tradition which developed over the course of the past three millennia from magical and religious beginnings—constantly incorporating new ideas and findings while simultaneously retaining older beliefs—and which was, with greater or lesser degrees of alteration, adopted by China's neighboring countries—Japan, Korea, and, Vietnam. The theoretical and practical reality of this medicine in the tenth century differed from that of the first century and, likewise, the nineteenth century from that of the tenth century.

Second, the term "Chinese medicine" covers the contents of the relevant literature from the People's Republic of China (PRC) as well as the daily reality of traditional Chinese medicine as practiced there. A type of "Chinese medicine"

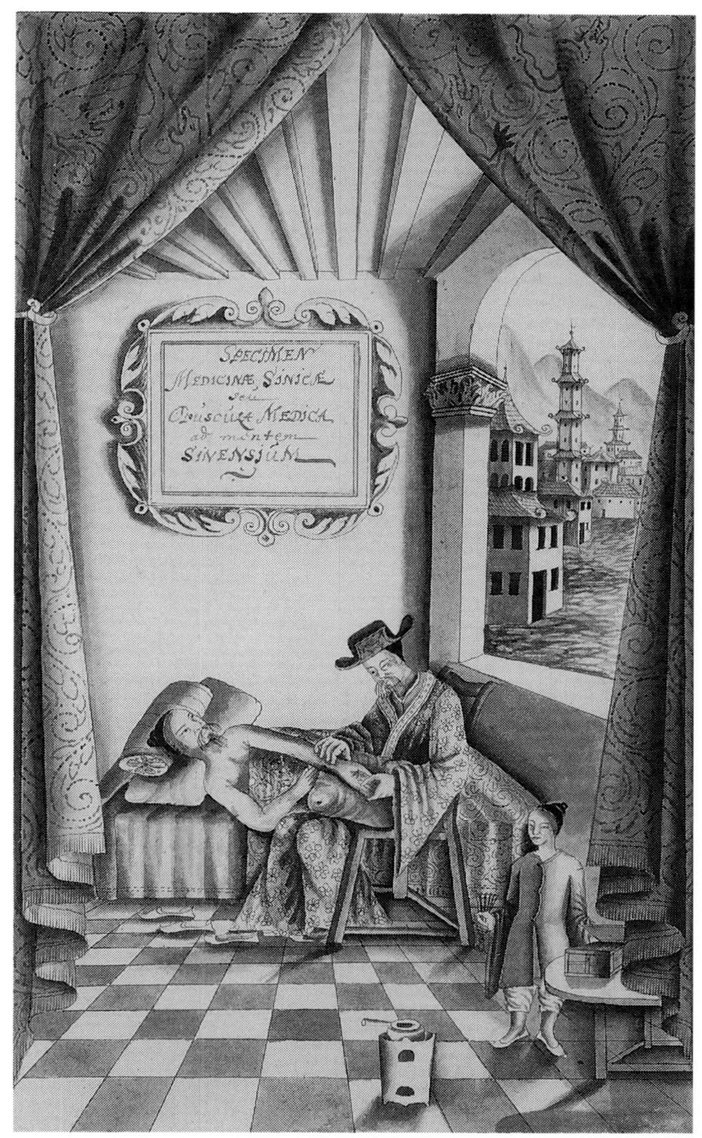

1. A Chinese doctor feels the pulse of his patient. In the foreground on the right, an assistant has readied needles for acupuncture. A stove indicates that a medicinal decoction may be prepared. Frontispiece of the *Specimen Medicinae Sinicae sive Opuscula Medica ad mentem Sinensium* by Andreas Cleyer, 1682. Staatsbibliothek, Berlin.

was developed in the PRC in the 1950s in contrast to "Western" medicine and as an alternative to it, and which at the same time has abandoned all of the traditional aspects of Chinese healing that appear to the authorities to be no longer justifiable on the grounds of materialistic and scientific criteria.

Third, numerous European and American writers and clinicians use the term "Chinese medicine" to describe their interpretations of traditional Chinese medicine based on their training with Chinese, Japanese, Vietnamese, Ceylnese, European, or American teachers as well as on their own sometimes different understandings arising from personal experience.

Finally, it should be pointed out that, about 150 years ago, the scientifically oriented medicine of Europe found entry into China, and that it dominates medical care there today. In recent decades, Chinese physicians and scientists have made important contributions to the development of "Western" medicine; these also should be regarded as a component of "Chinese medicine" today.

At present, research has not yet been done on broad areas of the history of medicine in China prior to the twentieth century or on the acceptance of what in China is called "Western medicine". Only a few of the roughly thirteen thousand medical texts which have been composed in China over the past two millennia, and which are still available in libraries and private collections, have been translated into Western languages. Even the question of converting traditional Chinese medical terminology into Western terms has not been settled; a standardized system of German or English equivalents agreed upon by all translators of Chinese medical texts does not yet exist. Thus, our knowledge of Chinese medicine cannot be compared to the body of literature concerning the history of Western medicine and should be regarded as preliminary.

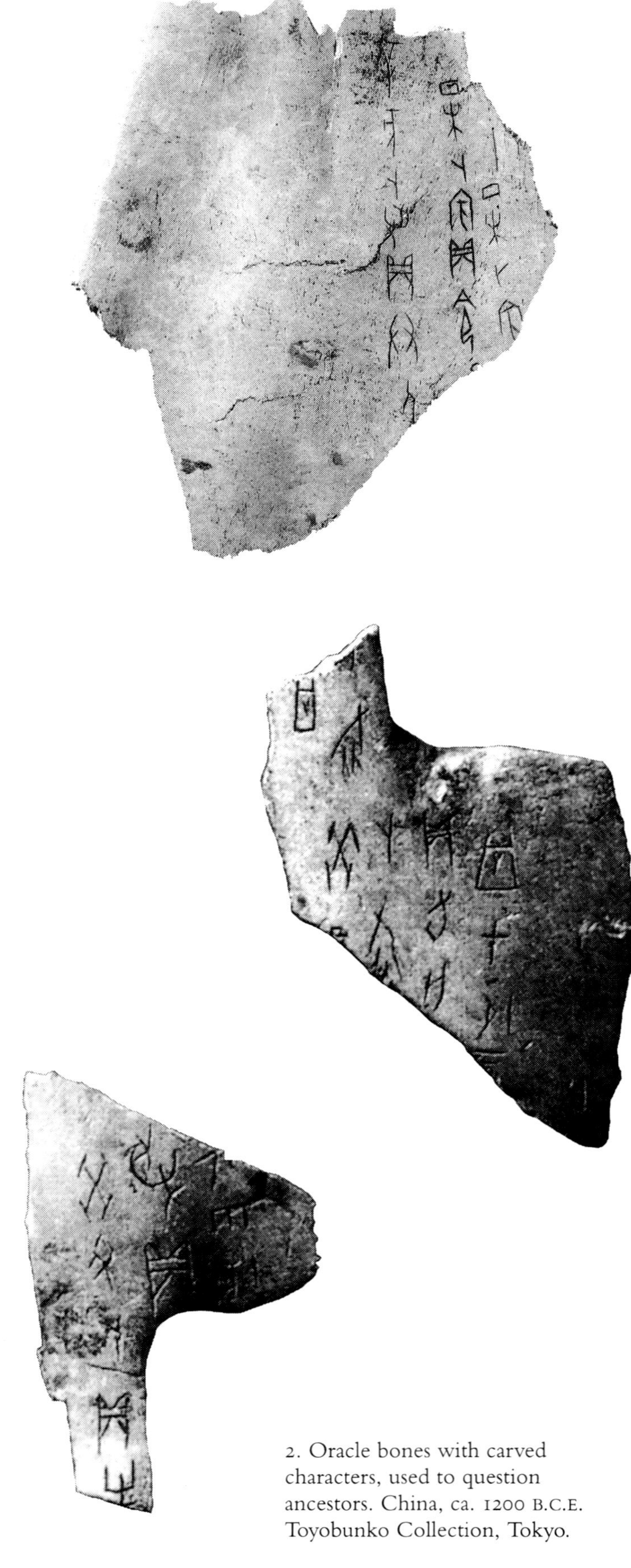

2. Oracle bones with carved characters, used to question ancestors. China, ca. 1200 B.C.E. Toyobunko Collection, Tokyo.

## I. Ancestral Healing

The oldest Chinese records of a systematic procedure against misfortune (systematic in the sense of being legitimated by an explanatory set of ideas) date from the eleventh century B.C.E. We can deduce from these records, in the form of divinatory inscriptions on tortoise shells and animal bones, that early Chinese healers were not yet cognizant of the distinctions between different forms of misfortune which seem so self-evident today. Apparently it was thought that individual physical afflictions stemmed from the same causes as other types of misfortune that affected the entire community. A crisis in the relationship between the living members of the community and their still present, but no longer living, ancestors could lead to stomach or tooth ache as well as to failure in military conflicts, a drought, or a bad harvest. Therefore, curing such misfortunes did not require an expert whose attention was focused solely on the body or on some other limited arena of human suffering. Ancestral healing was socially conceived and was concerned only with restoring harmony between living and non-living members of a community. Both two groups had rights and obligations, the observance or non-observance of which determined fortune and misfortune.

It appears that, at least in the pre-scientific period of healing and medicine in China, the symbolism of the natural and social environment time and again played a decisive role in the formulation of notions about health and illness. Until the recent past, clear relationships could be pointed out between the origin, nature, correct treatment, and appropriate prevention of physical and psychological suffering of an individual on the one hand and social crises on the other. However, for two-and-a-half thousand years China consisted of a heterogeneous society, in which various groups with different social realities coexisted and thus also internalized divergent conceptions of crisis and harmony. Hence, it should not be surprising that a traditional Chinese medicine in the sense of a homogenous system of ideas with corresponding therapeutic practices did not exist until the twentieth century.

Traditional Chinese medicine refers, therefore, to a broad spectrum of partly contradictory beliefs about illness and health which extends from magical, religious, and demonological etiologies to insights which could have grown out of experiences incomprehensible to us today (such as large areas of materia medica, but also massage and blood-letting) and scientific discoveries.

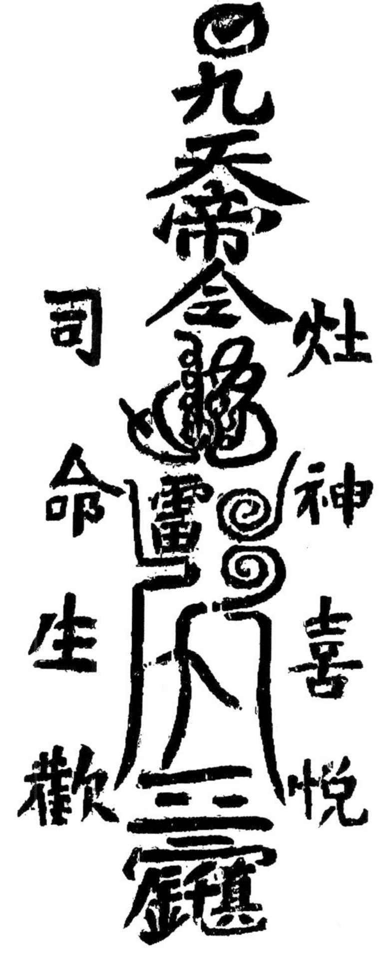

3. Demonological, exorcistic formula for the Command of the Ruler of the Nine Heavens to suppress a now unidentifiable disaster. The altogether eight characters on the right and left sides state: "The Stove God is in a cheerful mood; the Director of Fate gives pleasure." Since Chinese antiquity, there has been the belief that the Stove God ascends to heaven once a year in order to report on the good and bad deeds of the members of the household in whose stove he resides. Heaven sends down good or bad fortune accordingly. Print from a nineteenth- or early twentieth-century wood-block.

The history of Chinese medicine is not so much a succession of ever newer theoretical explanatory models and corresponding practical therapies, but rather a constant enrichment of already existing knowledge. The notion of progress, at least as an ideal, which has determined the history of medicine in the West—whereby previous knowledge is considered to be obsolete and discarded as it "progresses"—is viewed in China as an amplification of knowledge in which old views are never considered to be outdated and are continuously updated. Chinese culture seems to have hesitated to a greater extent than that of the West to commit periodically to a very specific explanatory model which could serve, for a time, as the sole basis for truth and truth-finding.

## II. Medicine and Demonism

The above-mentioned ancestral healings of the Chinese Shang period (17th–11th centuries B.C.E.) may have been supplemented with practical knowledge from areas such as pharmaceutics, but in available sources such empirical practices appeared much later, since the middle of the last millennium B.C.E. By that time, a new conceptual system—demonologically based medicine—had emerged that, although not obliterating ancestral healing, pushed it to second rank. In contrast to ancestral healing, demonologically based medicine was not rooted in the conviction that harmony between the living and the non-living members of society was possible. Demonism was based on the notion that, alongside the living, there existed a host of usually malevolent demons—believed to be former human souls—that, unlike the ancestors, could no longer be assigned to specific living humans within a familial relationship. Accordingly humans were constantly threatened by these demons and had to protect themselves in order to avoid numerous kinds of afflictions.

The transition from ancestral healing to demonism coincided with basic political transformations in China. Struggles over the succession to the throne in the eighth century and an ensuing instability of power led to centuries of increasingly brutal warfare during which formerly valid ethical norms for legislating the relations between rulers and their states as well as the conduct between individual humans were annulled. Over this long period of turmoil, when the survival of individuals depended mostly on their ability to protect themselves from external attacks via alliances with third parties or the strengthening of their own defenses, a health care system which based individual and collective well-being on similar criteria also gained plausibility.

Talismans were created to announce to the invisible, but potential demonic attackers, the powerful spirits with which their holders were aligned. If the attackers did not disappear immediately, exorcistic spells were cast to explain to those demons, who had penetrated an individual's body and were causing illness, the rapidity with which superior

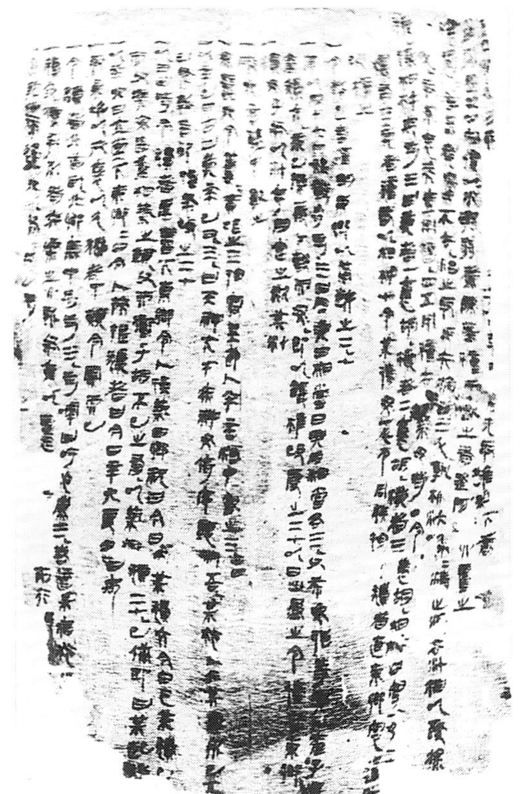

4. Excerpts from the Mawangdui textual fragment *Formulas for 52 Illnesses* (*Wushier bingfang* 五十二病方). Ink on silk, ca. 167 B.C.E.

powers would strike them if they did not disappear immediately. Medicinal substances which may have been therapeutically effective even before the emergence of the belief in demons were integrated into this paradigm and regarded as demon-killers, as was the practice of inserting needles into areas of the body where pain or swelling indicated the residence of a demon.

In the early 1970s, archaeologists discovered a funerary complex from 168 B.C.E., known as Mawangdui, near the city of Changsha in the central Chinese province of Hunan. Besides many other items, they found fourteen medical texts which provide a fairly precise record of the transformations which occurred in medicine towards the end of the Zhou period (1122–221), during the Qin dynasty (221–206), and at the beginning of the Han period (206 B.C.E.–220 C.E.), namely in the late third and early second centuries B.C.E.

Coincidentally, these so-called Mawangdui manuscripts (see chapter 2, p. 19), supplemented by discoveries in other burial and storage sites, also constitute the oldest known medical texts of China in general. Their unknown authors described prognostic and diagnostic principles and procedures, as well as various options for therapeutic intervention, that might have been based entirely in empiricism. These include, for example, gymnastic exercises, minor surgery for hemorrhoids, baths, compresses, cauterization with burning herb cones, massage, and, most importantly, the use of medicinal drugs.

Acupuncture, the treatment of illness with needles, is not mentioned in any of the Mawangdui texts; the earliest citation of this procedure is found not in a medical text, but in a historical one, the *Shiji* 史記 (Records of a Historiographer) by Sima Qian 司馬遷 from approximately 90 B.C.E. No serious indication exists that proves acupuncture was practiced in China before this time, much less that it was wide-spread. A careful reading of the *Huang Di neijing suwen* 黄帝内经素问 (*Inner Classic of the Huang Di: Elementary Questions*) suggests that at least until the second century B.C.E., blood-letting was the treatment of choice when Chinese doctors attempted to treat a "fullness" of the blood vessels. [5]

The most extensive Mawangdui document is a collection of formulas that is today called the *Wushier bingfang* 五十二病方 (*Formulas for Fifty-two Illnesses*). From this text, the coexistence of demonism, magic, and natural knowledge can be deduced—e.g. a host of exorcistic procedures, which supplemented a system of medicinal drugs based on more than 200 natural substances and objects from everyday life, complicated pharmaceutical procedures for preparation, as well as a differentiated knowledge of external and internal forms of application. In later centuries, the authors of large formulae collections also frequently dedicated one or more chapters to exorcistic techniques; however, in purely quantitative terms demonism assumed a peripheral role in the medical literature of the Imperial period. It was transmitted in its own literature and expressed by Daoism and popular religious currents.

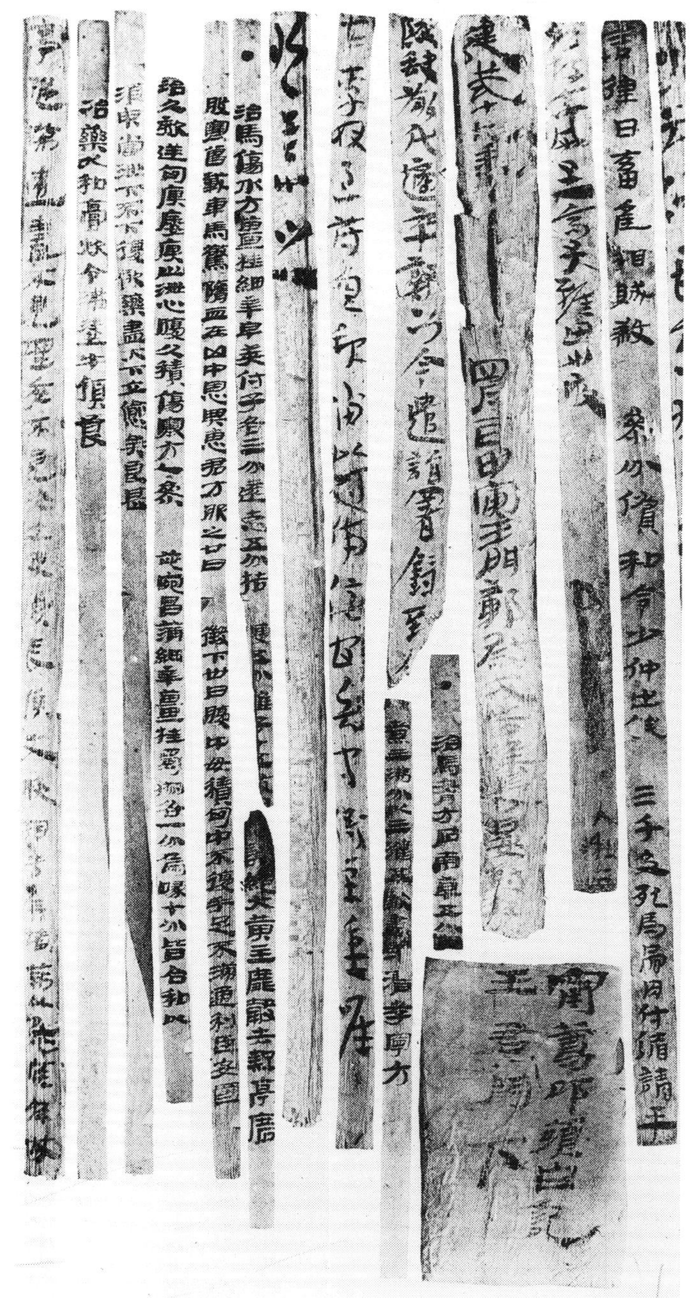

5. Formulae prescriptions on wooden slips, probably from the Eastern Han (25–220) to Jin (265–420) periods. These wooden slips were excavated in 1907 by an expedition under the direction of Sir Aurel Stein near Dunhuang on the Great Wall. They contain formulas for the treatment of humans, horses, and cattle.

It was during the period of the "Warring States" in the centuries before the unification of the empire in 221 B.C.E. that the theoretical foundations which subsequently contributed to the formation of an actual medicine in China during the following three centuries were developed.

As in Greece at that time, there were also efforts in China to categorize the totality of the material world and to explain the creation, existence, transformation, and passing of all phenomena through the mutual interaction of their categories.

A dualistic world view of obscure origins viewed all appearances as belonging to two opposite yet complementary poles which were constantly passing into, and emerging out of, each other—yin and yang. The early yin-yang philosophers considered all phenomena to be interconnected and engaged in constant transformation, e.g., day emerges from the night and again passes into the night, high tide follows on low tide and then recedes into low tide. This initial bifurcation of all phenomena was soon supplemented by a two-fold subdivision of yin and yang into yin-in-yin, yang-in-yin and yang-in-yang, yin-in-yang, and a three-fold subdivision of each into great yin, minor yin, ceasing yin, and great yang, brilliant yang, minor yang.

Another philosophy, that seems to have been originally distinct from the yin-yang world view, was based on a five-fold categorization of everything in existence and assigned the totality of all phenomena to the so-called Five Phases, i.e. five equal groupings of all material and immaterial appearances which were in various ways engaged in the constant dynamics of giving rise to each other, conquering each other, and controlling each other.

Although the yin-yang and Five Phases theories seem to have competed with each other at first, both were synthesized during the early Han period of the second and first centuries B.C.E. into a complex system of ideas that have since been transmitted as the natural law foundation of Chinese medicine. This aspect of Chinese medicine is called the Medicine of Systematic Correspondences because the body, with its anatomical components and physiological processes, was included in the yin-yang Five Phases system just like the entire social and natural environment surrounding it. In this system, all individual appearances were viewed as parts of a greater whole whose internal transformations were never to be considered in isolation but in correspondence with each other.

The unification of the empire and the subsequent transformation of economic relationships between its formerly isolated states gave rise to a totally new understanding of the structure and functions of the human body. For the first time in Chinese history, a complex politic body was formed in which various centers with different responsibilities con-

tributed to the welfare of the entire nation. The first
emperor of the unified China decreed the standardization
of writing, units of measurement, and track widths, and
ordered the construction of the North-South Canal in
order to link formerly separate cultural centers into a
homogeneous whole. The earlier self-sufficiency of these
centers was now replaced by an exchange of goods and
mutual dependency.

In turn, the image of the human organism, which presented itself to the thinkers of the time for elucidation of
health and illness, was also conceived in these terms. The
Mawangdui manuscripts had described eleven mutually isolated blood vessels in the body. Six of these vessels extended
upwards from the feet, some of them as far as the head; five
vessels extended from the hands through the arms into
either the chest or head. The authors of the Mawangdui
texts believed these vessels to be filled with vital vapors, the
so-called qi 氣. A surplus or deficiency of qi signified illness. An exchange between the vessels, however—let alone
a circulation—was unknown to these authors who associated only four of the vessels with an organ (e.g. the heart).

Contrary to this, texts written in the following two to
three centuries present models in which twelve functional
centers (the organs) are connected through a complicated
network of channels, through which circulates a constant
flow of blood and vapors to all regions of the body. The
functional centers are separated into two groups: the so-called
*zang* 藏 (depots) and the *fu* 府 (palaces or prefectures)—the
latter serving for administration and transportation. The first
group consists of the lungs, heart, spleen, liver, and kidneys;
in the second group are found the gall, bladder, stomach,
the large intestine, the small intestine, and the anatomically
unverifiable but so-called Triple Burner.

In a healthy organism, the qi enters continuously
through food and drink as well as through emanations from
the environment. The term qi has received as many layers
of meaning in the course of the centuries as the terms
*pneuma* or *spiritus* in Western medicine. In the context of
traditional Chinese medicine, the qi refers to minute material or immaterial "influences" which the organism absorbs,
transforms, transports to the individual functional centers,
utilizes as "constructive" or "protective influences," and
finally eliminates as waste.

Accordingly, illness can be triggered by human negligence or environmental influences. For example, a lack of
balance in the provision of all necessary influences, a surplus or deficiency of activity in the individual functional
centers, or an obstruction of the channel system connecting
these centers may cause problems which can otherwise
be prevented by a regular lifestyle that takes into account
the climatic differences during the course of the year.
Dietary measures which are intended to boost a deficit of
beneficial influences or drain excessive harmful ones treat
existing disturbances in the same way as the insertion of
a needle at specific body parts which are connected to particular internal organs.

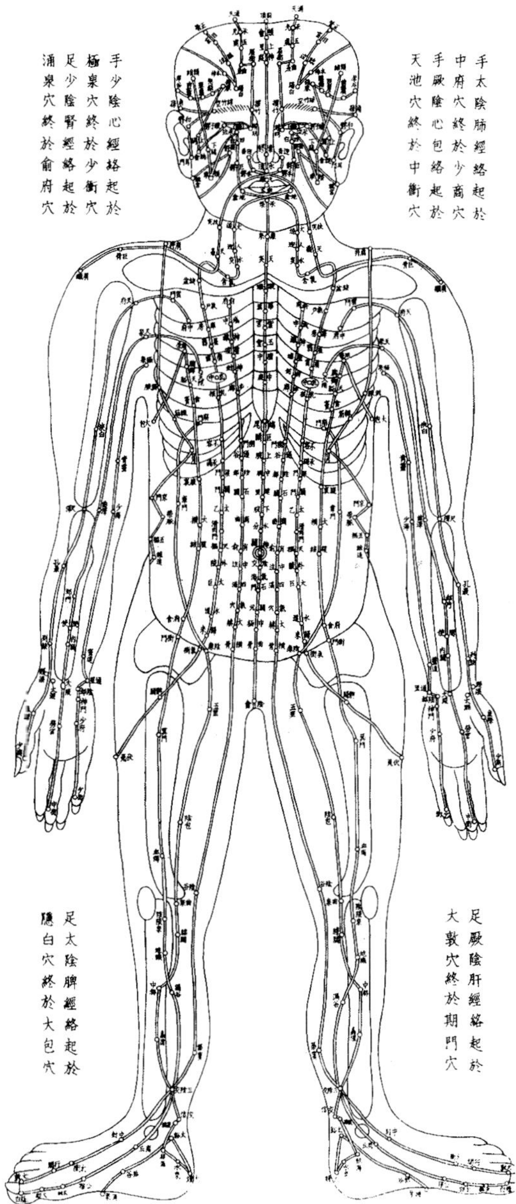

6. Illustration of the human
body marked with the course
of the conduits in relation to
the skeletal structure. Print,
early twentieth century.

This etiological and physiological model has always recognized an ontic-localistic as well as a functional-systematic notion of disease. The first is based on the idea that some, if not all, illnesses are caused by the invasion of tiny animals or harmful influences in particular areas of the body and can be attacked and eliminated there. Thus, when European bacteriology entered China in the late nineteenth and early twentieth century, it encountered conceptual preconditions which allowed for a matter-of-fact adoption of this new doctrine.

But traditional Chinese medicine has also viewed illness as a systemic disturbance particular to an individual and his or her physical constitution. Whereas the ontic-localistic diagnostic focus is on the type and location of the invader—and can therefore perform treatments without regard to the individual situation of the patient—the systemic view focuses on the individual patient and his particular lifestyle and is, in therapy, oriented towards the specific needs of the afflicted individual organism.

A fundamental principle basic to both viewpoints is the notion that "the Bad can never overcome the Good." This maxim expresses a renewed connection between medicine and ethical norms, which had already been characteristic of ancestral healing but had been rejected by demonism. A "good" lifestyle was again worthwhile, as seen in the now prominent social philosophy of Confucianism (which saw social harmony guaranteed primarily by the observance of behavioral norms appropriate for each social class), by Legalism (which saw social harmony guaranteed primarily by the observance of legal norms applied equally to everyone), and also by Daoism (which saw social harmony guaranteed primarily by the observance of regularities prescribed by nature). The lawless period of "Everybody-against-everybody" had been overcome, at least for the social elite. A lifestyle in accordance with moral norms promised not only social harmony, but also physical health for the individual.

## IV. Pharmaceutics

The rich pharmaceutical and pharmaceutical-technological knowledge of the Mawangdui texts suggests that the origins of these insights are much older still. Until the thirteenth century, the development of Chinese drug therapy seems to have been closely linked to Daoist circles, since Daoism stimulated an interest in investigating the connections between humans and the natural environment. In this area, an outstanding author worth mentioning—whose name and biographical details are known to us—is Tao Hongjing 陶弘景 (452–536), whose *Shennong bencaojing jizhu* 神農本草經集注 (*Shennong's Classic of Materia Medica Compiled and Commented [by Tao Hongjing]*) is the oldest extant Chinese pharmacopoeia.

Daoism is not a uniform doctrine, but instead developed as early as the last few centuries B.C.E. into a number of different currents which incorporated demonism, theistic

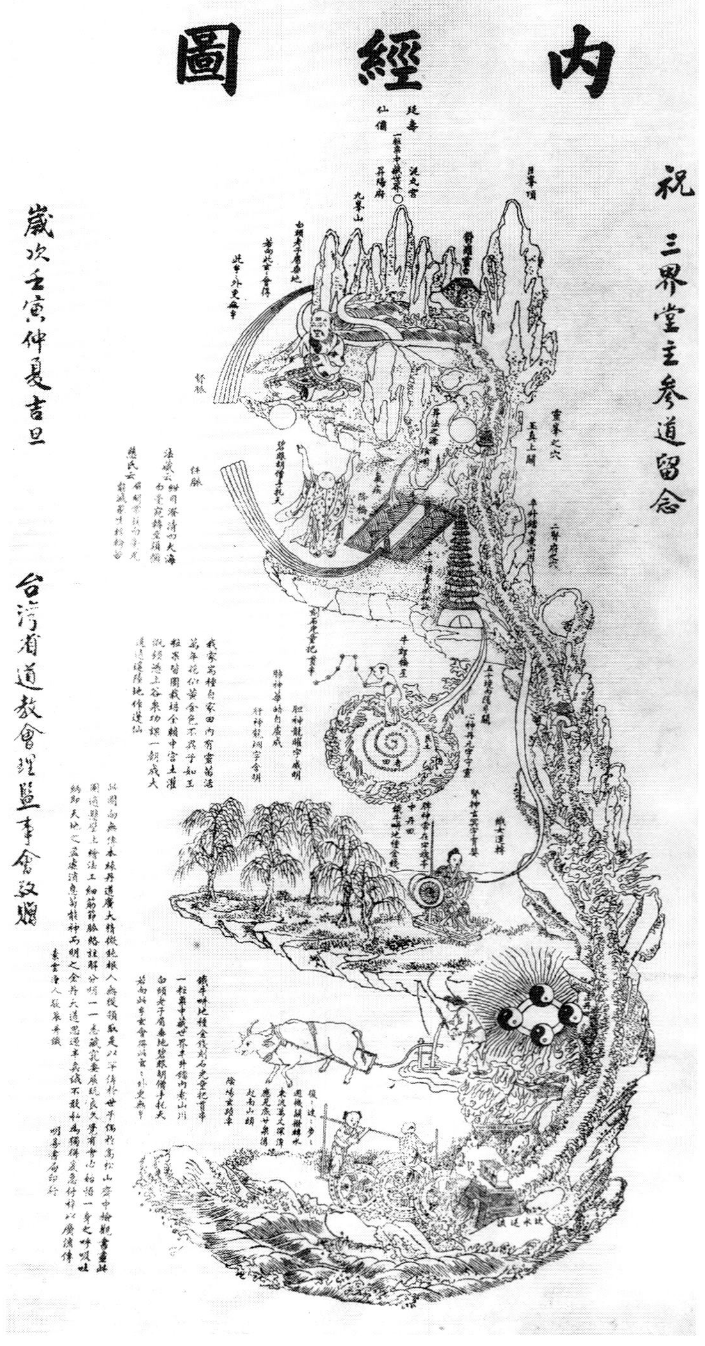

7. Allegorical representation of the physiology of the human body on the basis of Daoist ideas, *Neijingtu* 內經圖 (*Illustration of the Currents in the Interior*). Print with hand-written dedication, early twentieth century.

ideas, and finally some Buddhist notions. An early notion, documented in the work of the Daoist philosopher Zhuangzi 莊子, of the fourth to third centuries B.C.E., evidences a world view in which illness is regarded as meaningful—heralding the impending transition of a person from bodily existence to non-corporeal existence and soon thereafter, bodily rebirth.[6] But these elaborations by Zhuangzi remained an exception; for the Daoism of the Han period, the attempt to prolong earthly existence and, if possible, to transform it into "longevity without aging" became characteristic.

The quest for elixirs and herbs of immortality stimulated not only an involvement with natural substances, but also with chemical techniques of preparation. The first Chinese drug compendium, composed in the first or second century C.E. and now extant in a reconstructed version from about 500 C.E. by Tao Hongjing (see above), differentiated between 365 substances from the plant, animal, and mineral realms. These substances were ordered hierarchically into three groups. In an obvious parallel to the social ideas of the Daoists—where the duty of the ruler consisted of harmonizing the entire state system but not engaging actively in the business of leading the state—the highest and most noble group of medicinal drugs, the "lords," was used for the nourishment and prolongation of life and was therefore non-toxic. On the other hand, the lowest group of "assistants" was comprised only of drugs which, though poisonous, were appropriate for the treatment of acute illnesses. The middle group of "ministers" included substances of both types.

Over the course of the following centuries, the beginnings of materia medica that had been recorded in writing during the Han period developed into an extensive body of pharmaceutical literature which will be treated in detail below (see chapter 2, pp. 23–29). The same is true for the extremely diverse and multi-faceted literature of specialized subjects and medical theory. It should be pointed out here, that the theoretical framework which had been prepared in the doctrine of systematic correspondences since the Han period, was not abandoned in the literature of the Chinese elite until the arrival of Western medicine in the nineteenth century. On the other hand, however, an increasing splintering into various schools of interpretation within this framework becomes apparent from the end of the Song period (in the thirteenth century) onward. While all of the schools deduced their opinions systematically, from their observations and in relation to the content of the yin-yang and Five Phases theories, all of them lacked an objective criterion by which to convince others.

Therefore, no one school of thought of the second millennium was able to gain even temporary recognition as the dominant orthodoxy, and a coexistence of different approaches has characterized Chinese medicine since the fifteenth century. In a perspicacious analysis in his book *Yixue yuanliu lun* 醫學源流論 (*Concerning the Origin and Development of Medicine*) from 1757, the physician Xu Dachun 徐

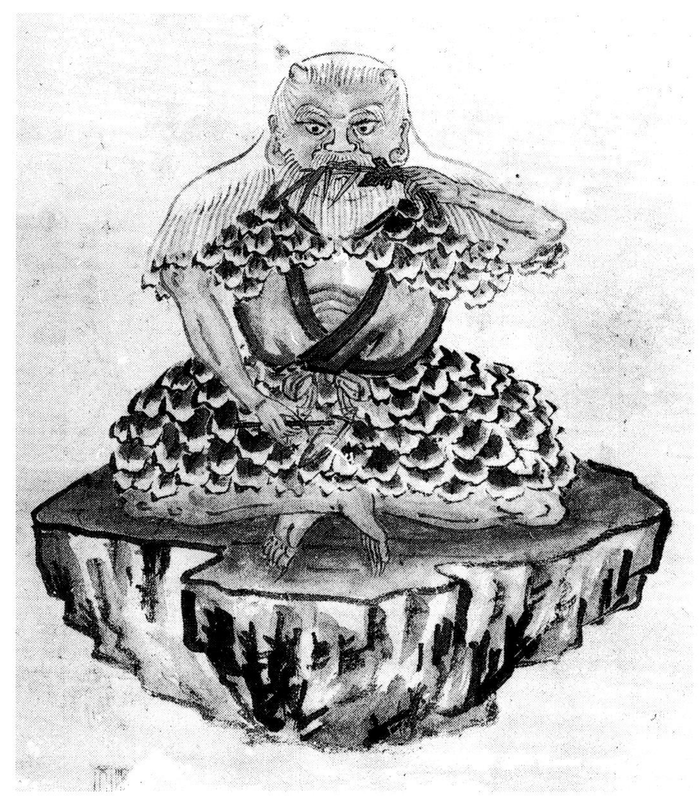

8. Shennong 神農, the ancestor of Chinese drug lore. The earliest literary source of the Shennong legend is the *Huainanzi* 淮南子, a text from the second century B.C.E. In which it is said that Shennong pitied the people of high antiquity who had often fallen ill due to their dietary habits: "He tried all herbs; in one day he found seventy that were toxic." Color drawing on paper, Japan, nineteenth or early twentieth century.

大椿 (ill. 70) finally regretted that the unequivocal tradition of Chinese medicine in the Han and pre-Han periods had been lost.[7] Clear attempts to view and present traditional Chinese medicine in a uniform framework like the one offered by Western medicine have been effective only since the founding of the People's Republic of China.

## "WESTERN" MEDICINE IN CHINA

In 1805, the feasibility of the smallpox vaccination, discovered by Edward Jenner, was introduced to the Portuguese colony of Macao by Dr. Pearson, a physician with the East India Company; in 1827, Dr. Colledge, also a physician with the East India Company, opened an eye clinic in Macao. The American missionary and physician Peter Parker founded the first clinic outside the colonial bases of the Western powers in the city of Canton in 1835. The activities of these individual physicians constitute the visible beginnings of a development which, within one and a half centuries, led to the predominance of a medicine in China that is to this day apostrophized as Western. By 1929, nine thousand Chinese physicians with Western training had been registered; in 1966, there were almost 160,000. According to Chinese accounts, 700,000 beds were available in hospitals for Western medicine in 1971.

At the beginning of the nineteenth century, European and American physicians in China did not express any superiority towards their Chinese colleagues who practiced traditional Chinese medicine and strove for an exchange of knowledge. A few decades later, however, this situation changed rather quickly due to the Western use of antisepsis, asepsis, anesthesia, and surgery, as well as the rapid expansion into specialized subjects, the development of bacteriology, and finally chemotherapy. For example, in the 1850s, the British physician Benjamin Hobson published a series of books in Chinese on the scientific foundations of Western medicine and on the most important special subjects. In his preface, he mentions the lack of anatomical knowledge and of a regulated education as the major causes of what he perceived to be the 'backwardness' of Chinese medicine (see chapter 2, p. 40f).

Beginning with the turn of the century, and particularly in the subsequent first three decades, the political powers in China—trying to restore their country's dignity and strength after defeats in the Opium War, the War against Japan, and the Boxer Rebellion—saw the only solution to this crisis to be adopting Western technology and science and therefore Western medicine. This position was reinforced not only by the increasing technological and military

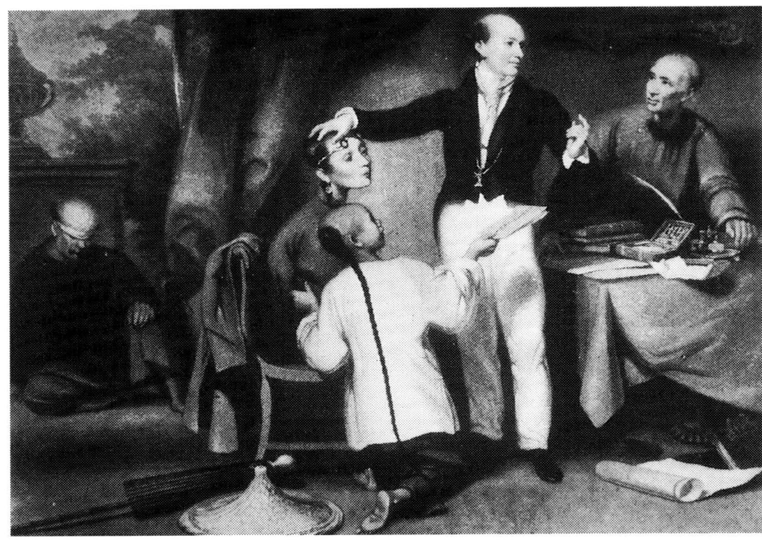

9. In 1927, Thomas R. Colledge, physician of the East India Company, opened an ophthalmic hospital in Macao. Engraving by William Daniel after a painting by George Chinnery. Royal College of Surgeons, London.

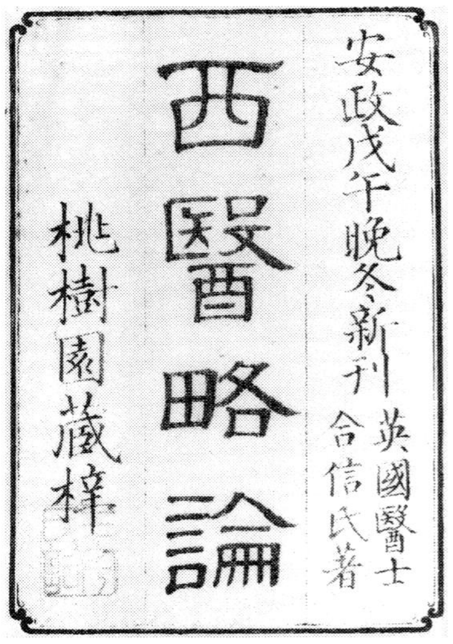

10. Title page of the *Outline of Western Medicine* by Benjamin Hobson and Guan Maocai. Japanese facsimile reprint of the original Chinese edition from 1857–58.

superiority of the European powers, but also by the example of Japan which had opened its doors successfully to Western civilization with the Meiji reforms of 1868. Until the 1940s, numerous Chinese reformers and intellectuals composed critical essays denouncing the traditional medicine of their country; in their often vitriolic sarcasm, these writings are not surpassed by even the most disapproving statements of present-day European and American representatives of Western medicine.

It was not until the 1950s, for pragmatic reasons (such as the limited number of physicians with a modern education) as well as political considerations in the People's Republic of China, that the contributions of traditional Chinese medicine received recognition. Attempts were made to unite Western and traditional medicine and to utilize the "advantages of both systems" by transmitting traditional knowledge to doctors of Western medicine in addition to their Western training. But these efforts remained as superficial and ultimately unsuccessful as the reverse attempts to offer an additional education in Western medicine to the representatives of the tradition.

Moreover, the 1950s and 1960s saw the rise of a novel occupational group, the so-called barefoot doctors. Some communes had privately decided to send younger members away to receive a basic education in primary healthcare in order to remedy the lack of physicians in the countryside. Upon their return, these initiates continued to work in their original occupations, but they also utilized their medical knowledge to provide the services of family planning, general hygiene, and the treatment of minor health problems. Their line of work included practical applications of modern Western treatments as well as traditional Chinese ones; theoretical knowledge was not included in their training.

Since the initiation of fundamental economic reforms and the opening of China to the outside world at the end of the 1970s, a policy of "three paths" has been in effect. First, Western medicine and traditional Chinese medicine should develop within their own frameworks. The third path is followed mainly by practitioners of Chinese medicine who use the results of the most recent diagnostic techniques from the West as the basis for their "traditional" treatments. In the last few years, eclectic-syncretistic approaches have become fashionable also in therapy. Thus, traditional drugs and formulas are supposed to round out or even improve the effects of chemotherapy or antibiotics.[8]

Not only are the theoretical problems that arise from integrating modern diagnostic and therapeutic categories into traditional Chinese medicine entirely unresolved (and in need of a solution probably only from the Western viewpoint), but even the basic attitude of Chinese society towards traditional Chinese medicine is still undecided.

The authorities of the People's Republic of China and the ideologues of the Communist Party have at no time

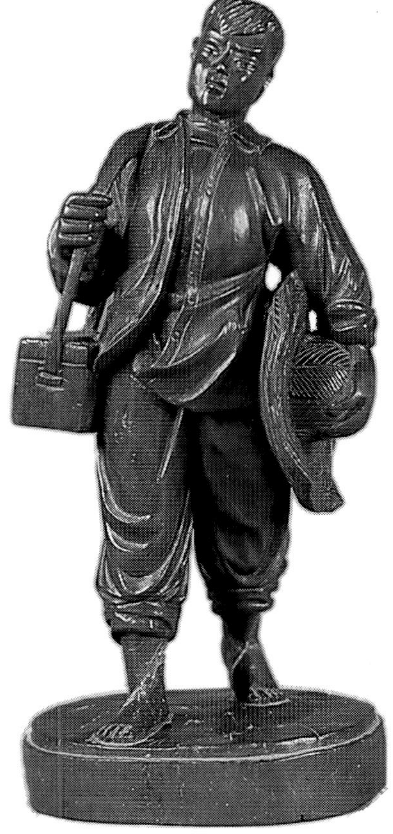

11. Barefoot doctor. Wooden figure, China, ca. 1957.

vouched for the safety of historical Chinese medicine. Recognizing the important role of traditional medicine in the public health policy of the People's Republic of China has always been connected to the demand for adjusting it to the social and scientific conditions of the Modern Age. The traditional Chinese medicine which is officially supported by the People's Republic of China is only a small remnant of the complex and multi-faceted medicine of the Imperial Age. All aspects of the tradition which refer to religious or otherwise metaphysical notions of the past that may appear absurd in light of current science (and which go back terminologically to the feudal hierarchy of the Imperial Age) have been deleted from textbooks. The significance of the remaining medicine is to a large extent based on the interest of European and American visitors to China who have invested a great deal of money and time since the 1980s into knowledge that has gained respect in the West to the same degree to which it has fallen into secondary status in China.

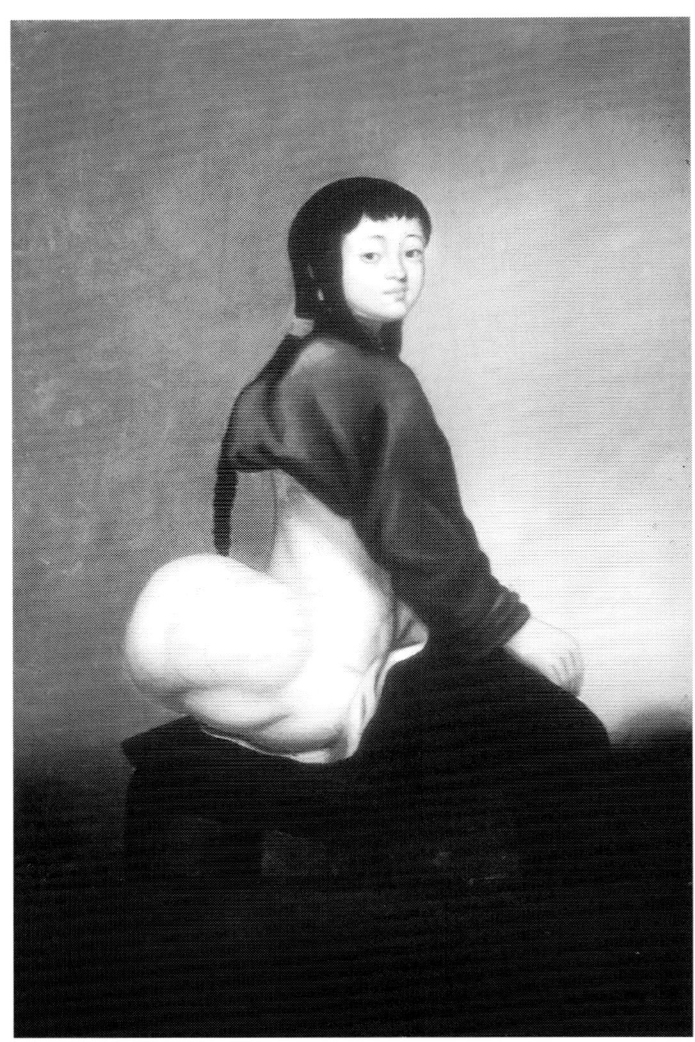

12. Surgical patient No. 3000 of Dr. Peter Parker in Canton. The tumor on the right hip of the twelve-year-old patient was successfully removed by Dr. Parker in two minutes and fourteen seconds on April 27, 1837. Painting by Lam Qua. Gordon Museum, Guy's Hospital, London.

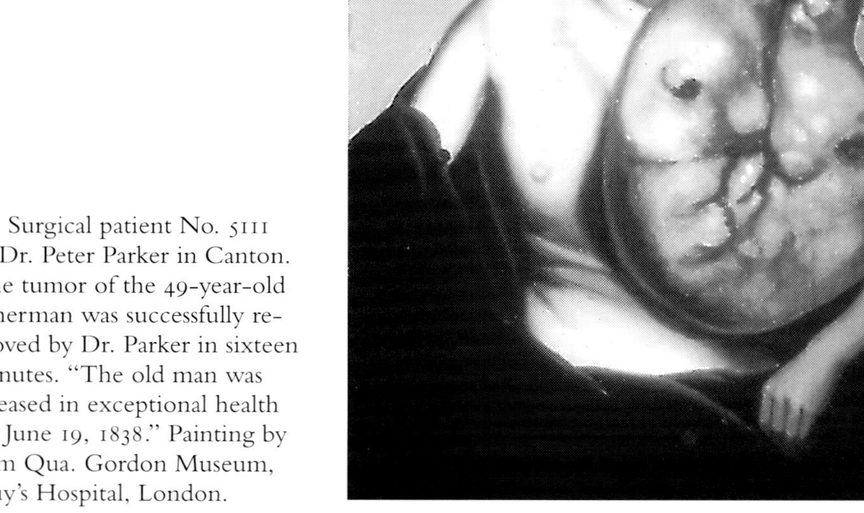

13. Surgical patient No. 5111 of Dr. Peter Parker in Canton. The tumor of the 49-year-old fisherman was successfully removed by Dr. Parker in sixteen minutes. "The old man was released in exceptional health on June 19, 1838." Painting by Lam Qua. Gordon Museum, Guy's Hospital, London.

# THE LITERATURE OF TRADITIONAL CHINESE MEDICINE AND PHARMACEUTICS

## THE MAWANGDUI TEXTS AS THE STARTING POINT FOR MEDICAL LITERATURE IN CHINA

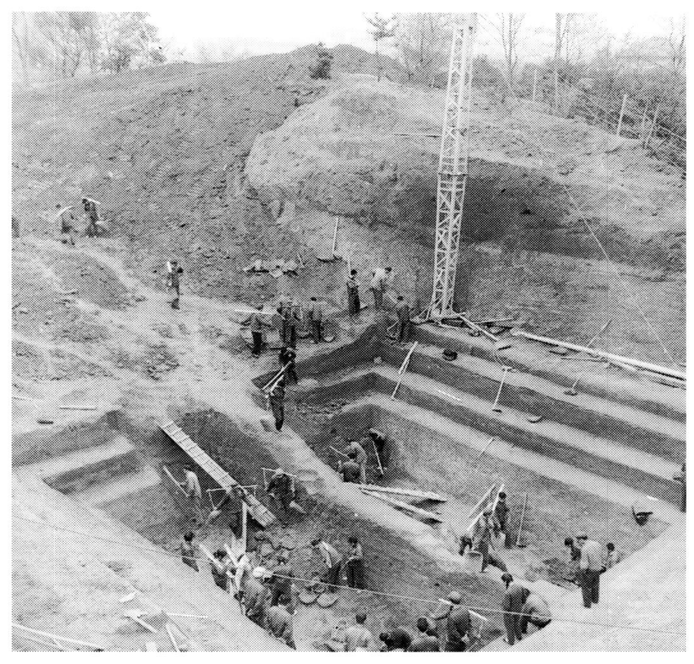

14. View of the unearthed Mawangdui tomb 3, 1973.

In a fortunate discovery, a tomb complex with largely untouched and well-preserved funeral gifts dating from 168 B.C.E. was unearthed in the beginning of the 1970s. It contained a total of fourteen texts of medical content, which provide a nearly straight path to the beginnings of Chinese medicine. Tomb 3 from Mawangdui 馬 王 堆 near Changsha, the capital of Hunan Province, contained objects which, presumably, had all been closely linked to the life of the Marquis Dai's family that was buried there. Whether or not these things had been placed in the tomb in order for the deceased to again have a complete household at their disposal is unclear.

There are no indications that the manuscripts were classified as antiquities in their time. In fact, they reflect the entire spectrum of medicine as it was practiced at the beginning of the second century B.C.E. by those with a formal education. Therefore, this constitutes a firm date from which the further development of medical theory and practice in China can be evaluated. This find is particularly significant for the historical classification of acupuncture and the *Inner Classic of the Yellow Emperor*, the *Huang Di neijing* 黃 帝 內 經 (see p. 30). The contents of the Mawangdui manuscripts prove the fallacy of formerly widespread assumptions regarding the biblical age of needle therapy and of this corpus of medical philosophy, the oldest in China to have been transmitted through the centuries. As the last link in a chain of evidence, the Mawangdui texts prove that the *Huang Di neijing* and acupuncture can only have originated afterwards. (see also pp. 23, 42ff.).

The American sinologist Donald Harper has completely translated and analyzed the fourteen Mawangdui texts, thereby making them accessible to other scientists who do not possess the necessary knowledge of the Chinese language.[9] The broad spectrum of their contents is as much worth our attention as is the diversity of theoretical approaches that can be deduced from the therapeutic advice recorded in them.

Manuscript I contains a total of five texts on a silk cloth, originally 24 cm wide and 450 cm long, and folded in more than thirty layers. Since only the edges of the folds were decomposed when the grave was opened, the vast majority of characters are still legible. Two of the texts describe the course of the eleven vessel tracts of the body that were known at the time and offer lists of ailments associated with the condition of these vessels. The only therapeutic option for influencing these vessels was believed to be cauterization, namely the practice of heating certain points on the skin above the vessels through the application of burning cones of herbs. Another one of these texts, in a slightly altered version, was also found in a tomb in a different location in China and can—on the basis of its contents—be regarded as a precursor to certain explanations in the *Huang Di neijing*. This shows that these texts were not an isolated occurrence, but belonged to a body of literature that was circulated among the literate elite.

The third text in manuscript I discusses pathological conditions of qi in the vessels and offers advice on how to open the vessels with a lancing stone. It also includes notes on how to diagnose the condition of the vessels by feeling the pulse at the bones. The fourth text contains a list of indications of death, recognizable primarily from the condition of the vessels. The fifth and final text is a collection of formulas titled *Wushier bingfang* 五十二病方 (Formulas Against Fifty-two Illnesses) by Chinese researchers because the 283 formulas that are still legible in it are organized into fifty-two indications (ill. 4). The majority of therapies are based on the application of pharmaceutical substances; in addition, cauterization, lancing stones, hot compresses, fumigation, baths, minor surgery, massage, and cupping are also discussed. Furthermore, forty formulas contain exorcistic spells and magic-religious measures, frequently used in addition to treatments with drugs or other practices.

Manuscript II is a silk cloth approximately 50 cm wide and 110 cm long that contains three texts. The first text offers macrobiotic advice concerning dietetics. It recommends, in particular, the ingestion of a plant called *shiwei* (that is unidentifiable today), rather than grains. The text further includes advice on breathing exercises for fixed times of the day and year, during which the adept are specifically instructed to avoid five types of atmospheric qi and ingest six preferable types of qi. A second text in this manuscript is largely identical with the second text in manuscript I. Manuscript II also contains a list of forty-four

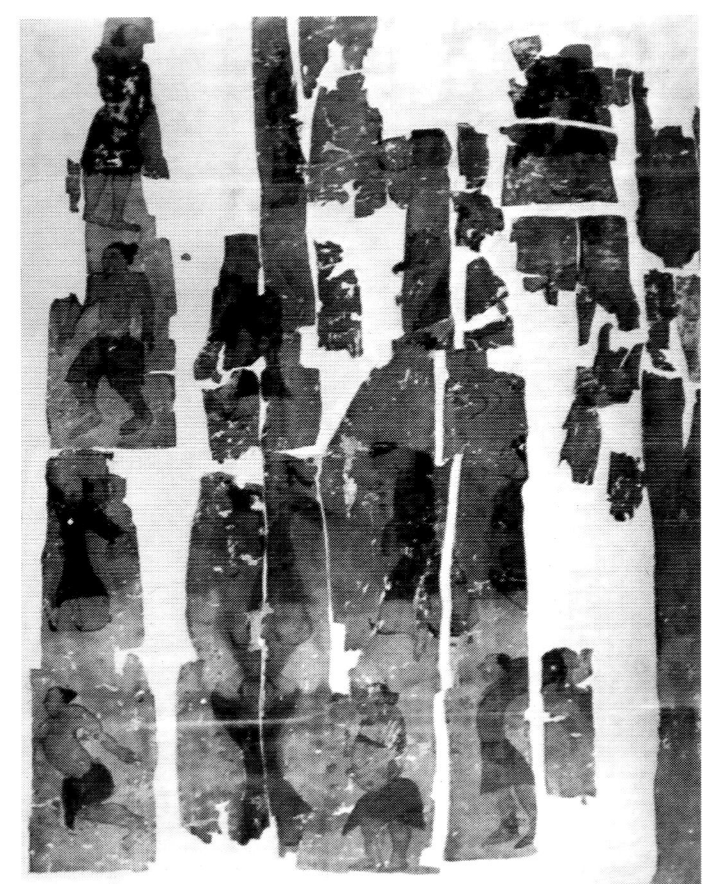

15. Excerpt from Mawangdui manuscript II with drawings of individuals engaged in physical exercises. Condition at the time of the tomb's opening, 1973.

drawings depicting figures engaged in physical exercises, partly for the treatment of certain ailments and partly for the preservation of good health, as the captions explain.

Manuscript III only contains one text with numerous formulas of various objectives. The silk cloth on which it is written is 24 cm wide and in worse condition than the others; the original length can no longer be estimated. The medical and magical formulas promise such results as a strong constitution, the renewal of black hair or else—like a kind of antique doping—the acceleration of a runner's speed. Several formulas serve as the foundations for sexual practices.

Manuscript IV, 24 cm wide and of undetermined length, is also quite badly damaged. The only text on this cloth is a collection of formulas for different indications, such as an illustrated technique for burying a placenta, drug formulas for the treatment of snake bites, and formulas for the preparation of vaginal suppositories.

Manuscript V is a silk cloth that is approximately 49 cm wide and equally long. The entire content of this manuscript is related to birth. In the upper half, there are two drawings: one for prognosticating a child's fate and the other for determining the most advantageous location for burying a placenta. Lastly, the text explains conception and offers advice for the treatment of the fetus during pregnancy.

Manuscript VI consists of bamboo slabs and contains two texts. The first one presents the answers of ten macrobiotic experts to certain questions. The second explains sexual practices for the purpose of treating illness and preserving health.

Manuscript VII consists of eleven wooden slabs that are ca. 23 cm long and 1.2 cm wide, as well as fifty-six bamboo slabs that are ca. 28 cm long and 0.5 cm wide. The text on the wooden slabs contains spells of the kind that were common in the early Han period. It also offers methods of squashing an opponent in court, separating a married couple, seducing a seemingly unattainable person, or quieting screaming children. The text on the bamboo slabs is mostly concerned with sexual practices. [10]

This "gift" from the Han period to contemporary culture, so rich in content and informative in many perspectives, marks the beginning of a literary tradition that equals the history of Western medicine. Supplemented throughout the centuries with individual texts (13,000 preserved and innumerable lost at the end of the Imperial period in 1912), this body of literature eloquently expresses the search of the upper class for an appropriate theory to explain, and effective clinical procedures to heal illness and prevent premature death.

In general, one can distinguish between two different approaches in Chinese medical literature, one of prevention and early treatment and one of therapy. Many authors dedicated their writings to the preservation of health and the treatment of illness in its early manifestation. They applied notions from the yin-yang and Five Phases theories to the

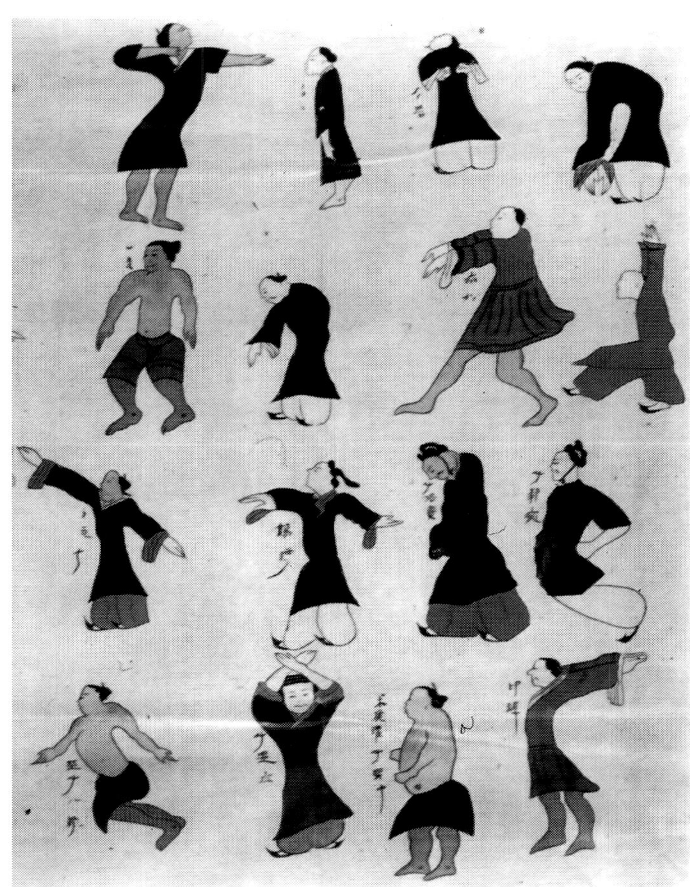

16. Excerpt from Mawangdui manuscript II. Reconstruction of the original drawings (compare ill. p. 20).

conduct of one's life and the cause and treatment of illnesses. For two millennia, these authors focused primarily on training their readers to recognize the first indications of illness, i.e. that point in time when, in their opinion, a stimulation with needles at body points that were determined by theory or known from experience could still cause a reversal of the pathological process. On the basis of such approaches to early treatment, a literature was, of course, developed which discussed needles for the treatment of more problematic and manifest illnesses, a method which the authors of antiquity had viewed as a purely professional blunder.

But what else, other than the needle, cured illnesses? An answer to this question can be found, for example, in Sun Simiao's 孫思邈 *Qianjin yifang* 千金翼方 (*Additional Formulas Worth a Thousand Pieces of Gold*) from the seventh century:

> Wei Fan said to Bian Que: The physical basis has to be secured by food; the only way to heal an illness is with drugs. If one does not know the appropriate foods, one will be unable to reach the fullness of one's life; if one is unaware of the properties of drugs, one will be unable to use them to remove illnesses. This means food is able to expel the bad and to satisfy the depots and palaces (i.e. the functional centers in the body). Drugs are able to calm the mind and nurture [human] nature in order to thereby strengthen the four qi. Anybody's son, therefore, has to know of these two things. Thus, if the father of a gentleman has fallen ill, then [the son] must first place his stakes on food to cure him. If the treatment with food is unsuccessful, then he has to place his stakes on drugs. A filial son, thus, has no choice but to possess in-depth knowledge of the properties of foods as well as drugs.[11]

Acupuncture is not taken into consideration here. The authors of almost all works on materia medica and prescriptions self-consciously emphasized the power of drugs in the treatment of illness, thereby continuing until the present the tradition of giving primary significance to pharmaceutics which had arisen from undocumented beginnings. In fact, Chinese pharmaceutics—including the dietetics mentioned in the quotation above—carried the main responsibility for the treatment of acute illnesses in the entire history of Chinese medicine. In contrast to the literature on health preservation and the treatment of illnesses in their early manifestations, prescriptions literature, and even more so, pharmaceutical literature, remained largely free of theory, with the exception of Zhang Ji's 張機 works (ca. 200 C.E.). Systematic efforts to also submit drug usage to a strict theoretical framework were begun only in the late Sung period, (twelfth and thirteenth centuries). After about three centuries, however, the social and ideological environment which had made these efforts possible disappeared, and the theoretically based application of drugs was paralyzed in the status quo of the Yuan period.

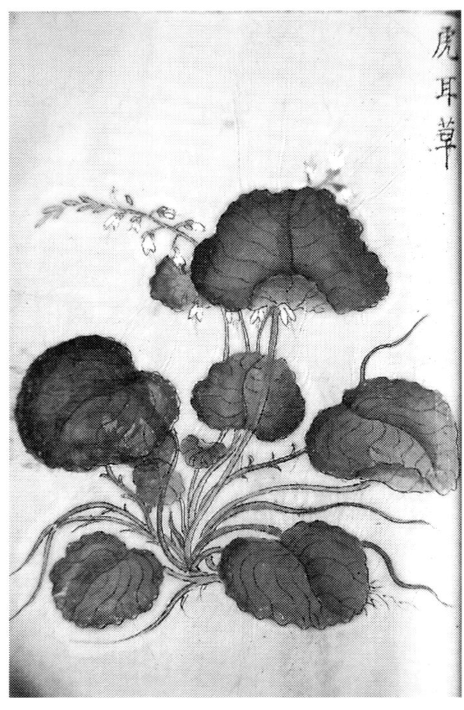

17. Drawing of the plant *hu'ercao* (*Saxifraga stolonifera* [*L.*] *Meerb.*) from the *Lü chanyan bencao* 履巉巖本草 (*Materia Medica of the Mountain Cliff Wanderer*), 1220. Ming period copy. Academy of Chinese Medicine, Peking.

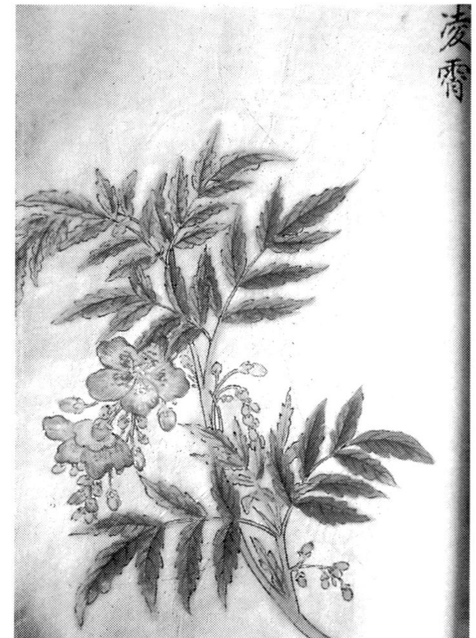

18. Drawing of the plant *lingxiao* (*Campis grandiflora* [*Thonb.*] *Loisel.*) from the *Lü chanyan bencao* 履巉巖本草 (*Materia Medica of the Mountain Cliff Wanderer*), 1220. Ming period copy. Academy of Chinese Medicine, Peking.

The visible beginnings of this development are found in the Mawangdui text *Wushier bingfang* from the second century B.C.E., the first preserved collection of prescriptions in Chinese medical literature. The range of the drugs mentioned is diverse, including vegetable, animal, and mineral sources and objects from every-day life. The variety of possible applications suggests that this tradition was already well-established at the time the text was written down.

Pigs' fat, boys' urine, gall, human spermatic fluid, animal blood, chicken eggs, water from rinsing rice, turtle brain, and wagon grease, as well as "fat from the human head" are carrier substances that were described as binding agents and solvents for external drugs, as binding agents for pills, as mediums for sitzbaths and medical ablutions, as well as substances for the preservation of moisture.

Both the pharmaceutical refining of drugs and their further processing into various types of drugs prove the advanced state of pharmaceutical art and pharmaceutical knowledge in the early Han period. Yet it took two more centuries until the knowledge of individual drugs required its own literature. The first drug compendium was composed in the first century C.E., the *Shennong bencaojing* 神農本草 經 (*Shennong's Classic of Materia Medica*) with 365 separate monographs, which formed the basis for a long line of sequential writings.

Texts on prescriptions and materia medica probably constitute the majority of medical literature in China. Hardly one of these many thousand works, however, has yet been analyzed, in terms of its content, from a Western perspective, much less translated. So far, only a first survey exists of the history of materia medica, the smallest and most accessible aspect of this literature.[13] Accordingly, Chinese and also non-Chinese authors between the Han dynasty and the end of the Imperial period composed about 300 texts on materia medica that are known or preserved today in the form of complete works, titles, or textual fragments. Some of these books discussed narrowly defined topics of pharmaceutics, others attempted a comprehensive survey of pharmaceutical knowledge.[14]

One of the great early pharmaceutical encyclopedias that first contained several hundred—and since the tenth century over one-thousand—drug monographs is the *Xinxiu bencao* 新修本草 (*Newly Revised Materia Medica*) by Su Jing 穌敬, Li Ji 李勣, et al., from the year 659 with 850 drug monographs. This text constitutes the first inventory of Chinese drugs to be initiated and ordered by a government in China. While the text of this work has largely been preserved till today, the illustrations that were attached to the individual drug descriptions have been irretrievably lost.

The *Kaibao xin xiangding bencao* 開寶新詳定本草 (*Newly Tested and Defined Materia Medica of the Kaibao Period*) by Liu Han 劉翰 et al., from the year 973 containing 983

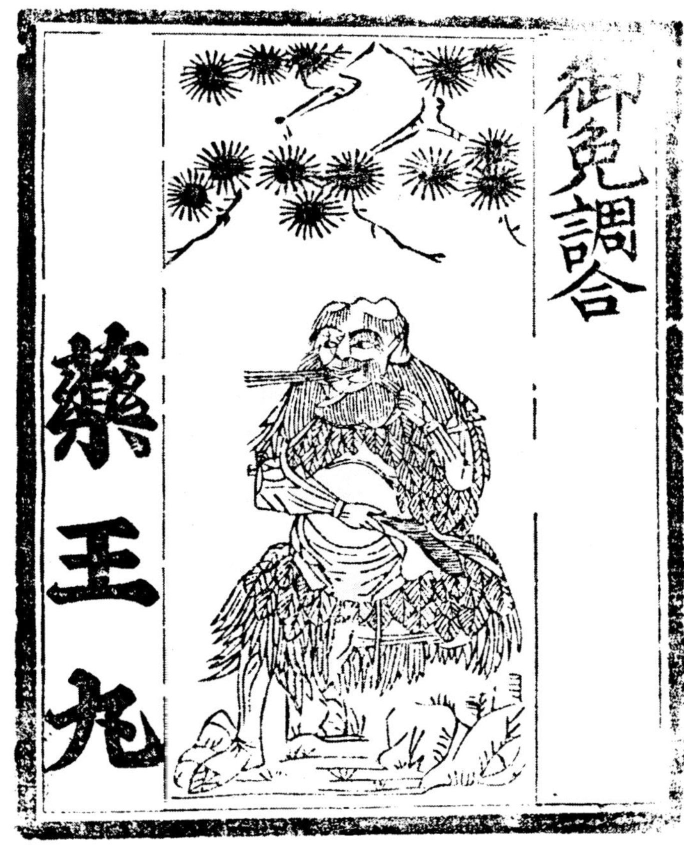

19. Shennong, the ancestor of Chinese pharmaceutics. Advertisement for "Medicine King Pills, manufactured under licence." Wood-block print, Japan, early twentieth century. See also plate 31.

monographs, was the first printed materia medica in China. The *Jingshi zhenglei daguan bencao* 經史證類大觀本草 (*Annotated And Topically Ordered Materia Medica of the Daguan Period, Based on the Classics and Historical Writings*) by Tang Shenwei 唐慎微 from 1108 with 1,744 monographs, is the first of these comprehensive works which has been completely preserved until the present.

The most famous encyclopedically arranged materia medica of traditional Chinese medicine is the *Bencao gang mu* 本草綱目 (*Materia Medica Arranged In Monographs According to Topics*) from 1596 (ills. 21, 22). The author, a physician by the name of Li Shizhen 李時珍 (1518–1593), described approximately 1,900 drugs in 52 volumes and needed more than three decades for the composition of this impressive work. Even today it still constitutes a storehouse of natural knowledge but has so far been translated, in its entirety, only into Japanese.

Such comprehensive encyclopedias were always complemented by smaller works whose authors limited themselves to specific questions. Specialized works treated, for example, drugs of certain regions, such as the *Hu bencao* 胡本草 (*Materia Medica of the Hu Countries*) by Zheng Qian 鄭虔 (from the eighth century) which deals with the medicines of the peoples neighboring China on the northwest, while others were concerned with only one substance, like the *Renzhen zhuan* 人參傳 (*Chronicle of Ginseng*), written by Li Yanwen 李言聞 around the year 1500.

The authors sometimes dealt exclusively with pharmaceutical technology, such as Pang Anshi 龐安時 in his eleventh century work *Xiuzhi yao fa* 修治藥法 (*Procedures of Drug Processing*), or detailed the effects of mineral springs, such as in the *Shiwu bencao* 食物本草 (*Dietetic Materia Medica*) by Lu He 盧和 from the sixteenth century. Alternately, they attempted to convey a manageable survey of overly extensive encyclopedic works, such as Wang An 汪昂 did in his *Bencao beiyao* 本草備要 (*Complete Survey of the Essentials of Pharmaceutics*), with 400 monographs, from the year 1682.

## FORMULARY LITERATURE

Besides the *Wushier bingfang* from the Mawangdui discoveries, the work of Zhang Ji 張機, an author from the late Han period, is also quite significant. Zhang Ji composed the *Shanghan zabing lun* 傷寒雜病論 (*Treatise on Cold Damage and Various [other] Illnesses*), whose content was probably divided as early as the third century by Wang Shuhe 王叔和, and at the latest, during the Song period in the eleventh century by editors in the Office for Medical Literature. The resulting works are known as the *Shanghan*

20. Initial lines of Xia Liangxin's 夏良心 preface to the *Bencao gang mu* 本草綱目 (*Materia Medica Arranged in Monographs According to Topics*) by Li Shizhen: "The gentlemen used the medical teachings in order to preserve life; they applied them within a greater framework in order to assist the world. Therefore, medicine was called a humanitarian skill, and in later times even regarded as an art. Bureaucrats hardly ever talk of it, and merchants don't loose any words about it! When the sages of antiquity did not reside at court, they surely lived among physicians and fortune tellers. How could anyone possibly regard medicine with disdain? For doctors, materia medica was rake and hoe, bow and arrow. The greatest and the smallest animals and plants form an overwhelming diversity; they are dispersed in (mountains and marshes...)." *Bencao gang mu*, second edition, 1603. Staatsbibliothek, Berlin.

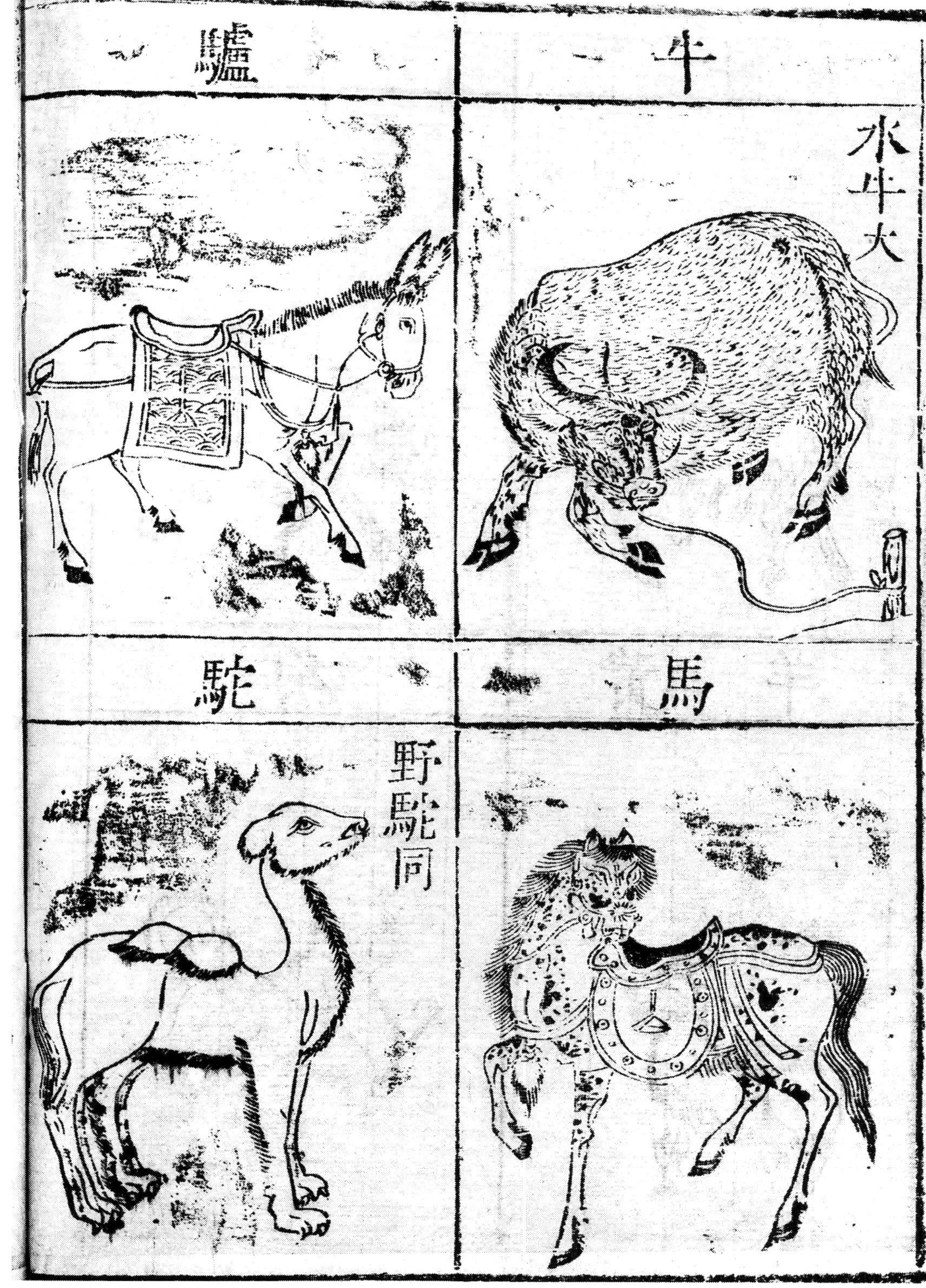



21. From right to left: Ox (large water buffalo), donkey, horse, and camel. Illustrations to the chapter on animal medicines from the *Bencao gang mu* 本草綱目 (*Materia Medica Arranged in Monographs According to Topics*), 1596. Undated edition, publisher Benlitang 本立堂, from the Qing dynasty (1648–1912).

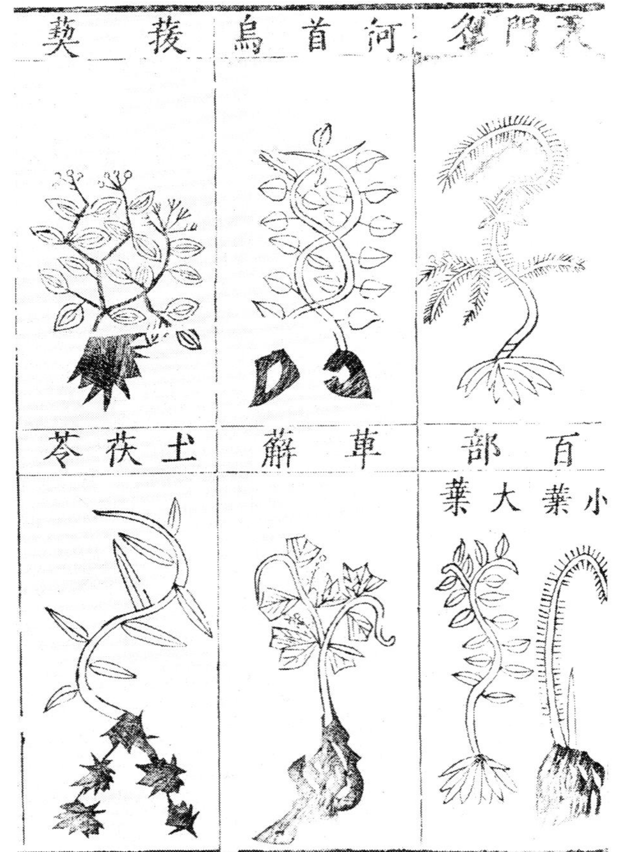

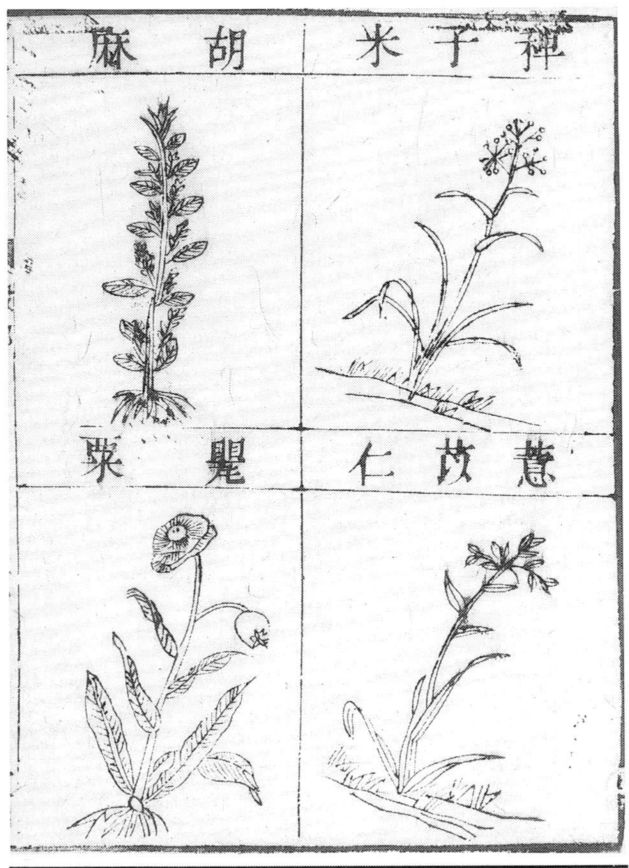





*lun* 傷寒論 (*Treatise on Cold Damage*) and the *Jingui yaolüe fang lun* 金櫃要略方論 (*Discussion of the Essential Formulas from the Golden Trunk*), two texts of a similar content but different structure.

Zhang Ji was the first author of a formulary in China to demand that drugs be applied on the basis of yin-yang theories. Unfortunately, he approached his readers too early with this concept and further complicated his position by limiting himself to a single etiology, the illnesses caused by "cold damage." It was many centuries before another author again considered it worthwhile to publish formulas against a single illness in book format. It was not until the reinterpretation of Confucianism during the Song dynasty, exactly one millennium later, that the spirit of the times allowed for the mutual approximation of such aspects of Chinese culture that had heretofore been attributed to either Daoism or Confucianism. The first long-lasting and systematic attempts to link knowledge about the effects of drugs with the medical concepts of the yin-yang and Five Phases theories originated in this conciliatory climate. Also, the *Shanghan lun*, which had barely been able to exert any influence in the preceding millennium, was rediscovered during the Zhang-Ji renaissance of the late Song, Jin, and Yuan periods (from the

22. From right to left: *tianmendong* (*Asparagus cochinchinensis* [*Lour.*] *Merr.*), *heshouwu* (*Polygonum multiflorum Thunb.*), *bajia* (*Smilax china L.*), *baibu* (*Stemona japonica* [*Bl.*] *Miq.*), *beixie* (*Dioscorea hypoglauca Palib.*), and *tufuling* (*Smilax glabra Roxb.*). Illustrations to the chapter on tuber and rhizome drugs from the *Bencao gang mu*, second edition, 1603. Staatsbibliothek, Berlin.

23. From right to left: *baizimi* (*Echinochloa crusgalli L.?*), *huma* (*Sesamum indicum DC.*), *yiyiren* (*Coix lachryma-jobi L.*), and *yingsu* (*Papaver somniferum L.*). From *Shiwubencao huizuan* 食物本草會纂 (*Selected Dietary Materia Medica*), 1691, edition from 1803.

twelfth to the fifteenth centuries). Numerous reprints and commentaries were created and in Japan, the thoughts of Zhang Ji constituted the most solid foundation for the application of Chinese formulary knowledge.

Important formulae collections were also produced during the Tang period such as the works of Sun Simiao 孫思邈 (581–682 ?) (see pp. 88–95) and the *Waitai biyao* 外臺秘要 (*Essentials from the Outer Terrace*) by Wang Dao 王燾 (670–755). While Sun Simiao may have incorporated his medical experience as a physician into his work, Wang Dao's information was derived from his position as a compiler in the national Central Library for more than 20 years. Out of personal interest, he used his position there to compose a comprehensive survey of formulary knowledge from past centuries until his own times.

The Song period again produced two works that summarized all formulary knowledge. In a grand project under the direction of the medical official Wang Huaiyin 王懷隱, officials of the Imperial Hanlin Academy merged unpublished folk recipes with all previously published formularies into the 100-chapter *Taiping shenghui fang* 太平聖惠方 (*Formulary of the Sages' Grace from the Period of Great Peace*) printed in 992.

The first two chapters of this voluminous book are dedicated to diagnosis and the general foundations of formulary art. Chapters 3–7 discuss all illnesses of the functional centers of an organism, while chapters 8–14 contain formulas for illnesses caused by cold damage. Chapters 15–59 contain formulas for various internal afflictions (including eye, mouth, tooth, and throat problems). Chapters 60–68 are devoted to so-called external illnesses, chapters 69–81 to gynecological illnesses, and chapters 82–93 to pediatric illnesses. Chapters 94 and 95 consist of the "Regulations from the Trove of Knowledge of Hermits and Alchemists." Chapters 96–98 are dedicated to dietetics and the treatment of illnesses with food. Finally, chapters 99 and 100 offer a list of acupuncture and cauterization points.

The *Taiping shenghui fang* was created as part of the comprehensive public health measures of the Song governments, which were probably a reaction against the massive migration of the population from the countryside and the creation of large cities where the traditional family structures had become unable to offer protection. In June of 1076, the Chinese government decreed, for the first time, that pharmacies of ready prepared drugs be established, and it arranged for the publication, in 1078, of the *Taiyiju fang* 太醫局方 (*Formulary of the Imperial Office of Medicine*), a collection of standard formulas designed to be sold in these pharmacies. [15]

In 1136, the government approved a specific trademark for all products that were distributed by these pharmacies, in order to distinguish their drugs from counterfeit ones sold at pharmacies not nationally supervised. [16] For centuries to come, this measure laid the foundations in China for the marketing of ready prepared medications with various therapeutic aims by pharmacies. It was not appreciably

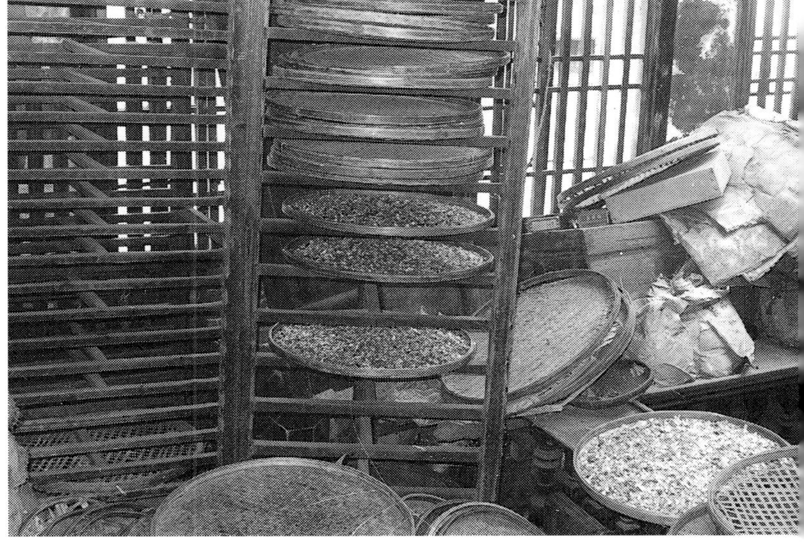

24. Wooden rack for drying plant-based medicinal drugs, which lay on flat wicker baskets in the shade. Photograph of a pharmacy in Taipeh, 1970.

different from the mass marketing of specialty or manufactured products by European pharmacies and pharmaceutical industries since the 19th century.

The primary focus of the complex formulary literature in China was not the design of individual formulas that were based on a diagnosis of an individual patient's health and were rooted in theory. Rather, the aim was to offer knowledge about drug combinations that could affect certain signs of illness, regardless of an individual's constitution. Accordingly, formulae collections such as the *Taiping huimin hejiju fang* 太平惠民和劑局方 (*Formulary of the Offices for the Compilation of Formulas for the Assistance of the Public in the Taiping Period*) were organized according to states of discomfort and illnesses that were widely known among the educated. Thus, they were ultimately directed against claims by professionally practicing physicians. For example, Zhu Zhenheng 朱震亨 (1282–1358), one of the Four Great Masters of the Jin and Yuan Period, who had composed many texts on medical theory himself, wrote in a critical commentary to the *Taiping huimin hejiju fang*, that was later printed as an appendix to this formula collection:

> These pharmacy formulas are published as a book so that one can design formulas according to signs of disease. This means, in order to apply drugs, one does not need to visit a doctor, and one does not have to prepare anything extra. One buys something, and there is instant success. Pills and powders effect the curing of illness and pain in a simple manner. An attitude of love towards the public has reached visible perfection here! Thus, the formulas that proved effective for our ancestors were collected here in order to apply them to uncountable illnesses of the people of our age. Where is the difference between someone who carves a notch in [the rim of his] boat in order to [later] find his sword [that has fallen into the water at this place] and someone who sets out to find a thoroughbred horse based on a drawing? It should be quite difficult indeed to score a hit in this way! [17]

Yet another impressive literary testimony to the public interest in the distribution of formulary knowledge is the *Shengji zonglu* 聖濟總錄 (*Comprehensive Record of the Sages' Help*) from the reign of Zhenghe 政和 (1111–1117). As in the two texts mentioned above, the authors of the *Shengji zonglu* endeavored to include not only all published knowledge, but also folk recipes in their work. In addition to almost 20,000 formulas, the reader of this book will find detailed information about the theoretical foundations of Chinese medicine. Obviously, this includes astrological and demonological knowledge; thus the *Shengji zonglu* contains one of the largest collections of exorcistic characters believed to be medically effective. Only the editions of the People's Republic of China have relinquished the reproduction of this integral aspect of traditional Chinese medicine.

In the history of Chinese medicine in the pre-Republican era, the interest of various Song governments in the health

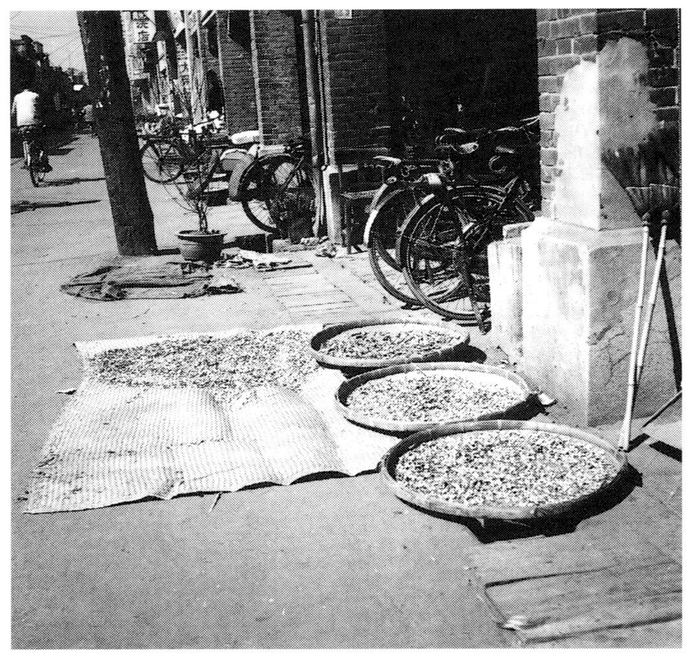

25. Plant-based medicinal drugs drying on flat wicker baskets in the sun. Photograph in front of a pharmacy in Taizhong, Taiwan, 1970.

of the general population remained an exception. Public welfare pharmacies are still documented until the beginning of the Ming period in the fourteenth century, but do not appear in the chronicles afterwards. This also marks the end of the era of the great pharmaceutical works and formularies whose publication had been sponsored by the government. In the following six centuries, many authors continued to compose sometimes quite extensive formularies, but hardly any of these gained fame comparable to those of the Tang and Song periods.

The conclusion of the Imperial period brought an end to the tradition of classic materia medica and formularies. A few authors with a classical education, such as Cao Yingfu 曹穎甫 (1866–1938), continued to compose commentaries on the ancient texts in traditional style, but Western medicine had become so important since the beginning of the twentieth century that even these works could no longer avoid dealing with the new information. This led to the development of a separate style of literature whose authors strove, with changing emphasis, to preserve as many of the traditional ideas as possible by relating them to scientifically oriented medicine.

26. Depiction of a pharmacy open to the street. The characters above the workshop state: "In this pharmacy, decoctions that respond to illness conditions are manufactured according to the rules." A board positioned to the left of the building states: "In this pharmacy, genuine medicines from [Si]chuan and Guang[dong] are sold." In the room on the left, an assistant sits in front of an instrument for cutting drugs. A wooden rack is located in the back corner for drying plant-based drugs in the shade. Three flat wicker baskets for drying plant-based drugs in the sun lie to the right of the pharmacy. From the *Qingming-shanghetu* 清明上河圖 (*Up River [to the Capital] After the Spring Festival*). Excerpt of a drawing, 1248. See also figure 54.

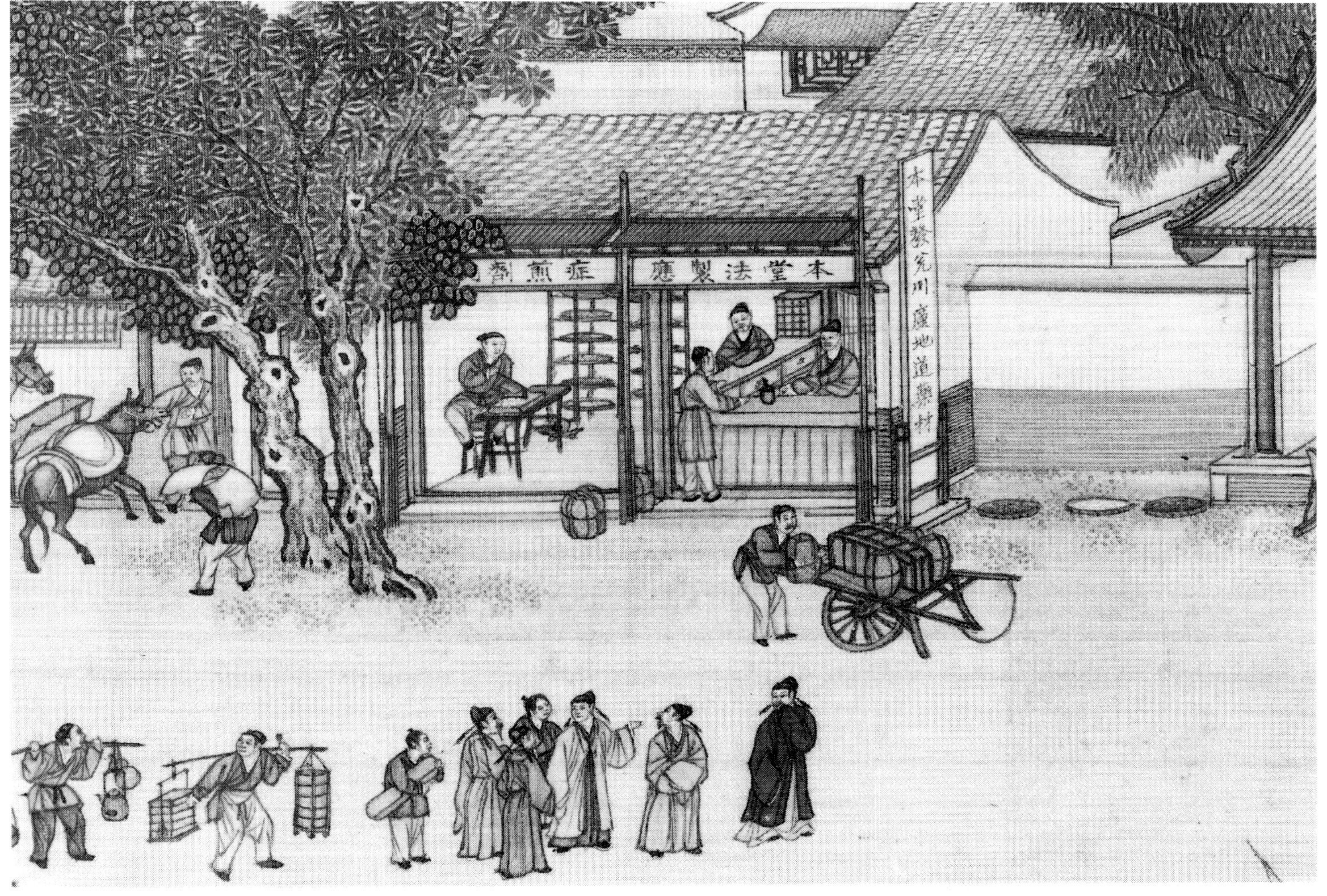

## I. *The Classics of the Han Period*

While the roots of a literature of medical theory in Chinese medicine are obvious, the literature's chronology is not quite as clear as that of pharmaceutical and formulary literature.

The *Huang Di neijing* 黃帝內經 (*Inner Classic of Huang Di*), with its two parts *Suwen* 素問 (*Elementary Questions*) and *Lingshu* 靈樞 (*Divine Axis*), is the great foundation from which Chinese medical theory departed. This corpus was undoubtedly composed from textual fragments of various authors and times. It is still unclear when the individual fragments were written or when they were included in the larger text.[18] Current research suggests that the oldest core of the *Huang Di neijing* dates from the second century B.C.E., but that other ideas mentioned there, e.g. that illnesses are caused by "wind," might be even older.[19] Aside from these parts, which are insignificant to the total text, the main content of the *Huang Di neijing* dates from subsequent centuries. The *Huang Di neijing* contains statements about the human organism which are based on ideas that developed after the unification of the empire under Qin Shihuangdi. One such idea is that the human body is a complicated mechanism composed of a limited number of functional centers ("depots" and "palaces"). These centers look after their own duties, but also contribute constantly to the whole in order to ensure general well-being. The connection between the depots and palaces is maintained by a system of primary and secondary conduits of different ranks. Ultimately, it is the passability of these conduits which guarantees—in imitation of the economic realities of the unified Chinese empire—the transport of all kinds of goods within the body. Likewise, their obstruction can cause all kinds of crises and, therefore, illnesses.

Based on yin-yang and Five Phases theories, the relationships of these functional areas within the body and with the conditions of the macro-environment can be recognized; it is the role of medicine to maintain the body's ability to function, and to protect it from harmful external influences, by observing these relationships. The *Huang Di neijing* mentions fire, summer heat, drought, humidity, cold, and wind as climatic elements of the universe whose influence on the body must be considered, in addition to five emotions that may arise in the organism itself and cause internal problems

The use of medicinal drugs is almost completely ignored in the *Huang Di neijing*. Therapy focuses exclusively on the vessels.[20] It is obvious that the older layers of the *Huang Di neijing,* which date from the first centuries near the turn of the Common Era, were still influenced by instructions to

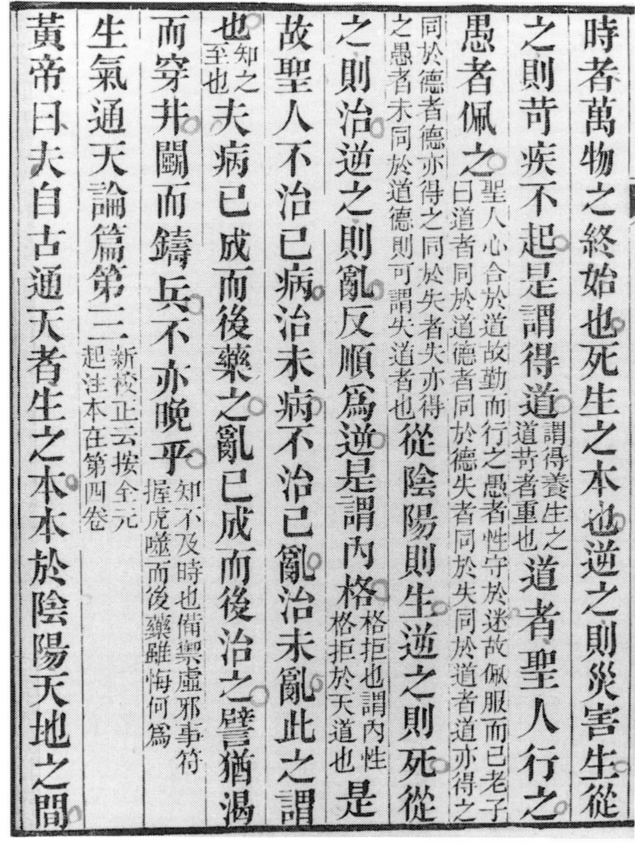

27. "If one follows [the natural course of] yin and yang, then [one can] live; if one goes against it, then [one must] die. If one follows it, then order [arises]; if one acts against it, then disorder [arises]. To turn against conforming, this is 'to act against it'; this is the so-called 'inner rejection.' Therefore, when [it is said], 'The sages did not wait to impose order until an illness had already erupted; they ordered there, where an illness had not yet arisen. They did not wait to impose order until disorder had already arisen, they ordered there, where disorder had not yet arisen,' this is explained [by the elaborations above]. Therefore, if an illness has already arisen and one treats it medically only afterwards, or if disorder has already arisen and one imposes order only afterwards, then this is comparable to digging a well only after one is already thirsty, or to forging weapons only after a fight has already started. Would this not also be too late?!" Textual fragment from the first chapter of *Huang Di neijing suwen* 黃帝內經素問 (*Inner Classic of Huang Di, Elementary Questions*), with insertions of later commentaries. Text ca. first century B.C.E. to second century C.E.; commentaries earlier than sixth century C.E.

treat illness by blood-letting. Through a process that has yet to be explained, blood-letting might have developed into acupuncture for, at a still undetermined point in history, the crudely tapered stone that had been used to open blood vessels gave way to a fine needle. The visible blood that was removed gave way to invisible qi that would be regulated.[21] The vessels themselves, clearly visible points of intervention for blood-letting under the surface of the skin, gave way to so-called conduits, a system of connections between the individual functional centers that cannot be proven anatomically and was, for the most part, assumed to run deep within the limbs inside the body.

Although the *Huang Di neijing* contains all these layers, it is historically worthwhile to consider what it does not contain. The foundational text of Chinese acupuncture largely neglects the specific points on the skin at which to insert the needles. Only a few chapters, and in particular the commentaries by Wang Bing 王冰 from the Tang period, introduced this innovation into the *Huang Di neijing*.

A third of the *Huang Di neijing suwen* is exclusively devoted to a separate teaching of 'five periods and six qi.' The seven extensive *Suwen* chapters practically comprise a book within a book. They attempt to order the apparently disordered climatic changes over the course of the years, and to define those illnesses that are likely to arise from various climatic conditions.

The text of the *Huang Di neijing* that is available today, and which has served as the basis for all reprints and commentaries since the Song period, went through its final revision in the editorial rooms of the Imperial Office for Medical Literature in the eleventh century. Only in a temple library in Japan have substantial fragments of an earlier eighth-century edition been preserved in the *Huang Di neijing taisu* 黃帝內經太素 (*Great Elementaries from the Inner Classic of Huang Di*) by Yang Shangshan 楊上善.

An unknown author in the second century C.E. tried to arrange the heterogeneous content of the *Huang Di neijing* into a strict system and, at the same time, draw diagnostic and therapeutic conclusions from the circulation of blood and qi mentioned there. The *Nanjing* 難經 (*Classic of Difficult Issues*), as this work is titled, founded the tradition of pulse diagnosis in Chinese medicine. It was recognized as the most important source of ancient medical theory until the Mongol period (thirteenth to fourteenth century). It was only in the context of the literary fundamentalism of the Ming and Qing periods that it was no longer understood how later authors could have tried to improve the *Huang Di neijing*. During that time, the *Nanjing* was demoted to the status of a mere commentary on the *Huang Di neijing*. This erroneous evaluation continues to be found in all Chinese history books of the twentieth century.[22]

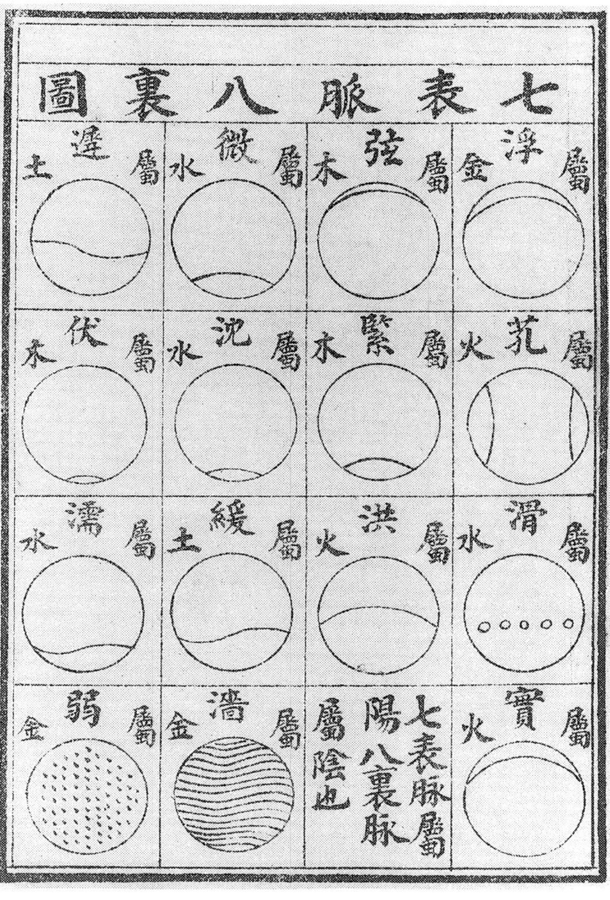

28. Schematic representation of fifteen pulse variations, including their classifications within the categories of the Five Phases theory. From right to left: "Floating on the surface, belonging to [the phase of] metal; like a bow-string, belonging to [the phase of] wood; weak, belonging to [the phase of] water; slowed down, belonging to [the phase of] earth; hollow, belonging to [the phase of] fire; firm, belonging to [the phase of] wood; deep down, belonging to [the phase of] water; hidden, belonging to [the phase of] wood; smooth, belonging to [the phase of] water; extensive, belonging to [the phase of] fire; gentle, belonging to [the phase of] earth; damp, belonging to [the phase of] water; filled in, belonging to [the phase of] fire; rough, belonging to [the phase of] metal; weak, belonging to [the phase of] metal." From *Tuzhu nanjing maijue* 圖注難經脈訣 (*Commented and Illustrated [Edition of the] Classic of Difficult Issues and Pulse Doctrine*), 1683. Undated edition, publisher Guangyi shuju, 上海廣益書局, Shanghai ca. early-twentieth century.

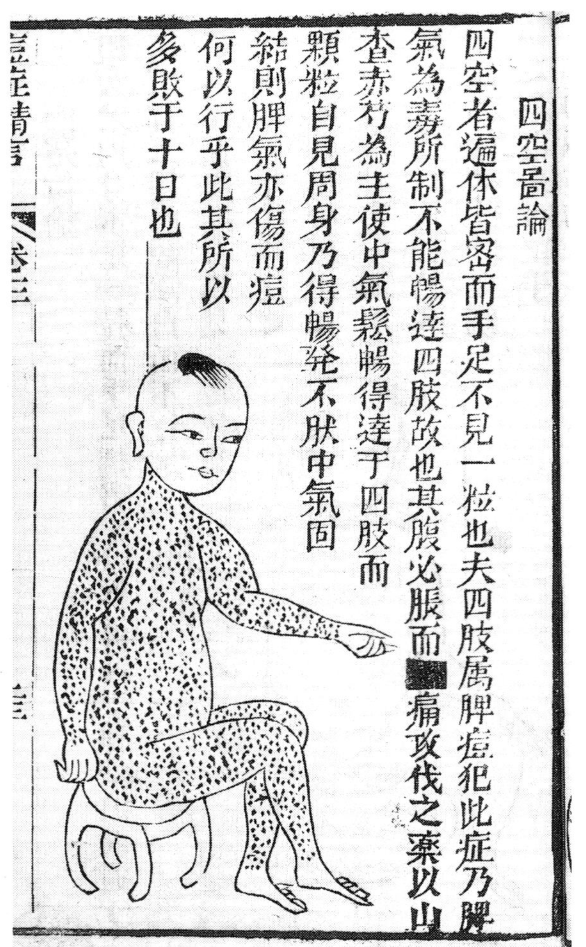


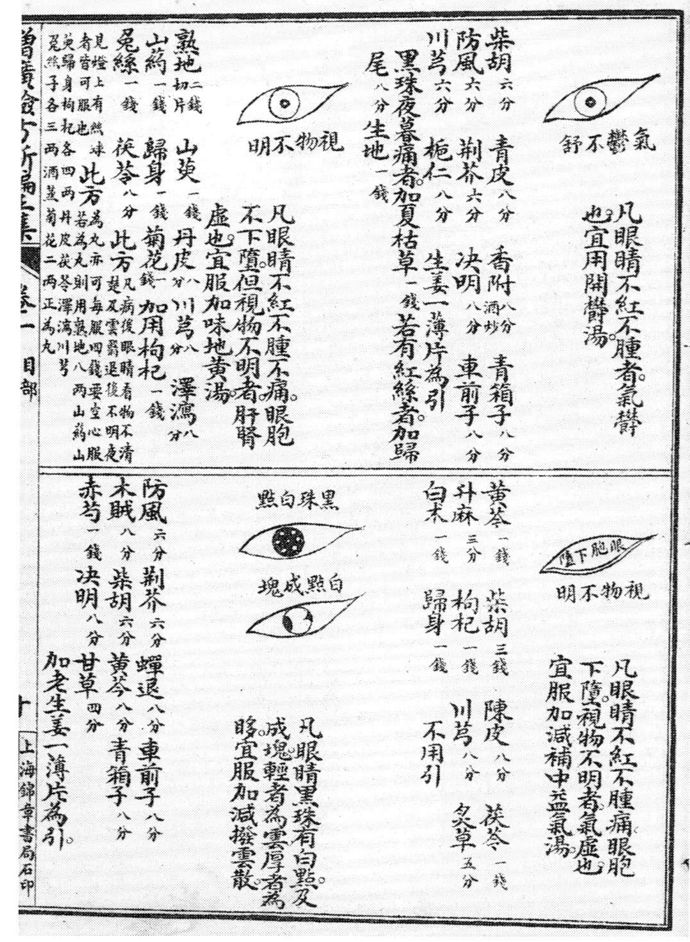


---

29. Text and illustrations to the disease type "Four Open Spaces": " 'Four Open Spaces' means that the entire body is densely covered [with smallpox pustules], and only on the hands and feet, not a single grain is visible. The reason is: The four limbs are connected to the spleen. If [the spleen] is attacked by smallpox, then this condition arises. This means, the qi of the spleen is held back by the [smallpox] poison and is unable to penetrate [into the hands and feet]. [In this condition,] the abdomen is permanently swollen and painful. The counter-attack is lead by the drugs *shanzha* (*Crataegus pinnatifida Bge.* and other types of *Crataegus*) and *chishao* (*Paeonia lactiflora Pall.* and other types of *Paeonia*). They cause the central qi to flow freely, thereby allowing it to reach the four limbs, so that the pustules also appear there. The entire body is penetrated thoroughly, and the swellings are gone. If the central qi congeals into a knot, then the qi of the spleen will also suffer harm; how, then, could the pustules pass through [the body]? This is the reason, why [patients] commonly die on the tenth day." From *Douzhen jingyan* 痘疹精言 (*Essential Statements on Pox and Pustule Disorders*), 1753. Edition n.p., publisher Jijintang 集錦堂, 1824.

30. Upper right: "Suppressed qi does not flow freely. If the eyes are neither reddened nor swollen, then the qi is suppressed. [As therapy,] the 'decoction which liberates what is suppressed' is recommended." Upper left: "Objects are seen out of focus. If the eyes are neither reddened nor sore and if the eyelid also does not droop down and one merely sees objects out of focus, then it is a [qi]deficiency of the liver and kidneys. [As therapy,] the '*dihuang* (*Rehmannia glutinosa* [*Gaertn.*] *Libosch.*) decoction, supplemented with [a few] substances' is recommended." Lower right: "Objects are seen out of focus. If the eyes are neither reddened nor swollen, if the eyelid droops down, and if things are seen out of focus, then this is a deficiency of qi. [As therapy,] one should take the 'adjusted decoction which replenishes the center and increases the qi.'" Lower left (top): "White dots on the iris." Lower left (bottom): "White dots turn into bulbs. If there are white dots on the iris and they turn into bulbs which appear as clouds in light cases and as opaqueness in severe cases, then [as therapy,] one should take the 'adjusted powder that disperses the clouds.'" Information in each case appended with detailed formula prescription. Illustrations and text from the section "Eyes." From *Yanfang xinbian* 驗方新編 (*Newly Compiled Proven Formulas*), 1846. Undated edition, publisher Jinzhang shuju 上海錦章圖書局, in Shanghai.

## 2. The Literature of Medical Specialties

A substantial body of literature was developed in the centuries after the beginning of the Han period, whose content and lines of development remain completely unresearched. This corpus contains practically all of the subjects that may also be found in the history of European medicine. Examples of titles from various specialized fields include the *Maijing* 脈經 (*Classic of Pulse*) by Wang Shuhe 王叔和 from the third century and the *Zhenjiu jiayijing* 針灸甲乙經 (*Classic of Needling and Cauterization [with the Chapters] A, B, [etc.]*) by Huangfu Mi 皇甫謐 (214–282). The *Zhubing yuanhou lun* 諸病源候論 (*Treatise on the Causes and Signs of All Illnesses*) from 610 by Chao Yuanfang 巢元方 is the oldest known etiological work in China, while the *Xi xuan jilu* 洗冤集錄 (*Collected Records of the Washing Away of Wrong-doings*) by Song Ci 宋慈, from 1247, is the oldest specialized forensic text in the world. Under the name of Sun Simiao (581–682), and on the basis of earlier ophthalmological texts that were heavily influenced by Indian knowledge, an unknown compiler of the fifteenth or sixteenth century composed the ophthalmological classic, *Yinhai jingwei* 銀海精微 (*Essential Subtleties of the Silver Sea*).[24] The fields of gynecology and pediatrics have produced their own literature since the Tang period.[25] An essential pediatric compendium that has been reprinted until the present is the *Youyou xinshu* 幼幼新書 (*New Writings about the Little Ones*) by Liu Fang 劉昉 from 1132. One exception from this variegated canon is anatomy, a subject that even after initial impulses from outside of China failed to be developed further.

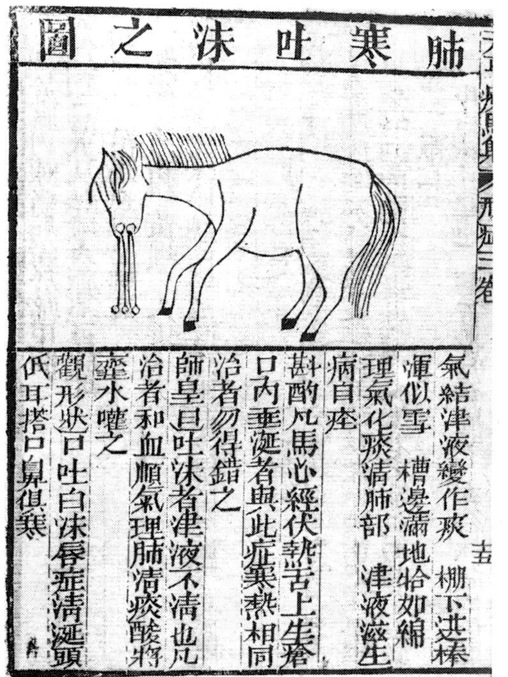

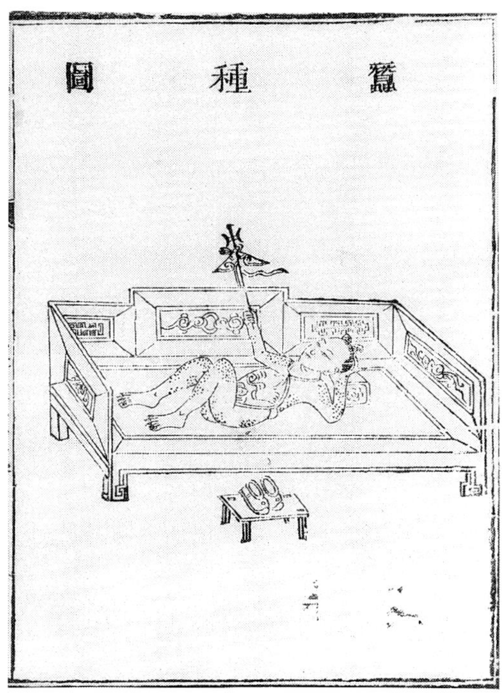

31. Text and illustration to the horse disease "foam spitting due to coldness of the lungs." In *Quantu niumatuojing* 全圖牛馬駝經 (*Complete Illustrated Classic of Cattle, Horse, and Camel [Diseases]*), *Yuan Heng liaomaji* 元亨療馬集 (*Collection of Horse Diseases by [Yu Ben]yuan and [Yu Ben]heng*), 1608. Edition n.p., publisher Sanyitang 三義堂, 1889.

32. Illustration to the skin disorder resembling 蠶種 (silkworm eggs). From *Yucuan yizongjinjian* 御纂醫宗金鑑 (*Imperially Decreed Golden Mirror of Medical Ancestors*), 1742. Edition n.p., publisher Jiangxi shuju 江西書局, 1876.

### 3. Theoretical Literature Since the Song Period

It is possible to retrace the historical development of the theoretical foundations of medicine in the eyes of the Chinese literati class through books whose authors dealt with theoretical considerations. An increasing array of differing viewpoints and procedures can be found since the thirteenth century. Although the secondary literature of China and, even more so, of Europe and America, seems to suggest nowadays that Chinese medicine has remained unchanged over the last two thousand years, the historical development suggests otherwise.

Numerous physicians attempted in their writings to harmonize their personal observations and practical experiences with the theoretical foundations of the classics. In so doing, they reached extremely diverse conclusions. The dynamic growth of Chinese knowledge and ideas that is comparable to Western developments followed a different pattern than that of Europe in at least one aspect. The attempt to construct general theories recognized by the majority, if not all, of a discipline's members is a purely European phenomenon. At no point in traditional Chinese medicine is there a scientific evolution in the sense of Thomas Kuhn, or the replacement of one style of reasoning with another in the sense of Ludwik Fleck.[26] Since Kuhn and Fleck based their theories about the progress of knowledge only on European conditions, their statements cannot apply to China. When a Chinese doctor proposed a new theory he found followers, but there was no need to tenaciously dispute which theory was the best, that is, most convincing, one and should therefore be accepted as the current state of knowledge and the only valid guideline for medical practice. Such an attitude is unknown to this day among representatives of traditional Chinese medicine in China and abroad. Anyone may found their own school by mixing personal reflections with historical excerpts, nowadays generously including diagnostic and therapeutic aspects of scientifically oriented medicine.

The whole range of theoretical approaches since the Song period has only begun to be surveyed, because only a minute number of medical texts of the second millennium have so far been classified or at least provisionally analyzed by content. Liu Wansu 劉完素 (1110–1200), for example, reached the conclusion that illness was generally caused by the body overheating; Zhang Congzheng 張從正 (1156–1228) regarded illness as the result of an invasion of pathogenic influences in the body that were to be countered primarily by "attack and purgation." Li Gao 李杲 (1180–1251) realized that functional disturbances of the spleen and stomach (both organs were believed to be responsible for digestion and metabolism) caused most illnesses; he therefore demanded a strengthening of these two functional centers.

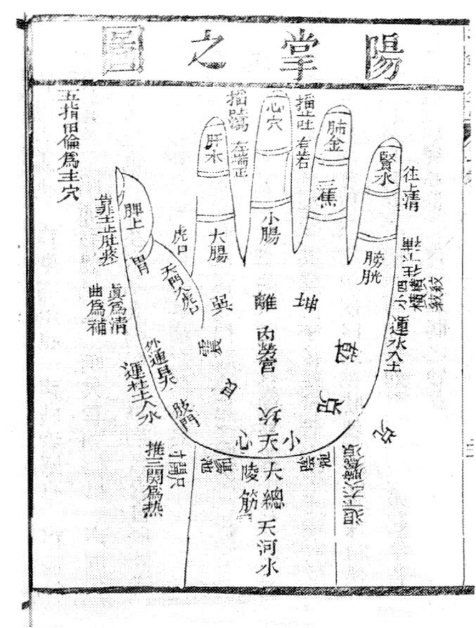

33. Depiction of the left inner hand with information about the classifications of the phalanges in the categories of the Five Phases theory and the associations between the areas of the hand and the trigrams of the *Classic of Changes, Yijing* 易經. From *Xiao'er tuina guangyi* 小兒推拿廣意 (*Expanded Significance of the Push and Pull Massage for Small Children*), 1676. Undated edition, publisher Xuegushanfang 江陰學古山房, Jiangyin, Qing dynasty.

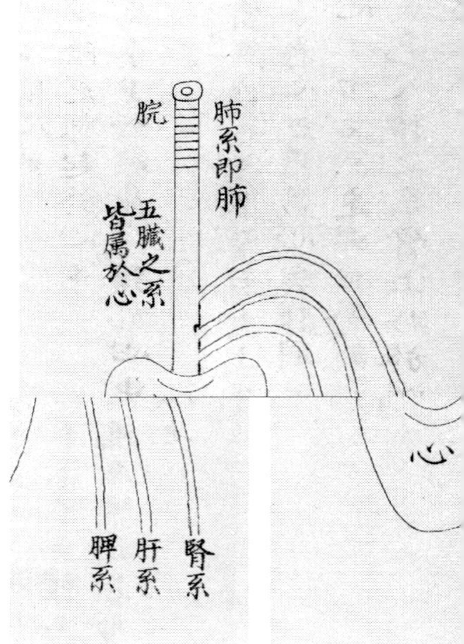

34. Depiction of the heart with an extended exit tube ("connection to the lung, proceeds to the lung"), from which three narrower exits branch off (from right to left: "connection to kidney," "connection to liver," "connection to spleen"). Private medical handbook, undated manuscript.

Paul U. Unschuld

# Medicine in China

Historical Artifacts and Images

© Prestel, Munich · London · New York, 2000

ISBN 3-7913-2149-8

## ERRATA

Due to an unforeseen error in the printing process, three images (figs. 34, 37, and 38) were reproduced incorrectly. For your convenience the complete images are shown again here.

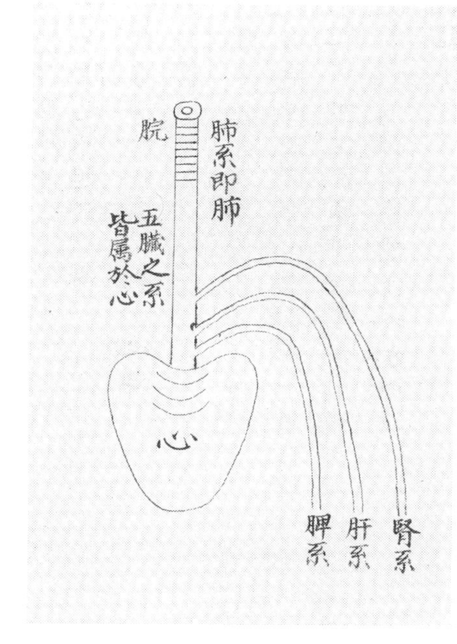


34

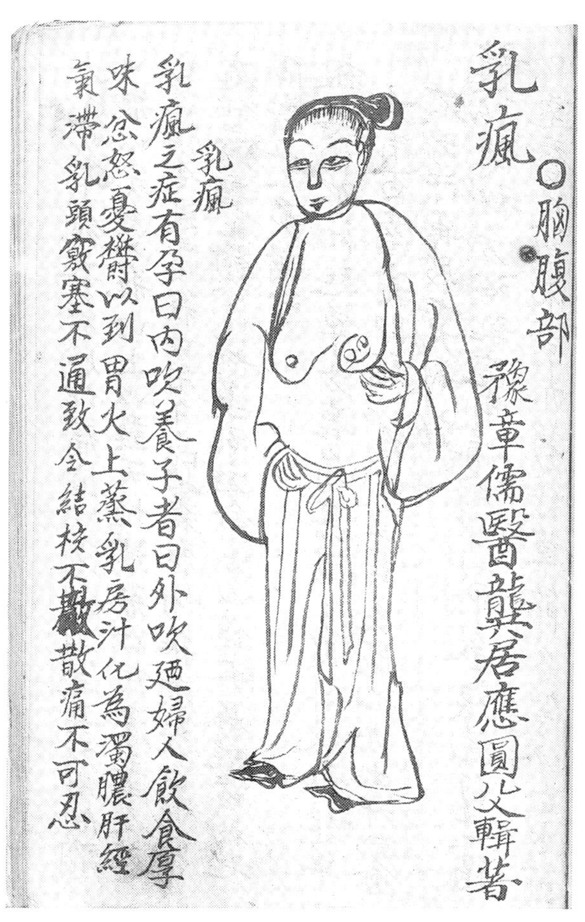


37

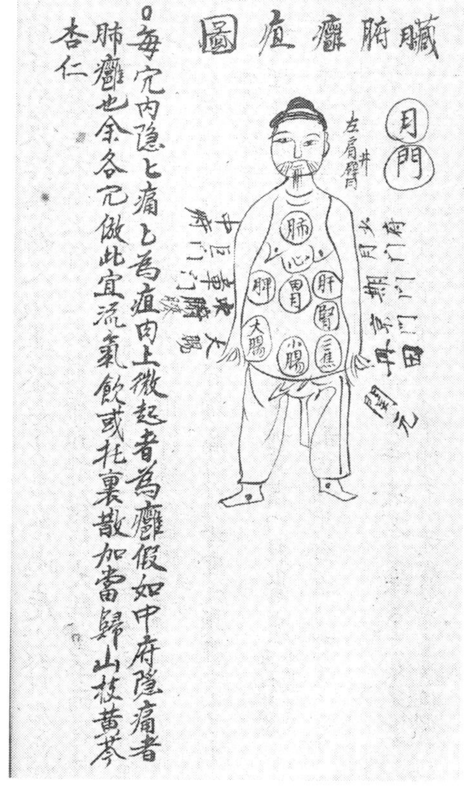


38

The Ming and Qing periods brought with them an even greater splintering of opinions. No writer was able to part with the ancient yin-yang and Five Phases theories, but within this conceptual cage the authors of medical literature turned in many directions in order to understand the body and its illnesses. Some dealt only with the internal functions of the body, others with the external pathogenic influences on the body. Some retraced the centuries in order to find answers in the past, others walked completely new paths in order to find their bearings in real, morphological facts. The Chinese official Wang Qingren 王清任 (1768–1831), for example, happened to acquire an interest in anatomy and then spent decades of his life showing the discrepancies that he—but no one else—perceived between the claims of ancient authors about the internal body and empirical facts. The book that he finally published one year before his death was entitled *Yilin gaicuo* 醫林改錯 (*Correction of Mistakes in Medicine*).[27]

When Western medicine eventually entered China in the nineteenth century—in a developmental stage that was identical to what is referred to as Western medicine today only in its methodology—it did not encounter a homogeneous system of ideas and practices, but rather a medical system that was quite unstable and was splintered into numerous factions. The very recent European discoveries regarding pathogenic germs, and their medicinal or surgical removal, were in China received as the solution of a riddle that had already been pursued for centuries.

The theory of hostile germs—that they should be kept out of the body as if a military enemy or, if they had already penetrated, to be destroyed or expelled as had been newly developed in the West—had been a core aspect of Chinese literati medicine for two millennia. Military metaphors have made sense in Western medicine only for the last hundred years, since the victorious advance of bacteriology and, subsequently, immunology. In China, the expression that "the use of drugs resembles the advance of soldiers" had been self-evidently implicit, and frequently explicit, since the Han period.[28] Only the culturally defensive attempts of twentieth-century China to stress a completely autonomous medical tradition, combined with Western wishful thinking about a fundamentally different medicine in China, have created an artificial chasm between Western and Chinese medicine which is not historically justified in its current state.

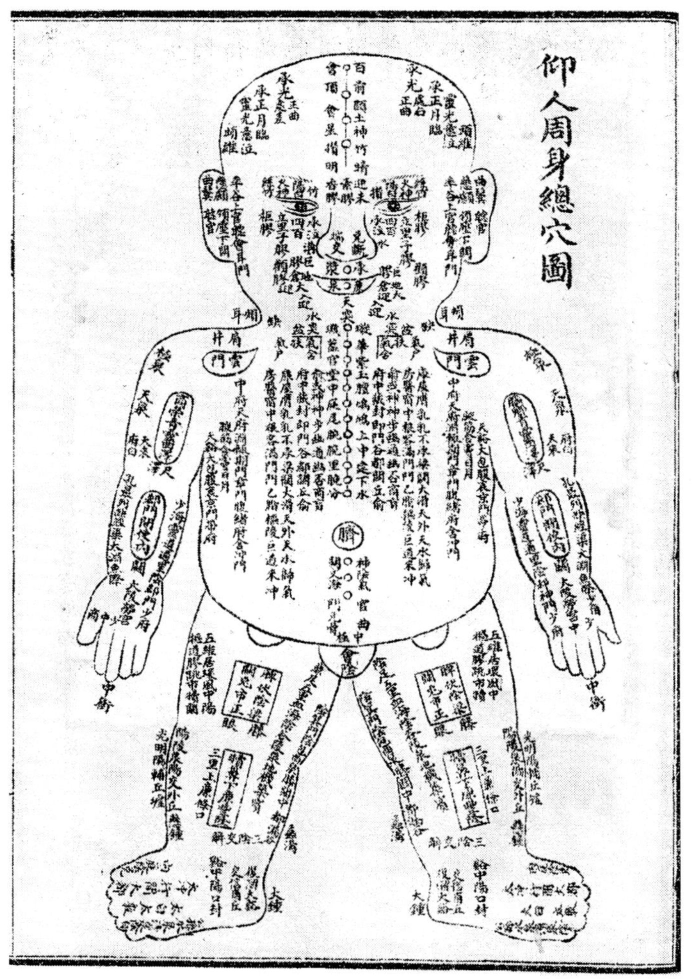

35. "Site plan of all openings [for needling] of the entire human body in frontal view." From *Zengbuhuitu zhenjiudacheng* 增補繪圖針灸大成 (*Expanded and Illustrated Great Compendium of Acupuncture and Moxibustion*), 1601. Edition dated as "republic" by the publisher Guangyishuju 廣益書局.

### The *Chuanya*

Until the nineteenth century, only a small fragment of the population in Europe was able to take advantage of the (questionable) skills of physicians who had been educated in the universities. Similarly, physicians in China who were able to read the literature and apply it in medical practice constituted a minority whose only beneficiaries were the formally educated elite.

It is largely unknown what kind of knowledge the healers of the masses possessed and in which ways they treated the illnesses of their clients. Like their European counterparts, the formally educated elite generally did not consider it worthwhile to listen to the words of folk doctors. In the history of Chinese medicine, we are not yet aware of exceptions like Paracelsus or his contemporary Vesalius, the two most influential innovators of European medicine at the verge of the modern period who did not hesitate to contact the less-respected healers of the lower classes.

A single parallel is a text that offers a small window on everyday medicine in China, clearly different from that of the upper classes. In the eighteenth century, the physician and author of several scholarly texts, Zhao Xuemin 趙學敏 (ca. 1720–1805), composed the *Chuanya* 串雅 (*Stringing Together the Refined*), based on the notes of an otherwise unknown itinerant physician named Zong Boyun and other sources from folk medicine. The fate of the book shows that Zhao Xuemin did not address a topic of widespread interest. First published in 1851, the book had few buyers; regardless, a second edition appeared in 1890.

The reader of the *Chuanya* first notices that yin-yang and Five Phases theories are largely absent from this work. This is not too surprising: only the literati class of the Imperial period lived in an environment where ideas about the constant predictability of processes in the universe and in the human organism made sense. The elite of the Imperial period followed an ideology according to which it was every individual's duty and advantage to fit into the social order. This was the only way to ensure a straight procession to the highest offices, or at least to existential security.

Fundamentally different from this was the world of the peasants. Not even the greatest physical struggles could protect them from losing the fruits of their labor—if not their lives—in unpredictable disasters. Such disasters could be caused by climatic conditions such as droughts or floods, but all too frequently they were caused, instead, by the less supernatural interventions of a corrupt government. It is hardly surprising, therefore, that among the individuals in this strata of society, repeatedly forced to suffer, the experience of the unpredictable power of individuals—be it officials who extorted unbearable taxes or spirits who caused

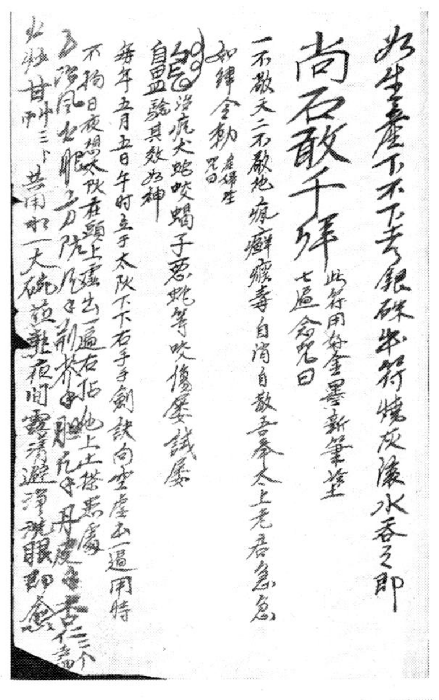

36. Juxtaposition of demonological, magical, and empirical-pharmaceutical cures: "If, during a birth, [the child] ought to be discharged, but is not, then one should write a talisman in silver cinnabar, burn it into ashes and [have the woman] ingest these [ashes] with boiled water. [The talisman says] as follows: 'Thousandfold respectful greetings to the keeper of the stone.' One should write this talisman seven times in good gold ink and with a new brush. Simultaneously, one should pronounce the following spell: 'First, no veneration to Heaven. Second, no veneration to Earth. Wind disorder, freshness disorder, phlegm, and poison may dissolve and disperse on their own. I am ordered by the Old Sire in Highest Height. Quick, quick, this is like an order.' When the birth has happened, the spell is: (An exorcistic character follows here). This cures rabid dogs, snake bites, as well as bite injuries by maggots and evil snakes. Numerous attempts have led to equally numerous successes. The efficacy is miraculous. One should position oneself under the sun each year on the fifth day of the fifth month at the *wu* hour (11–13th hours). The right hand is pointed downwards. The [left] hand should execute a sword gesture in open space and write [this talisman] once. When one [has to] use it, one should not take note of whether it is day or night. One should visualize the sun above one's head and write [the talisman] once into empty space. The right hand should grasp the ground and smear the dirt on the affected area. Five. Formula for the treatment of Wind Fire Eyes. *Fangfeng* (root of *Saposhnikovia divaricata* [*Turcz.*] *Schischk.*), 1 qian; *jingjie* (herb of *Schizonepeta tenuifolia Briq.*), 1 qian; *danpi* (root bark of *Paeonia suffruticosa Andr.*), 1 qian; *xingren* (seed stones of *Prunus armeniaca L.*), 2 qian; remove the oil. Fire dried *gancao* (root of *Glycyrrhiza uralensi Fisch.*), 3 qian. Bring all [drugs] to a boil with a large bowl of water. Cleanse the eyes with pure night dew. This brings relief." Private medical handbook, undated manuscript.

droughts or floods—was prevalent, whereas the elite were influenced by ideas about the constant and predictable processes of a greater order. Consequently, yin-yang and Five Phases theories held persuasive powers only for the latter. By contrast, the accommodation of superior powers, characterized the social and medical "healing" of those who depended on them.

The *Chuanya* distinguishes between three categories of drugs, one that rises in the body, another that sinks and a third that interrupts the progression of an illness or a physical context (such as a tooth loosening). The group of "interrupting" drugs is likewise divided into three groups, depending on whether the aim of such an interruption is to hit the body at a specific "golden point," to deploy an effect that would penetrate the entire body "like a fishing net being dragged through a creek," or to cause results that would radiate outwards in all directions in the organism "like a club with spikes on all sides." In addition to these medicinal effects, apparently based on mechanistic metaphors, the *Chuanya* mentions numerous exorcistic drugs in order to fight pathogens that could disturb or harm the body or the senses from the outside and might occasionally penetrate into the body. It is not difficult to imagine how readily European ideas of bacteriology were embraced when they entered China in the late nineteenth century.

Besides the internal drugs described in the first four chapters, the *Chuanya* also records many other therapeutic practices which presumably cover the entire spectrum of therapeutic intervention of itinerant and popular physicians. Individual paragraphs are devoted to the following therapeutic measures: exorcistic characters, exorcistic techniques, raising the dead, life-saving measures (e.g. in the case of a fractured skull or sudden heart pains), needling procedures (acupuncture), burning procedures (moxibustion), fumigation procedures, plasters, steams, ablutions, heat compresses, and breathing techniques.

The skills of the itinerant physician were apparently not limited to the treatment of human patients, but also had to be applied to veterinary medicine (including the treatment of sick silkworms) and the treatment of affected plants. Appropriate formulas form the second to last entry in the *Chuanya*. The concluding paragraph is entitled "Playing with Drugs." Here, we find "procedures to avoid intoxication from the consumption of wine," "procedures to etch pictures into mirrors," "procedures to remove ink characters from documents," "pills to suppress hunger and thirst," "pills to make demons visible," "procedures to create dreams at will," and, lastly, a "procedure to create a wooden dog that can walk automatically."


Medical Manuscripts


Compared to the printed literature of Chinese medicine which is so voluminous and, at the same time, almost completely unresearched, the unprinted literature has been

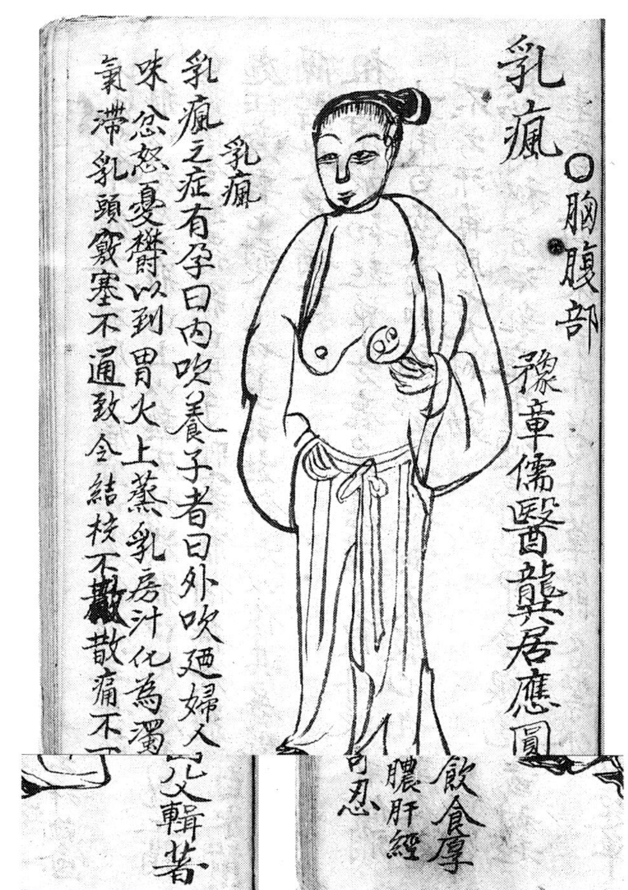

37. Text and drawing to "breast wind disorder": "Section Breast and Abdomen. Composed by the Confucian scholar physician Gong Ju[zhong], Yingyuan, from Yuzhang. Breast wind disorder. The condition breast wind disorder is called 'blown from the inside' in a pregnant woman, and 'blown from the outside' in a nursing mother. The cause lies in the fact that a woman ingests liquids or solids of extremely strong taste or that she is angry or sad. In such cases, the fire of the stomach rises up and heats the breast chamber. The juice [of milk contained therein] is transformed into cloudy puss. The qi of the liver conduit blocks the nipple. Thereby the opening is obstructed. Knots are formed which can no longer be dispersed. The pain is unbearable." Private medical handbook, undated manuscript.

entirely neglected. In Europe, there are countless manuscripts of medical texts from the centuries before the introduction of printing; Scholars of classical philology and *Fachprosa* have studied many of these sources but are still far from exhausting them. There are no known manuscripts, with the exception of the Mawangdui texts and a few other discoveries from Han-period tombs, that predate the first printed medical texts from China, which were produced there half a millennium earlier than in Europe. Not one manuscript from subsequent centuries has been investigated yet, much less edited, possibly because of the assumption that only important texts were printed and, therefore, deserve priority.

This might, in fact, be a false conclusion. Those texts were printed which, in the eyes of the publisher, promised to draw the attention of a larger audience and, therefore, to make a greater profit. In this, the contents of the printed works certainly met their expectations and the ideology of the literati class. The *Chuanya* was, after all, published half a century after its creation, but the small number of sales of this text, so full in content and insights from our perspective, might have caused other publishers not to consider this kind of title.

The collection of medical manuscripts in the Unschuld Collection of the Museum for Völkerkunde Berlin (Dahlem) includes very diverse materials. They range from texts that were available in printed form but were copied manually by students or physicians for lack of finances or because the printed texts were not available any more, to private formulae collections and unpublished theoretical papers, to personal documents that had always been intended for private use only. Among the last category is a phrase book from an itinerant physician. It offers insights into psychological methods for increasing sales and the ethical standards of a traveling drug salesman/doctor which are more informative than those from any other known source (see pp. 75–78).

Similarly, many other primary sources among the medical texts which are in manuscript form in Chinese libraries and private collections are likely to offer insights into aspects of Chinese medicine that have been conveniently ignored in the printed literature.

Even Zhao Xuemin, usually so open-minded towards marginal topics, wrote in his introduction to the *Chuanya*, that he had not included those practices from the records of Zong Boyun in his book which he classified as "inhuman." Thus, he declined to reproduce in their entirety techniques by which itinerant physicians had "planted" illnesses into healthy clients in order to make a profit from the subsequent treatment of these illnesses. He only included a few examples of these procedures in the *Chuanya*, "in order to prove their existence."[29]

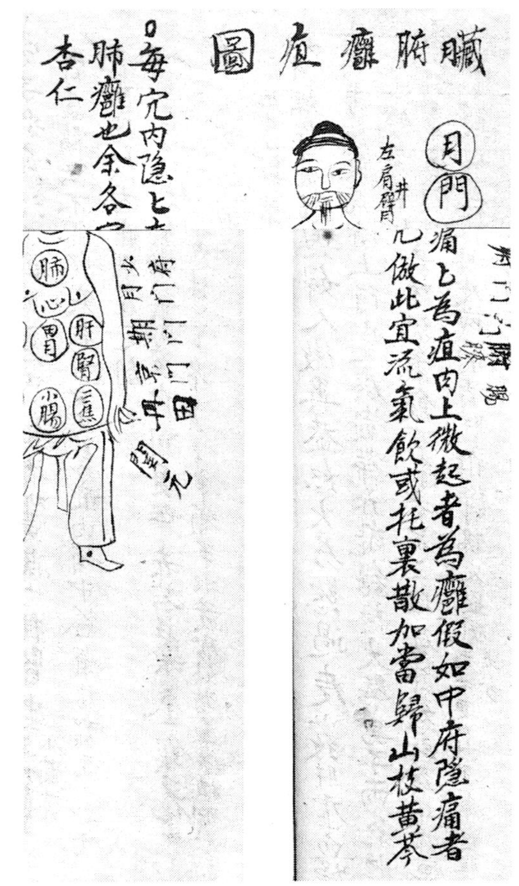

38. "Site plan of the abscesses and ulcers related to the depots and palace [organs]. Wherever there is pain under a [skin] opening without any visible sign, an ulcer [of a depot or palace organ] is located there. If the flesh rises up somewhat, then it is an abscess [in one of the organs]. If there is pain in the 'middle palace' without any visible sign, it is a lung abscess. The same also applies for the other points. [For the treatment,] the 'potion which makes the qi flow' or the 'powder which picks up the interior' are recommended, with the addition in each case of *danggui* (root of Angelica sinenis [Oliv.] Diels.), *shanzhi[ren]* (seed stones of Pittosporum glabratum Lindl.), *huangqin* (root of Scutellaria baicalensis Georgi), and *xingren* (seed stones of Prunus armeniaca L.)." Private medical handbook, undated manuscript.

# 5. Western Medicine in Chinese Texts

The first European medical text to be composed and published in Chinese was probably a small anatomical treatise by the Jesuit Johann Schreck (1576–1630).

Schreck was educated in medicine and mathematics and was particularly devoted to botany. He entered the Jesuit order in 1611 and then responded to an invitation by fellow monks, who were already in China, to apply his knowledge there for the benefit of spreading the Christian faith. While in Hangzhou he was forced to wait for permission to continue his journey to the capital, but he used this break to compose a short introduction to anatomy in Chinese. To be sure, after his arrival in Peking, his expertise was demanded primarily for the composition of mathematical and astronomical texts, since the Chinese court was convinced of the superiority of Western knowledge only in these areas. Therefore he put his short anatomy aside; only after his death, did Adam Schall pass on the manuscript to a native, Bi Gongchen 畢拱辰, who was interested in anatomy and subsequently published it under the title *Taixi renshen shuogai* 太西人身說概 (*Explanations of the Human Body from the Far West*).

It had only been a few decades before Schreck composed his manuscript, that Andreas von Wesel, known as Vesalius, had raised anatomy to a completely new level with his *De Humani Corporis Fabrica Libri Septem*, the influence of his text is clearly evident in Schreck's smaller outline. The first volume begins with a description of the skull bones and the skeleton, followed by comments on the cartilage, ligaments, meat fibers, wide tendons, glandular tissue, fatty tissue, blood vessels, tendons, skin, flesh, and muscles. The second volume discusses in dialogue form the physiology of the sense organs, the brain and sensation, the occurrence of language and movement, as well as the significance of the brain as the center for the perception of the environment.[30]

There is no obvious explanation for the fact that the anatomy and morphology of the human body was largely ignored in China in the long centuries between the composition of the fairly detailed information in the *Huang Di neijing* and *Nanjing*, that had probably been based on influences from abroad, and the turning point in the nineteenth century. Pointing to such factors as the Confucian focus on an unharmed body is not enough since in Europe, anatomy had to face similar and vigorous resistance from Christianity. It is notable that, regardless of the many social nonconformists in China, the cultural context was still so closely knit that, even among these outsiders, no one looked for a way into the real physical structures of the human body. Influenced by Indian ophthalmology, Chinese ophthalmological texts described the structural connections between the eye and the brain. Not one scholar or doctor in China, however, closely examined the actual shape of these structures.

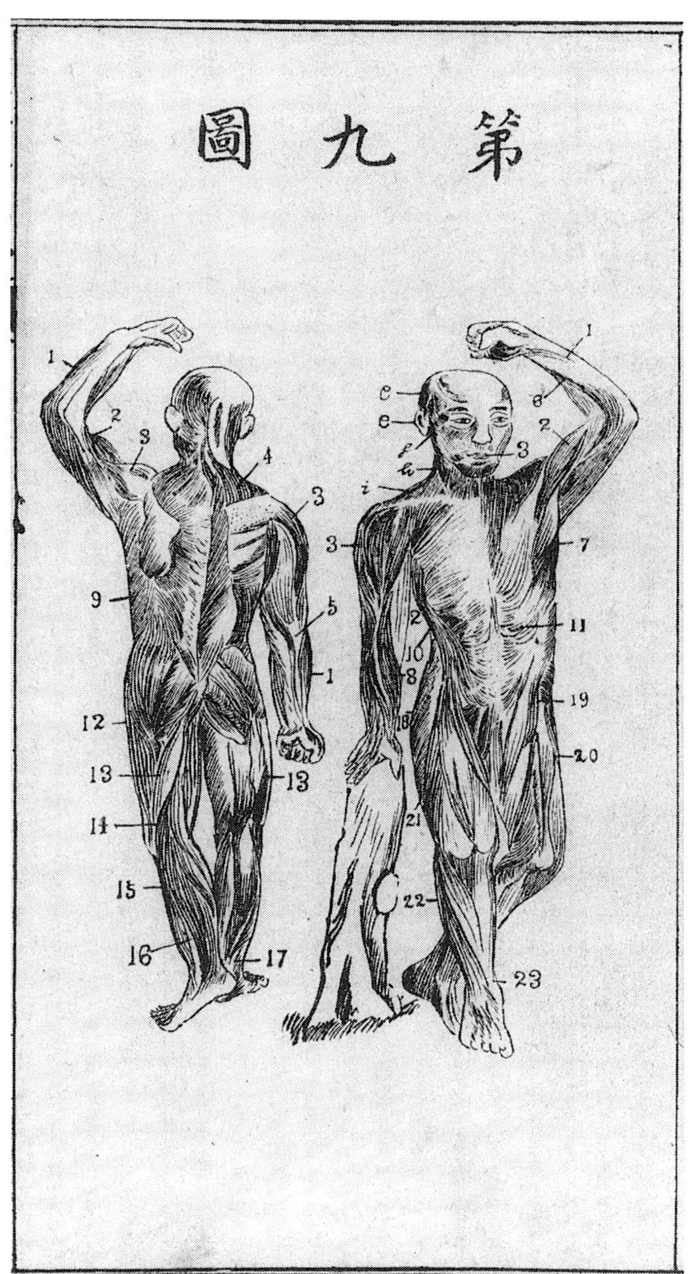

39. The muscles of the human body. From *Xinyixue tushuo* 新醫學圖説 (*Illustrated Explanations of the New Medicine*), edition n.p., n.d., late-nineteenth, early twentieth century. Society for Medical Research 醫學研究社.

It is paradoxical that vivisections and autopsies were performed in Europe throughout antiquity, the late Medieval and early Modern periods to gain detailed morphological knowledge, many centuries before the diagnostic, physiological, and, most importantly, pathological ideas that were related to such knowledge were developed. In China, conversely, the inside of the organism had been known as a site of war-like entanglements since the Han dynasty, and it was common sense to speak of the location of an illness and the path that an evil took inside the body after it had penetrated from the outside. While the theoretical foundations practically suggested the step towards morphology, no Chinese doctor ever is known to have opened up the body, prior to the 19th century, to investigate the depots, palaces, conduits, and other structures that were described in their texts.

Thus, Johann Schreck's *Taixi renshen shuogai* was not granted a long-lasting influence. There was no fertile ground in which the seed could have germinated. Two centuries later, Wang Qingren's isolated work, the *Yilin gaicuo* from 1830, would have probably not changed this, had it not been for the almost simultaneous large-scale introduction of Western medicine in combination with the economic and colonial interests of the Imperial powers in China. European and American physicians who took the time to look at traditional Chinese medicine focused their criticism primarily on what they considered to be its greatly outdated anatomical knowledge.

The British physician Benjamin Hobson was the first European who attempted, against this background, to introduce the Chinese public to Western science through a series of text books in the 1850s. Together with a Chinese collaborator named Guan Maocai 管茂材 in Shanghai, he published a four-volume work, in Chinese, on anatomy (1851), the *General Foundations of Western Medicine* (1857), *Internal Medicine* (2 volumes, including pharmaceutics, 1858), and *Gynecology and Pediatrics* (1858). A paragraph from Hobson's *Xiyi luelun* 西 醫 略 論 (*Survey of Western Medicine*) from 1857 illustrates the general attitude of Western doctors towards Chinese medicine:

The human body, the organs, and the entire organism, are comparable to a clockwork. If one fails to open it and take it apart, it is impossible to know how it functions and for what reasons it might fail. Therefore, Western countries permit the autopsy of dead bodies. If a person dies in an institution for old, insane, or deaf and mute people, and there are no relatives to claim the body, then the Bureau of Medicine is entitled to open the body for the purpose of instructing students. As soon as this autopsy is concluded, someone is ordered to dress and inter [the body] according to the regulations. As a result, all Western physicians know the secrets of the organs and blood vessels. Chinese students of medicine lack [an experience] of this kind. Old physicians with years [of practical experience] still fail to recognize the shape of the organs. Even when they are faced with an unknown and incurable symptom, they never find out where the origin of the disease was located. I wish China would create a Bureau of Medicine that would grant permission to medical scientists to

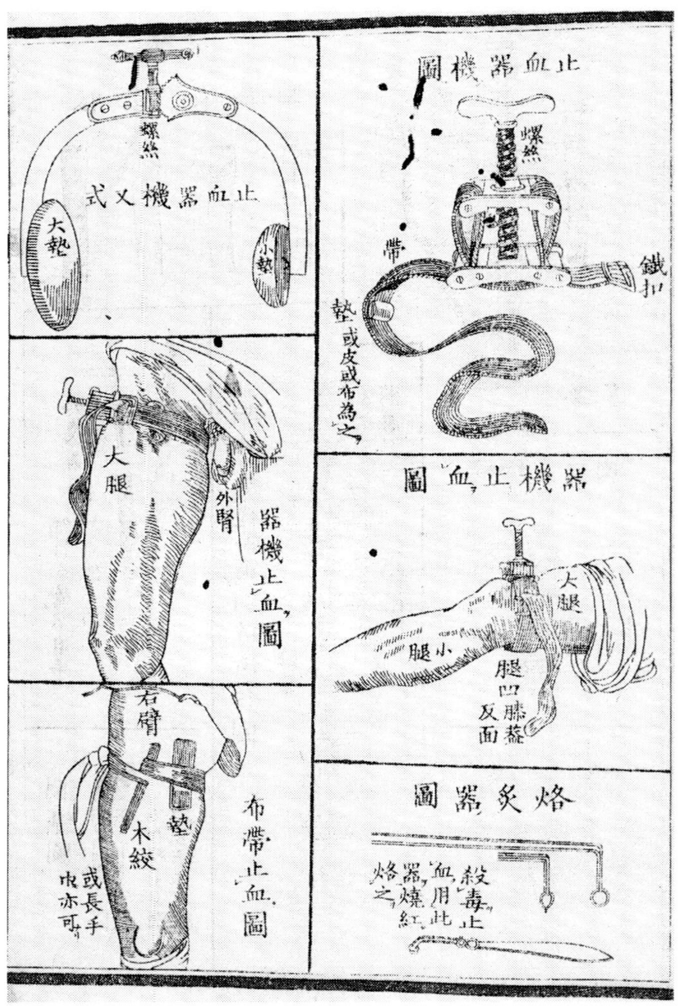

40. Hemostatic equipment from *Xiyi luelun* 西 醫 略 論 (*Survey of Western Medicine*) by Benjamin Hobson and Guan Maocai, 1857. Japanese facsimile reprint, 1858.

dissect and examine criminals who had been sentenced to death. As a result, medicine in China would most surely make great progress from the past.[31]

From the mid- to late nineteenth century, the only obstacle to the dissemination of Western medicine in China was a lack of access to adequate education. There was no professional organization of traditional physicians in China that could have organized a concerted opposition to the new information. There was also no ideological reason, with the exception of anatomy, why Western medicine should have met with rejection in China.

The year 1880 marked the appearance of a Chinese edition of Gray's *Anatomy* in three volumes. Because one hundred volumes sold every year, a second edition appeared in 1889.[32] While the price of this book is no longer known, it was certainly not cheap, containing, as it did, 265 illustrations of which 65 were hand-colored. The small booklet *Quanti xuzhi* 全體須知 (*Important Knowledge about the Entire Body*) (1894) by John Fryer, must have been more reasonably priced (Fryer also co-authored the book *Falü yixue* 法律醫學 (*Forensic Medicine*) with 24 chapters in 10 volumes which appeared in 1899).

Parallel to the translation of Western authors into Chinese, was the appearance of Western knowledge in its own literature by Chinese authors attempting to unite Western and Chinese medicine. Tang Zonghai 唐宗海 (1847–1897) was one of the first classically trained physicians to compose a text of this *zhongxi* (Chinese-Western) medical literature. He announced that one should "value the old, but not blindly trust the old," and demanded that one should not "close one's mind to [the achievements of Western] medicine."[33] His *Zhongxi huitong yijing jingyi* 中西惠通醫經精義 (*Essential Contents of the Medical Classics in the Mutually Beneficial Confluence of Chinese and Western [Knowledge]*) from 1884 was reprinted at least seventeen times over the next five decades. Together with the publication of numerous other titles of this genre, it illustrates the relentless Chinese desire to harmonize their own tradition with what was no longer foreign knowledge.[34]

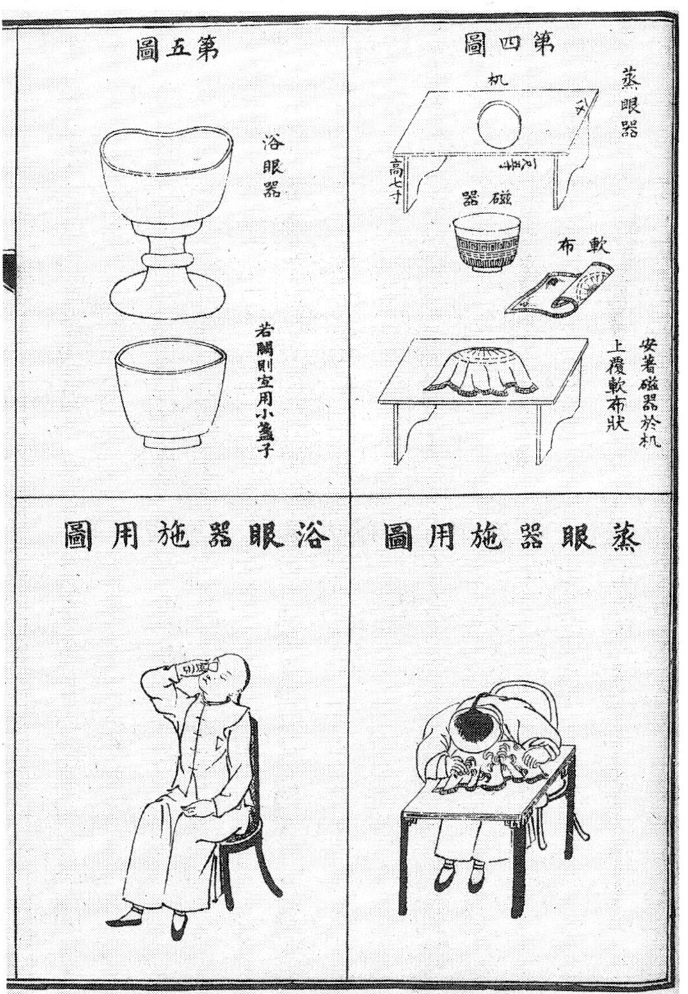


41. Instruments and techniques for steaming the eyes. Inserted into the *Yanke daquan* 眼科大全 (*Complete Ophthalmology*), 1642, at the beginning of the twentieth century. Publisher Dacheng shuju 上海大成書局, Shanghai, 1920.

# THE CHINESE PHARMACY

## DRUG USE AND CHINESE PHARMACOLOGY

It is traditional Chinese pharmaceutics, not acupuncture, that have played the primary role in the treatment of illness for the last two millennia in China. This aspect of Chinese medicine is revealed to us, practically without any mediation and in a highly refined stage of development, in the *Formulas Against 52 Illnesses* (*Wushier bingfang*) from the Mawangdui tomb complex. The Mawangdui formulas provide a multitude of techniques, differentiated by the aim and purpose of future application and indications (see p. 23), for processing a total of 224 natural and artificially created primary ingredients into different drug forms.

For two subsequent millennia there was a steady increase in the number of medicinally used natural substances described in pharmaceutical literature, culminating in a high point in the sixteenth century. Formulae collections and monographs on individual drugs preserved the corresponding information and, today, facilitate the analysis of what is practically an uninterrupted developmental history.

### *1. The Chinese Materia Medica*

The medicinal drugs of the *Wushier bingfang* are derived from a variety of sources, including 106 plants which were complemented by sixty-five animal, nine human, and fifteen mineral substances and ten implements from daily life.

While some of the basic plants were unknown in Europe, many, such as peaches ("expel worms from lesions in the skin"), dates (for a specific type of hemorrhoids), date stones (for urine retention and burning), or coltsfoot (for bites from rabid dogs) were well known in Europe and employed here in treating patients, too.

This is also true of animal preparations such as hare brain ("for frost bite"), hare skin ("helpful with burns when charred"), dried silkworms (for illnesses in the area of the reproductive organs), and beef (for a specific type of skin disease). Drugs of a human origin include the urine of newborn boys (for a specific kind of hemorrhoids, skin problems, and aconite poisoning), hair of the head (for injuries and skin problems), breast milk (for burns), sweat from the skin (for burns), and also male spermatic fluid

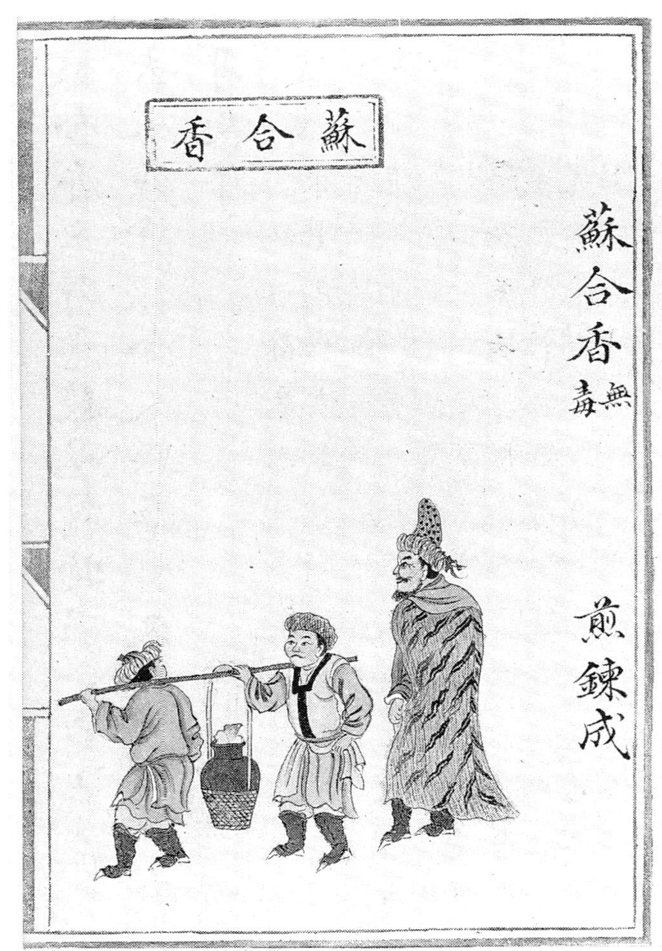

42. Illustration of the drug *suhexiang* (styrax). Text to the right: "Styrax, non-toxic. Gained by cooking and melting [procedure]." The drawing depicts a Western foreigner and two assistants bringing the drug to China, since styrax was imported from India for centuries. From *Yuzhi bencao pinhui jingyao* 御製本草品彙經要 (*Materia Medica Written on Imperial Orders, Containing the Essential and Important in Classified Order*), 1505. Identical copy of the original, nineteenth century or earlier. Staatsbibliothek, Berlin.

(for burns and various injuries). All of these substances were also used in European pharmaceutics until the seventeenth and eighteenth centuries under the category "dirt pharmacy."

The minerals of the *Wushier bingfang* were also not foreign to Europeans. Cinnabar and mercury were recommended for various skin problems and iron splinters were prescribed as an antidote for aconite poisoning. Salt is recommended for cramps following an injury, for leprosy, and urine retention as well as dysuria. Clear water floating above a suspension of mud whose particles have settled was given in the cases of infant colic and dysuria, but also for bites from rabid dogs. Dirt clots, finally, that accumulated on the bottom of a stove after wood had burned there for a long period of time, were also regarded as helpful for the effects of rabid dog bites.

While a real, natural, curative effect can be demonstrated or at least be assumed in these four drug categories, the application of substances from daily life seems to have been primarily based on magic. Examples include worn-out hemp clothing (for burns), tattered straw mats (for various injuries and warts), a woman's first menstrual cloth (for burns, a type of hemorrhoids, and other problems), jacket collars (for dysuria and urine retention), and wagon grease (for certain skin problems).

There was a continued increase in the number of drugs with known medicinal properties in the following two millennia. Many substances came from the different provinces of China, especially Sichuan, an area that is known to this date for its wealth of medicinal drugs. Other substances were imported to China from abroad and then integrated into materia medica there. Theriaca, for example, supposedly invented by King Mithridates of Pontus (124–62 B.C.E.), was one of the most coveted detoxicants of European pharmaceutics in the late Middle Ages and long into the Modern period.[35] This preparation of numerous ingredients was first described in China as *diyejia* 底野迦 in the Tang period text *Xinxiu bencao* 新修本草 from 659:

Diyejia. Taste: acrid, bitter. [Thermo-nature:] neutral. No toxicity. Controls all kinds of illnesses, the condition of being hit by evil, possession, bad qi, as well as abdominal obstructions. Origin: Western countries.

It is said that this drug is made from gall. Externally, it resembles pills that have been rotten for a long time. The color is reddish black. Foreigners import it occasionally. It is considered extremely valuable and expensive. It has proven its effectiveness in experiments.

Much later, in the encyclopedic pharmaceutical work *Bencao gang mu* 本草綱目 (1596) by Li Shizhen 李時珍, another drug was recorded that seems to have made its way from India to East Asia and was to become synonymous with the decline of China two-and-a-half centuries later: opium. (The first opium smoker is documented around

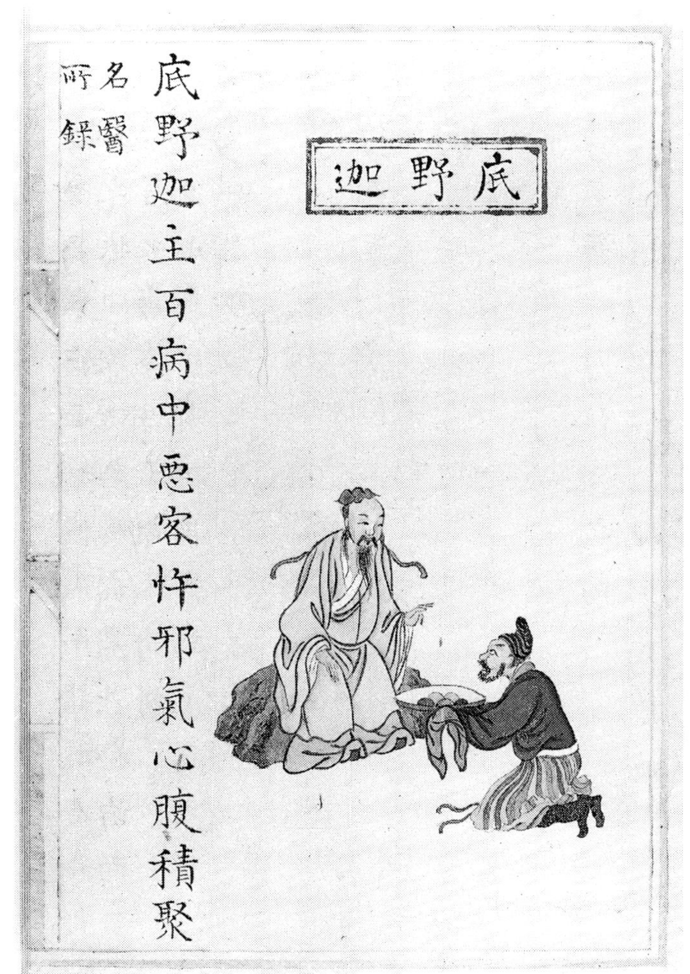

43. A foreigner presents a bowl of *diyejia* (theriaca) to a Chinese. From *Yuzhi bencao pinhui jingyao* 御製本草品彙經要 (*Materia Medica Written on Imperial Orders, Containing the Essential and Important in Classified Order*), 1505. Identical copy of the original, nineteenth century or earlier. Staatsbibliothek, Berlin.

1600.) As one of its uses, opium was recommended as a sexual stimulant.[36] In the *Bencao gang mu*, however, where the names *afurong* 阿芙蓉 or *apian* 阿片 were apparently used to transcribe the sound of the original Greek work "opion," the drug was indicated particularly for diarrhea.[37]

In the Modern period, a small number of Chinese drugs were also introduced into Western pharmaceutics: in 1887, the Japanese researcher Nagai isolated an alkaloid from *mahuang* 麻黃 (*Herba ephedrae*) which he called ephedrine.[38] Chaulmoogra oil, used in China since the fourteenth century for the treatment of leprosy, also became known in Europe in the nineteenth century, but has been recognized in scientifically oriented medicine, as ethylester,[39] only since 1920. Chinese angelica (*Radix angelicae sinensis*, Chinese: *danggui* 當歸) has been marketed as a gynecological preparation for several decades by a German pharmaceutical company. But the most famous Chinese drug, ginseng (*Radix ginseng*, Chinese: *renshen* 人參), although it is readily available for sale in Europe and the United States, has so far failed to leave the shelves of natural food stores and health shops and gain acceptance as a medicine.

Only a small number of substances, including rhubarb root and croton seeds, have been evaluated and applied to identical problems in both European and Chinese pharmacology. On the other hand, a medicinal drug like licorice root (*Radix glycyrrhizae uralensis*, Chinese: *gancao* 甘草), known in Western pharmaceutics for centuries and still taken in the form of a dried extract for the treatment of upset stomach, illustrates how the theoretical foundations of Chinese pharmacology led to classifications that were different from those in Europe. The pharmacological functions that this system attributed to licorice are completely incomprehensible from a modern scientific viewpoint and only make sense within the framework of Chinese theory. Thus, *gancao* is able to:

> ...replenish the qi of the spleen. The drug is used in cases of deficiency symptoms associated with the spleen in conjunction with shortness of breath and diarrhea. Furthermore, it moisturizes the lungs and ends coughing. It cools heat and conquers fire poison. The fresh drug is therefore used for carbuncles, ulcers, and throat infections, when they are caused by fire poison. For these purposes, it can be applied internally or externally. It alleviates cramps and pain. It is therefore used for painful cramps in the abdomen and legs. It alleviates and harmonizes the properties of other drugs. Because of its sweetness and other properties, it moderates cold and hot drugs in their functions. Since it penetrates into all twelve conduits, it is also able to direct other drugs to their destinations. Finally, it serves as an antidote to a number of toxic substances in either internal or external usage.[40]

Drugs were rarely used individually according to the theoretically based usage of traditional Chinese medicine. As a rule, several substances complemented each other in a

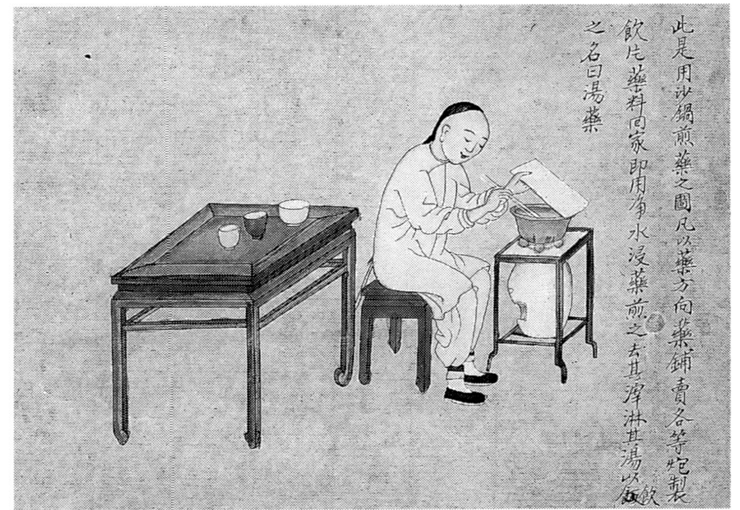


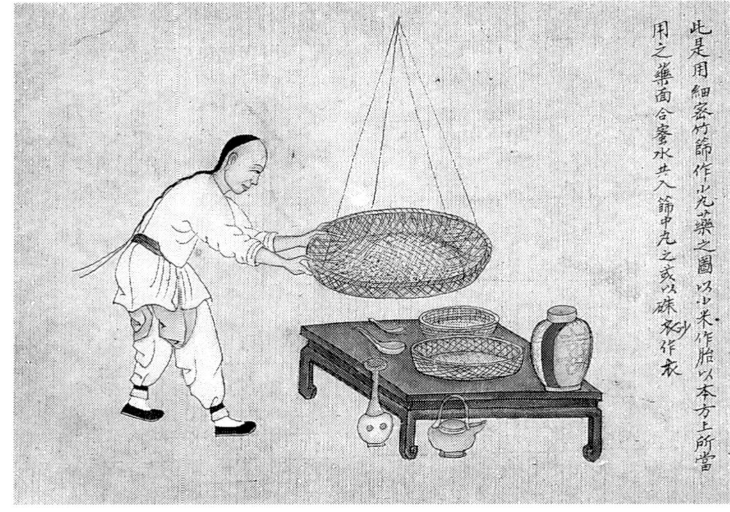


44. "This picture shows the boiling of medicine in a clay cooking pot. When one has purchased from a pharmacy medicinal drugs or pressed herbal tablets that have been processed according to a formula, one returns home and brings them to a boil in pure water. One removes the sediment and filters the decoction before drinking it. Its name is medicinal decoction." Chinese drawing, nineteenth century. Museum für Völkerkunde, Berlin.

45. "This picture shows the manufacturing of small pills by using a fine[ly woven] bamboo basket. The millet forms a kernel. The medicines indicated by the formula are added as powder together with honey-water [into the bamboo basket] and processed into pills [by swiveling the basket with the millet kernel]. Some [pills] are wrapped with *zhusha* (cinnabar)." Gouache, second half of the nineteenth century. Museum für Völkerkunde, Berlin.

broad spectrum of action. *Gancao*, for example, is administered with *dangshen* 當參 (*Radix codonopsitis pilosulae*) to treat lack of appetite, exhaustion, and diarrhea due to a deficiency of qi in the spleen. Together with *Herba ephedrae* and *Semen Pruni armeniacae* (apricot seeds, Chinese: *xingren* 杏仁), *gancao* treats pain and swelling in the throat. In conjunction with *Flores lonicerae japonicae* (Chinese: *jinyinhua* 金銀花), it is used to cure skin rashes that are caused by an excess of moisture. This list could be increased by many additional examples. A similar listing of such synergisms is recorded in the *Bencao gang mu* in chapters 2 and 3.

## 2. The Pharmaceutical Processing of Medicinal Drugs

What is most characteristic of Chinese pharmacology is not so much the diversity of its materia medica, which includes several thousand substances, but the combination of these substances on the one hand and their pharmaceutical preparation and processing on the other.

Not unlike Galenic pharmacology in Europe, the theory-based pharmacology of China ascribes specific qualities to each drug. These are their tastes—acrid, sweet, bitter, sour, salty, and neutral, and their thermo-natures—hot, cold, warm, cool, and neutral. The highly specific yin-yang classifications of these qualities allows for an explanation of the pharmacological effects of individual substances as diaphoretic, nauseating, releasing, harmonizing, warming, cooling, replenishing, or reducing.

It would greatly exceed the frame of this chapter and book to explain all of the subtleties of Chinese pharmacology as it developed over the thirteenth and fourteenth centuries. It is worth mentioning, however, that Chinese theoreticians not only created theories about the effects of yin-yang and Five Phases regularities on the human organism, but that they also tried to extend their application to the properties and actions of medicinal drugs.

This attempt certainly had practical consequences, since they aimed at refining the pharmaceutical technologies that had been known since the Han dynasty in order to meet all theoretical requirements. This means that it was the responsibility of those knowledgeable in pharmaceutics and in particular of pharmacists to increase, weaken, or completely modify the natural properties of drugs, first by pharmaceutical processing and, later, by preparing formulas in such a way that they reached specific points of action in the organism and exercised the desired pharmacological functions.

The following procedures are examples of processing forms that were described in drug compendiums from the Song period and the following centuries. They were meant to aid in the manufacture of medicinal drugs from raw materials and, sometimes, to modify already specified drug properties.[41]

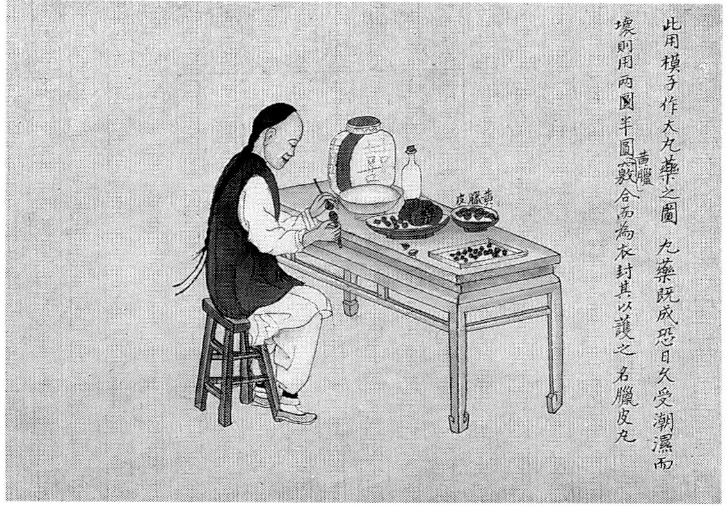


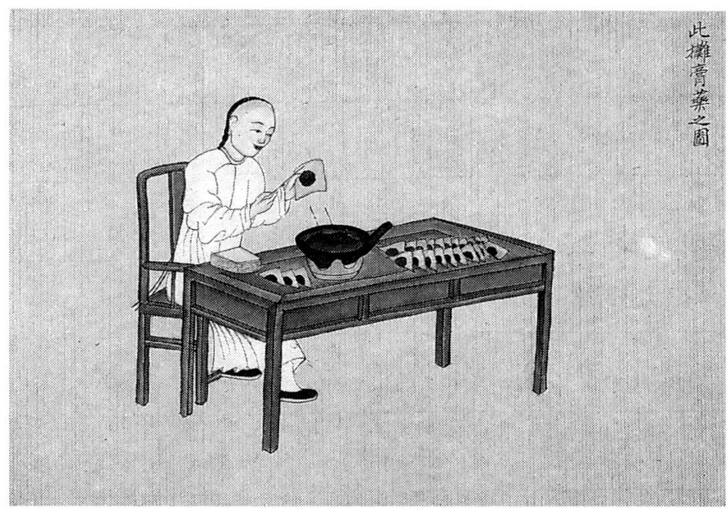


46. "This picture shows the manufacturing of large pill medicines with a mold. If pill medicines are stored for a longer period after having been manufactured, there is a danger that they will absorb humidity and rot. Therefore, one fills two open hemispheres with yellow wax, seals them, and, in this way, creates a protective cover [around the pills]. These are called wax cover pills." Gouache, second half of the nineteenth century. Museum für Völkerkunde, Berlin.

47. "This picture shows the manufacturing of ointment plaster medicines." Gouache, second half of the nineteenth century. Museum für Völkerkunde, Berlin.

*pao* 炮: Dry heat raw drugs directly above the flame or in a pot. Keep a distance between the flame and the pot.

*lan* 燀: Heat raw drugs directly in, or slightly above, the flame until a certain degree of charring occurs.

*bo* 爆: Dry heat raw drugs in a pot until they become brittle and crack or burst open.

*jiu* 灸: Heat raw drugs in various liquids such as wine, ginger juice, honey, etc. until done.

*wei* 煨: Cook raw drugs in hot ashes.

*chao* 炒: Roast raw drugs in a pot until their color turns yellowish. Stir and move drugs frequently.

*duan* 煅: Dry heat minerals and horn drugs in a pot or directly over the flame.

*lian* 煉: Heat metals for physical transformation, i.e. melting.

*zhi* 製: Transform the properties of raw drugs by chemical processes such as detoxification, or weaken the effects with water or wine.

*fei* 飛: Finely grind minerals and place in a mortar with water so that the impurities settle on the surface of the water and can be drained off. The heavy, pure sediment is then used for medicinal application.

*fu* 伏: Transform the effects by long storage.

*pang* 鎊: Finely shave bones and similar raw drugs.

*sha* 撼: Pound seed drugs, for example with the back of the hand.

*shai* 曬: Dry the raw drugs in the sun until they shrink and contract.

*pu* 曝: Briefly dry in the sun.

*lu* 露: Expose raw drugs to dew.

Different kinds of water—running water, boiled water, water that had been ladled and poured out again many times, or water from tree cavities—were associated with very specific properties that could be transferred to the raw drugs that were treated with it. This also applied to fires made from different fuels.

To be sure, there was only one school among the users of medicinal drugs which honored these theoretical rules and may have followed them, but it is impossible to determine the percentage of those who practiced a theory-based application of medicinal drugs in pre-modern Chinese

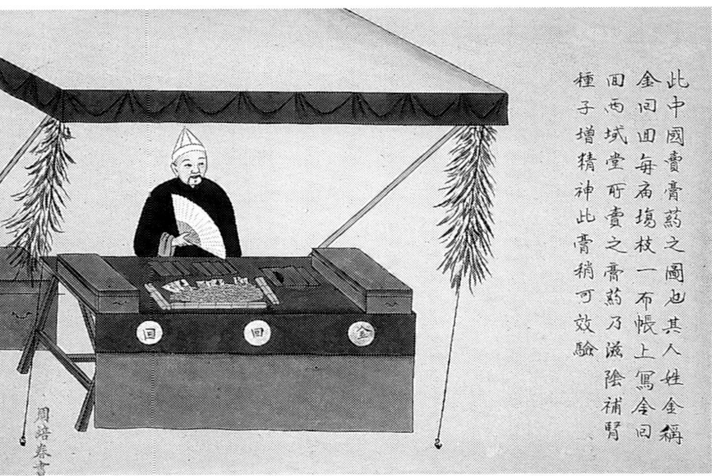



48. "This picture shows the sale of Chinese plaster medicines. The man's family name is Jin. He calls himself Jin Muslim. He sets up his stall in every market and writes on the curtain 'Jin Muslim's Pharmacy of the Western Regions.' The plaster medicines sold here nourish the yin [qi], replenish the kidneys, assist in producing offspring, and strengthen the spirit. These ointments can cause a certain effect." Gouache, second half of the nineteenth century. Museum für Völkerkunde, Berlin.

pharmaceutics. To this day, some of the fundamental principles are recommended for the processing and preparation of raw and medicinal drugs in the framework of traditional Chinese medicine.[42] More importantly, the preparation of different forms of medicines apparently continues to be convincing.

### 3. Frequently Prepared Forms of Medicines

The most common kind of preparation is the decoction. The Chinese technical term is *tang* 湯 and literally means "soup." Decoctions are solutions or suspensions which tend to get absorbed very quickly into the body and are therefore recommended especially for acute illnesses. In addition to water, wine (to strengthen the blood), vinegar (when the desired effect is contractive), milk (for a cooling effect), or even the urine of male infants (for the cooling of heat conditions) are used as extractive fluids.

Over the course of centuries, certain rules were formed about which substances should be boiled immediately, which ones should be added to the water later, which substances should be wrapped in a cloth before being exposed to the water, and which ones should be brought to a boil separately. Regardless, the cooking process is repeated two or three times, and, depending on the ailment, the resulting drug is usually taken two hours after meals (although it can also be taken before meals, especially if the ailment is located in the lower abdomen).

Pills, or *wan* 丸 in Chinese, are manufactured from powdered medicinal drugs in a binding agent, similar to traditional European pharmaceutics. The size of the pills varies depending on the illness; a pill might have the circumference of a cherry, or an even larger fruit, or it might be as small as the tip of a sewing needle. The desired effect is a mild and slow release of the medication, and depends greatly on the carrying agent. Water, honey, and wax are the most frequently used binding agents. A special variety are the so-called cinnabar pills, *dan* 丹 in Chinese. These are generally balls as large as walnuts, in which precious substances or minerals are imbedded. The name supposedly stems from the fact that cinnabar was originally used as a coating to protect the preparation and increase the effect of the pills for relieving certain irritations. Nowadays, a thick wax cover serves this purpose.

Medicinal powders, *san* 散 in Chinese, are the third most common type of medicine besides decoctions and pills.

The term *gao* 膏 refers simultaneously to three different forms of medicine. First it denotes syrups for internal application which are prepared by reducing watery drug extracts into thick concentrations and then mixing them with sugar or honey.

Second, the term *gao* refers to two kinds of plasters for external application that are used for the treatment of skin problems, painful "obstructions" in the joints and muscles,

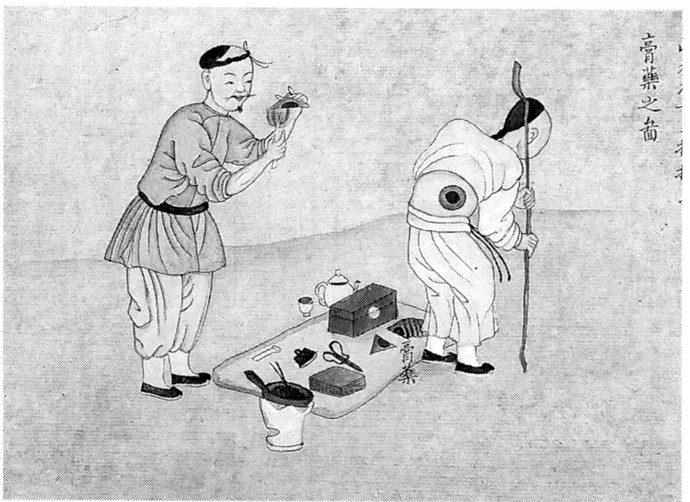

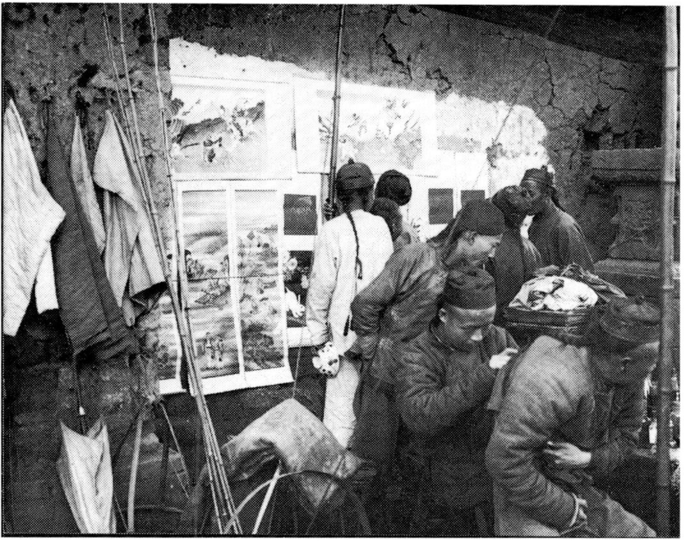

49. "This picture shows the display and sale of plaster medicines on streets and markets." In the foreground is a small stove with a pan for heating the plaster mixture which is then applied to a square piece of paper. Gouache, second half of the nineteenth century. Museum für Völkerkunde, Berlin.

50. Treatment of a patient's back by a doctor in an open market stall. Photograph ca. 1920.

fractures and sprains, and similar problems for which a treatment from the body's surface seems appropriate. The so-called plaster medicines (*gaoyao* 膏藥) are produced by gently heating or boiling medicinal drugs in oil, preferably sesame. The undissolved sediment is disposed of, beeswax is added, and the mixture is applied to paper or cloth. For the production of medicinal plasters (*yaogao* 藥膏), a powdered drug is added to a heated mixture of oil and beeswax.

In China, as in Europe, medicinal wines (*yaojiu* 藥酒), i.e. cold extracts of medicinal drugs in wine, have also been used since antiquity. [43]

## PHARMACIES: HISTORICAL TESTIMONIES

The preparation and processing of drugs in the two millennia of the Imperial period was located, to a limited extent, in the home kitchen, but primarily the pharmacy, although today, most pharmacies of traditional medicines now receive their drugs, already prepared, from central suppliers.

The Mawangdui manuscripts of the early Han period describe a sophisticated pharmaceutical technology, including all of the stages of collecting, processing, and preparing drugs from primary substances and raw materials (see p. 23), that is still known today. The practical application of traditional Chinese pharmaceutics, however, cannot be traced as far back in historical literature as pharmaceutical knowledge can.

The history of the Later Han refers to several individuals who traded medicinal drugs in the markets of Chang'an and elsewhere. An "old man suspended a gourd from the outside of his store in order to indicate that he diagnosed illnesses and sold medicines." [44] This is the first reference to a pharmacy in Chinese sources, and it illustrates an important detail of Chinese pharmaceutics: the gourd. Also known as the calabash or *hulu* 葫蘆 in Chinese, it remains the symbol of pharmaceutics in China to this day and therefore has continued to serve as an irreplaceable iconographic element for the representation of pharmacists (figure 109; plates 63, 102, 151).

Since the Han dynasty, a Director of Palace Medications, *shangyaojian* 尚藥監, was part of the medical bureaucracy in the imperial palace. This title was evidently not bestowed on a pharmacist, but on the palace physician (*taiyi* 太醫). Since the beginning of the Wei dynasty, there was evidence of a Palace Office of Pharmaceutics (*shangyaoju* 尚藥局) that continued until the Yuan dynasty. The officials were responsible for "composing medicines and making diagnoses" for the emperor. During the Tang period, a medicinal garden was established at the court where,

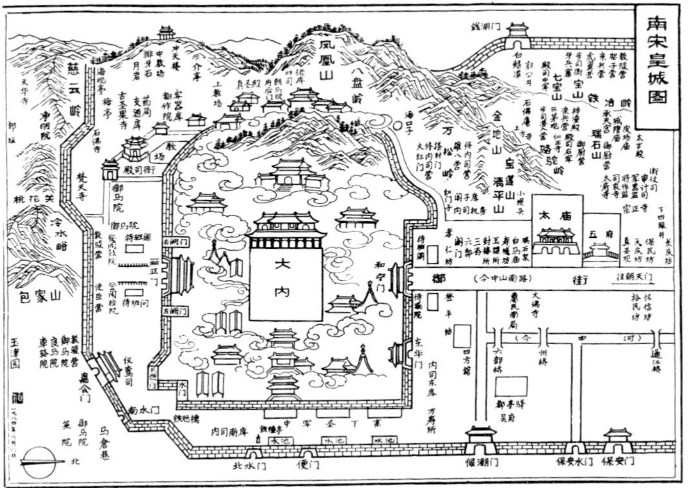

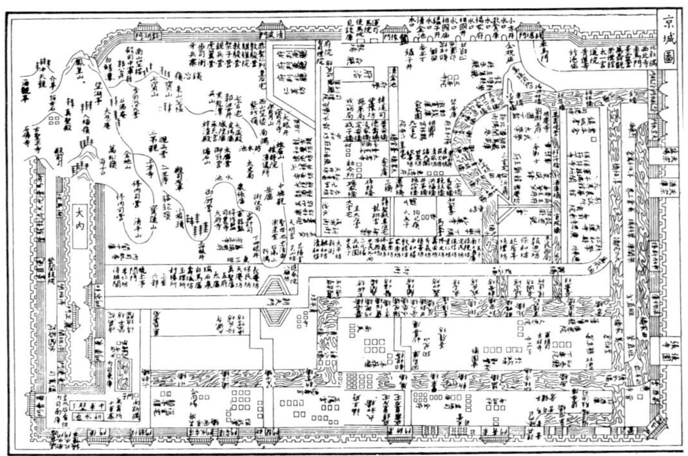

51. Map of the city of Hangzhou, during the Southern Song period from 1274, showing the locations of a 藥局 (Pharmaceutical Office) (upper left), and a 惠民南局 (Southern Office for Public Assistance), the latter possibly referring to 惠民藥局 (Pharmacy for Public Assistance) situated in the south. From *Xianchun Lin'an zhi* 咸淳臨安志 (*Xianchun Lin'an Chronicle*), 1867.

52. Map of Hangzhou, according to a model from 1274, showing the locations of an 施藥局 (Office for the Distribution of Medicines), an 慈幼局 (Office for Compassion towards the Little Ones), an orphanage opened in 1249, and a 惠民西局 (Western Office for Public Assistance) (center right), the latter possibly referring to the Pharmacy for Public Assistance situated in the west. From *Xianchun Lin'an zhi* 咸淳臨安志 (*Xianchun Lin'an Chronicle*), 1867.

depending on the season, basic ingredients were grown in order to be processed in fresh condition.[45] The sources also refer to several public pharmacies in private hands.[46]

An imperial pharmacy, *yuyaoyuan* 御藥院 or *yuyaoju* 御藥局, separate from the Palace Office of Pharmaceutics, was not established until the Song dynasty and was called *yuyaofang* 御藥房 during the Ming and Qing periods.[47] Probably in response to the problems that had been caused by the migration of peasants from the countryside to the cities, the rapid growth of cities, and the massive southward migration of the population in the Later Song period, the Song state, in the context of Wang Anshi's 王安石 reforms, also set up a system of state-directed pharmacies for the public welfare. This undertaking, unique in the history of medicine in China, had a dual goal: It attempted to ease the provision of the population with medicines and, at the same time, remove this vital area from the laws of the free market. The statutes even determined that pharmacies were to provide night service for urgent cases.

The first of these pharmacies, initially called *maiyaosuo* 賣藥所 (Store for Selling Medicines), was opened in Kaifeng in 1076. By 1103, the number of pharmacies had increased to seven. Five were known as Pharmacies for Processed Medicines (*shuyaosuo* 熟藥所), and two specialized in the pharmaceutical processing of drugs and were therefore called *xiuheyaosuo* 修和藥所. Each of these served as suppliers to pharmacies that combined the processed drugs according to certain formulas and delivered them to clients. In 1114, the term for the pharmacies was changed to *yiyaohuiminju* 醫藥惠民局 (Office for the Provision of the Population with Medicinal Drugs) and that for suppliers to *yiyaohejiju* 醫藥和劑局 (Office for the Composition of Medicinal Drugs). At the same time, such "offices" were also set up outside the capital in several other provinces. In 1142, the term for the pharmacies was again changed to *taipinghuiminju* 太平惠民局 (Office for the Provision of the Population in Great Peace).[48]

Despite the administration's good intentions, complaints about the commercialization of the government pharmacies arose quickly; the population sarcastically referred to the *huiminju* as *huiguanju* 惠官局 (Offices for the Provision of the Officials) and renamed the *hejiju* as *heliju* 和吏局 (Offices for the Harmony of Government Employees). In the early Ming period, the last of these pharmacies were still verifiable at least by name.[49]

The public pharmacies must have constituted only a small percentage of the stores where the population could purchase their medicines. The location of many pharmacies in Kaifeng can be deduced from the fairly detailed description by Meng Yuanlao 孟元老 in his *Dongjing menghualu* 東京夢華錄. Several of them specialized in the sale of medicines for specific ailments. We find references to pharmacies selling drugs for the treatment of mouth and throat problems, eye problems, pediatric and gynecological problems, and others. There were even pharmacies that were exclusively devoted to cosmetics.[50]

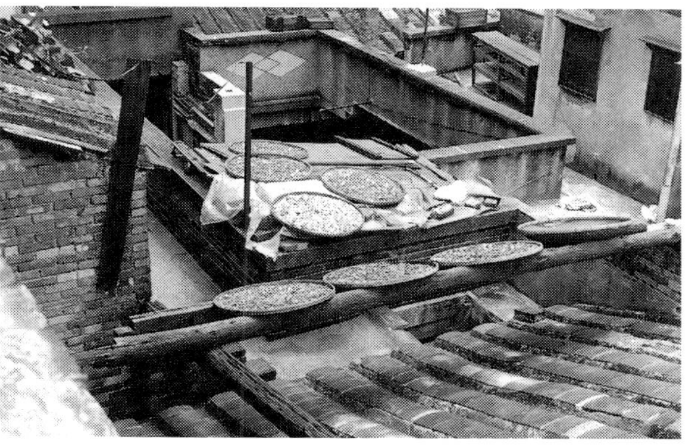

53. Sun drying of plant-based medicines in flat wicker baskets on a roof. Photograph from the roof of a pharmacy in Taipeh, Taiwan, 1970.

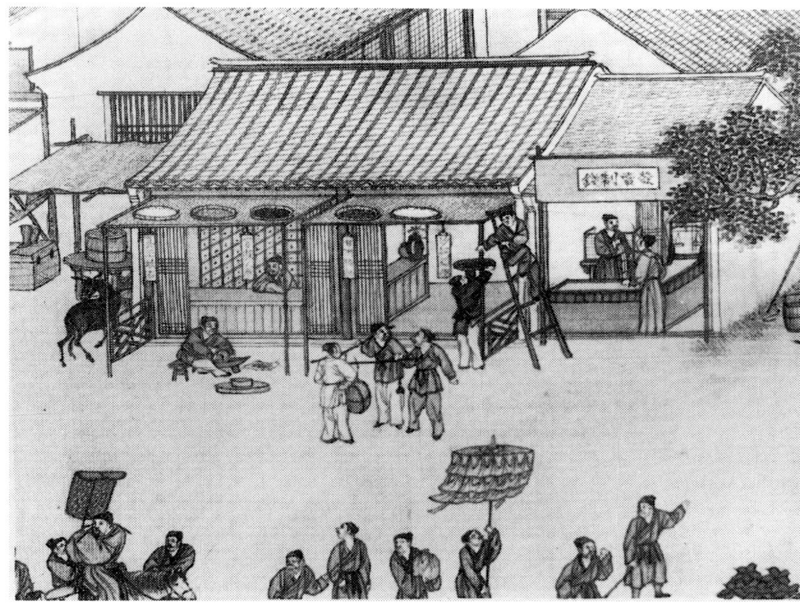

54. Drawing of a pharmacy open to the street. On the canopy, are plant-based drugs drying in flat wicker baskets. In front of the retail desk is an assistant operating the "drug boat," to chop drugs. Discernible at the left (from right to left) are two advertisements for ginseng and "autumn stone" (deposits on the bottom of urine collection jars). From the *Qingmingshanghetu* 清明上河圖 (*Up River to [the Capital] After the Spring Festival*). Excerpt of a drawing, 1248. See also figure 26.

Therefore, it is hardly surprising that the Song painting of a Chinese city, the *Qingming shanghetu* 清明上河圖, by Zhang Zeduan 張擇端 depicts two pharmacies (figures 26, 54). Their layout, depicted in great detail, does not differ at all from that of Chinese pharmacies which could still be encountered everywhere until the 1970s. The painting depicts stores that are open to the street; in figure 26, a client steps towards a retail desk where the pharmacist is waiting. Behind the pharmacist's back is a wall of shelving on which several hundred prepared drugs are stored, in a multitude of little drawers and on open shelves in containers of various sizes.

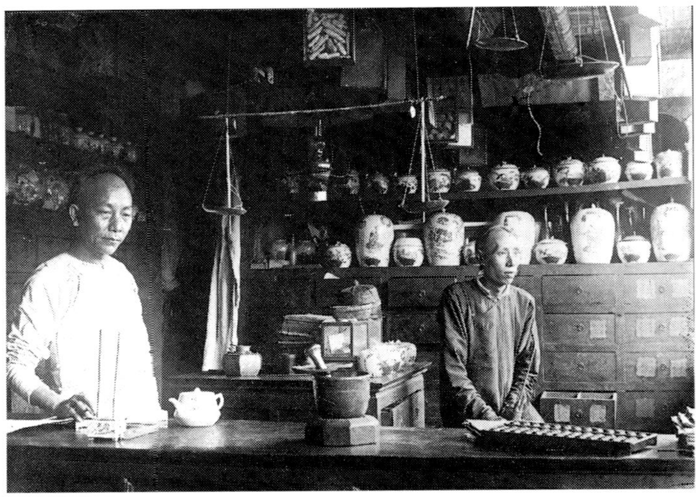

55. Pharmacist and assistant in a pharmacy in Yunnan, China. Photograph 1923.

## EQUIPMENT AND CONTAINERS

A few small implements, such as mortars for crushing and bowls for grating ingredients, are depicted on top of the retail desk (plate 69), and a "drug boat" made of wood or iron, to be worked with the hands or feet for the same purpose may be seen on the ground. Racks for drying raw drugs in the shade or, on the roof of the pharmacy in the sun, here look identical to those of the mid-twentieth century.

Because the pharmacy itself processed the raw materials that had been gathered in the wild or cultivated in medicinal herb gardens, it might have been common in Song times to have a back room set aside for such activities. All in all, the traditional Chinese pharmacy did not need a large array of technical resources, as seen in the painting: there were containers for drying raw drugs, for their subsequent preparation with liquids such as wine, vinegar, or boy's urine, for their pulverization and, where necessary, for their further processing into pills, plasters, or other kinds of medicines with binding agents. Individually prescribed medicines were, and still are, usually sold as processed substances which patients prepare themselves at home by boiling.

The implements are purely functional tools. Showy metal mortars, as were used in European pharmaceutics for many centuries, are unknown in China. Iron or brass mortars from South China have smooth linings that are slightly conically shaped towards their bases (plate 52). The pestle is made of rough-hewn wood with a metal tip. Northern Chinese brass mortars, however, come in many shapes and may even be decorated, e.g. with ridges (plate 51). A characteristic feature is the lid which is, like the mortar and the entire pestle, made from brass and meant to prevent the drugs from escaping while being crushed.

In contrast to metal mortars, porcelain ones are always richly decorated on their exteriors; in fact, older porcelains whose representations of scenery, dragons, flowers, or stylized

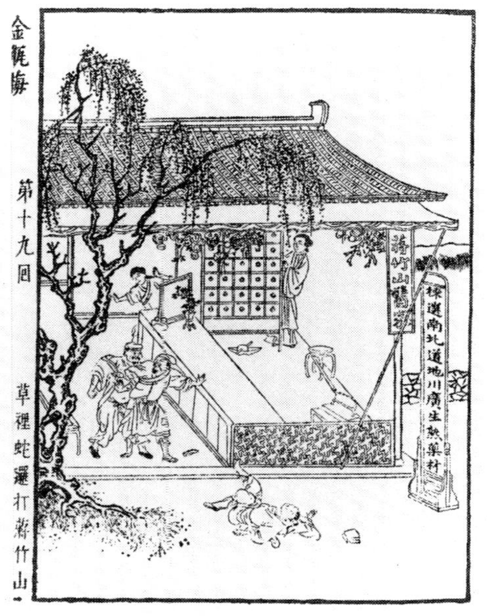

56. Illustration from the erotic novel *Jinpingmei* 金瓶梅 (*Plum Blossoms in a Golden Vase*) depicting a pharmacy open to the street. The sign to the right of the pharmacy says "Home of the physician Jiang Zhushan." The board on the street announces, "genuine raw and processed medicinal products, chosen in North and South, from [Si]chuan and Guang[dong]." On the floor in front of the drawers of drugs, is an "drug boat." The picture depicts the scene of an attack on the physician in his pharmacy. Undated edition of the *Jinpingmei*, first half of the seventeenth century. Staatsbibliothek, Berlin.

motifs have been preserved are considered to be irreplace-able and unique artifacts (plates 53–59). This does not apply to the porcelain grinding bowls that are also decorated; ranging in size from the minute to 25 cm in diameter, these mass-produced bowls can be categorized into only a few decorative types (plates 60–62). The most common motif is the peony, which also seems to have been very popular on vessels. Less frequent are landscape motifs or stylized orna-mentations. The pestles are crafted entirely from porce-lain—and consequently rarely preserved intact—or consist of a wooden handle (sometimes turned on a lathe, but usually smooth) with a porcelain tip.

## DATES AND NAMES OF CHINESE PHARMACIES

The *Tongrentang* 同仁堂 in Peking is the oldest pharmacy in China still in business. It was founded in the eighth year of Emperor Kangxi's reign (1669) by Le Xianchang 樂顯場, a former itinerant drug peddler who had come to Peking from Zhejiang and had initially wandered through the alleys with a rattle and vending tray.[51] The current establishment, on a side street of Qianmen Avenue south of the Square of Heavenly Peace, was opened in 1702 by the founder's son, Le Fengming 樂鳳鳴 and is regarded as one of the three most important pharmacies in China, along with the *Hu Qingyu tang* 胡慶餘堂 in Hangzhou and the pharmacy of Chen Liji 陳李濟 in Canton. Similar to pharmaceutical companies in Germany, which originated from pharmacies in the nineteenth century, the *Tongrentang* is known throughout China for the products of the affili-ated *Tongrentang* factory.

The names of Chinese pharmacies frequently contained allusions to the basic values of Confucian and Buddhist ethics. Thus, *tongren* in translation means "allowing to par-take in humaneness." Other examples are *shende* 慎德 (attention to virtue), *zhide* 至德 (utmost virtue), or *rende* 仁德 (virtue of humaneness). Some names were simply the sum of pleasant-sounding characters that attracted cus-tomers because of their aesthetic value, not because of their reference to medicine or illness. One example is the *Song-fentang* 誦芬堂 in Suzhou: *song* 誦 means "to recite," and *fen* 芬 "fragrant."

Other names pointed to the goal of medicine: *yongsheng* 永盛 (eternal abundance), *baoyuan* 保元 (preserving the original [qi]), *yishou* 益壽 (benefiting longevity), *shoukang* 壽康 (longevity and health), *wanquan* 萬全 (myriad heal-ings), or *baozi* 保滋 (protection and restoration). The alle-gorical term 'spring' for health also appeared in many phar-macy names, including *huichun* 回春 (return to spring),

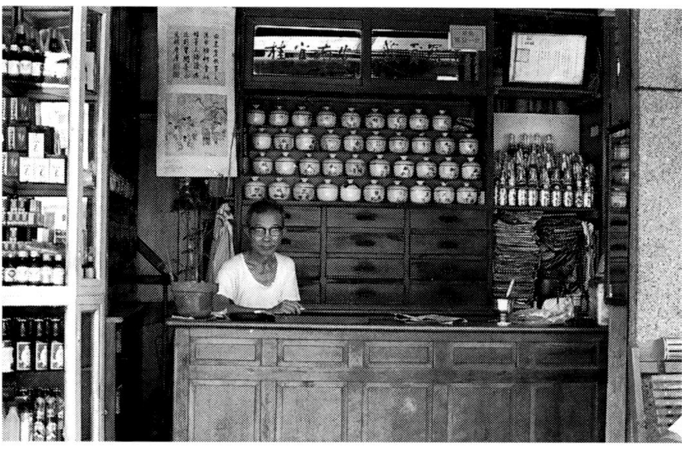

57. Drugstore of traditional Chinese pharmaceutics, open to the street. Photograph, Taipeh, 1970.

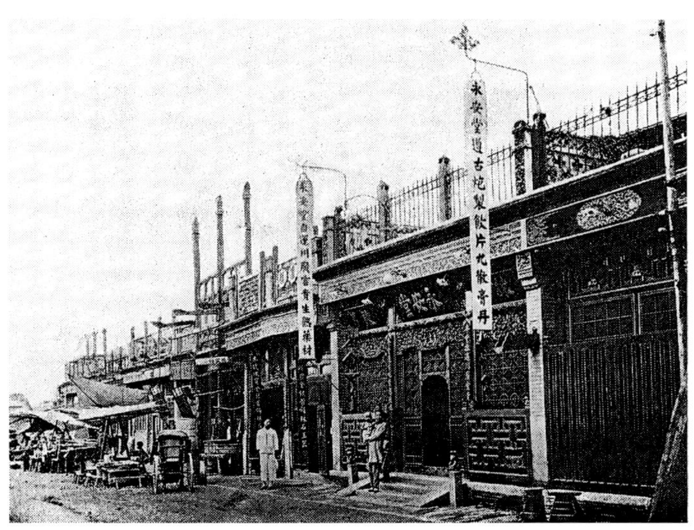

58. The facade of the *Yongan-tang* (Pharmacy of Eternal Peace) on a business street in China. The characters on the signs say (right), "Yongan Phar-macy. [Pressed Herbal] tablets for [the preparation of] potable [decoctions], pills, powders, ointments, and boli, manu-factured according to old instructions," and (left), "Yongan Pharmacy. Personally chosen raw and processed medicinal products from [Si]chuan, Guang[dong], Yun[nan], and Gui[zhou]." Photograph, Shanghai, 1926. From Louise Crane, *China in Sign and Symbol*.

*changchun* 長春 (long lasting spring), or *jichun* 濟春 (assisting spring). Names like *qingming* 清明 (clearing brightness) or *chongming* 重明 (renewing brightness) indicated a specialization in ophthalmology. Although the name of a former pharmacy in Peking, *Zhenyaotang* 針藥堂, literally translated, meant "Pharmacy for Needles and Drugs," until twenty or thirty years ago, it was rare that a pharmacy sold acupuncture needles. The term "needles" might therefore have referred to moxa sticks, called *leihuo shenzhen* 雷火神針 (spirit-like needles of the Leigong Fire), made out of mugwort, that were commonly used during the Qing dynasty instead of placing of burning *moxa* directly on the skin (plate 33).

Other names simply referred to the founder of the respective pharmacy, such as *Hu Qingyu tang* 胡慶餘堂 (Pharmacy of Hu Qingyu), *Feng Liaoxing tang* 馮了性堂 (Pharmacy of Feng Liaoxing), etc. Animal or plant names were, in contrast to Europe, not commonly used. The closest thing to the animal names so popular among German pharmacies was the golden phoenix as the trademark of the *Desheng tang* pharmacy 德生堂 in the market town of Chang'an, Haining County, near the city of Hangzhou (Zhejiang Province). All of the containers in which this pharmacy marketed its products carried the inscription "original establishment of the *Desheng* (Pharmacy) of Zhu Bunian 朱卜年 with the phoenix trademark," which was accompanied by a drawing of a phoenix (plates 112, 113).

The character *tang* 堂, used for "pharmacy" here, originally signified a "hall" for many purposes ranging from a legal court, to a store, to private living quarters; however in pharmaceutical names, it is occasionally replaced with the character *zhai* 齋 that conveys slightly higher expectations. *Zhai* is a scholar's living room, a library, or a study examplified by the *Yanglaozhai* 養榮齋, or "Scholar's Study for Nurturing into Blossoms," in Ningbo City, Zhejiang Province. Other characters that were used to signify the terms "store," "business," or "pharmacy" are *dian* 店, *guan* 館, *yaoshi* 藥室 and, recently, *yaoju* 藥局, as in: *Caizhilaodian* 採芝老店 (Original Soma Picking Store) in Hujun, Zhejiang Province; *Guangzhiguan* 廣芝館 (Soma Distribution Store) in Canton; and *Songlingyaoshi* 松齡藥室 (Pharmacy of Song Ling) and *Tongchunyaoju* 同春藥局 (Pharmacy for Partaking in Spring), in Wanzhou.

The good reputation of some pharmacies motivated subsequent generations, who were unable to continue the original establishments as direct heirs, to set up their own pharmacies, under the name of the pharmacies' founders. Thereby they created, in the course of time, competition under the same name of the founding house, and, by adding the claim "original establishment" (*laodian* 老店) to their companies names, some founding houses tried to elevate themselves above their off-spring with the same name.

59. Pharmacy delivery container of the "Pharmacy of the Virtue and Life of [Mr.] Zhu Bunian; original store with the phoenix as trademark."

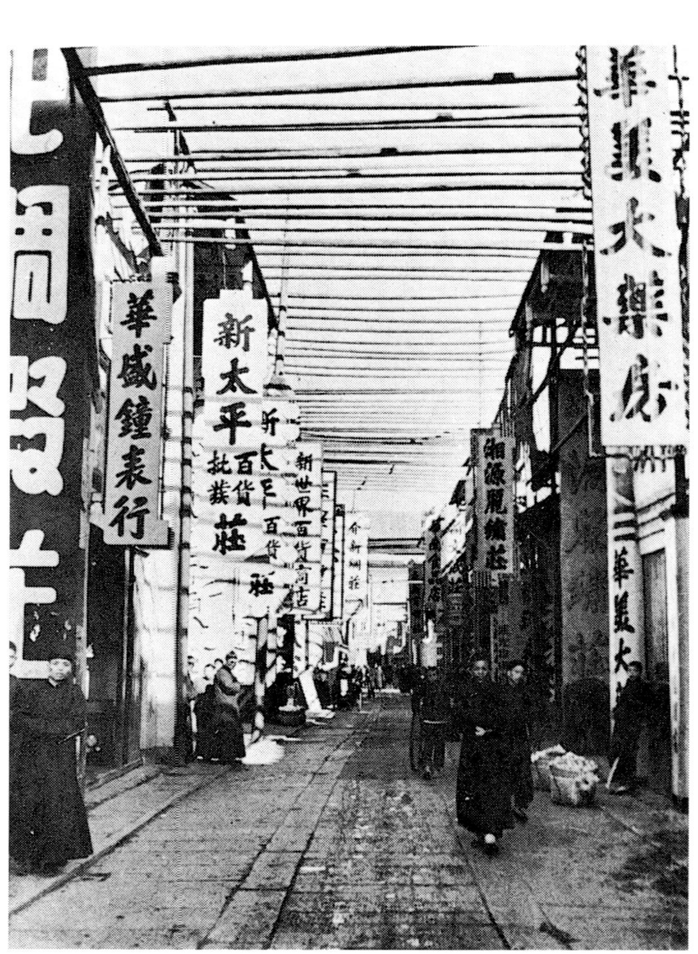

60. Street scene in Changsha/ Hunan. At the right edge of the picture is an advertisement for the Sino-American pharmacy. From Edward H. Hume, *Doctors East, Doctors West*, New York, 1946.

52

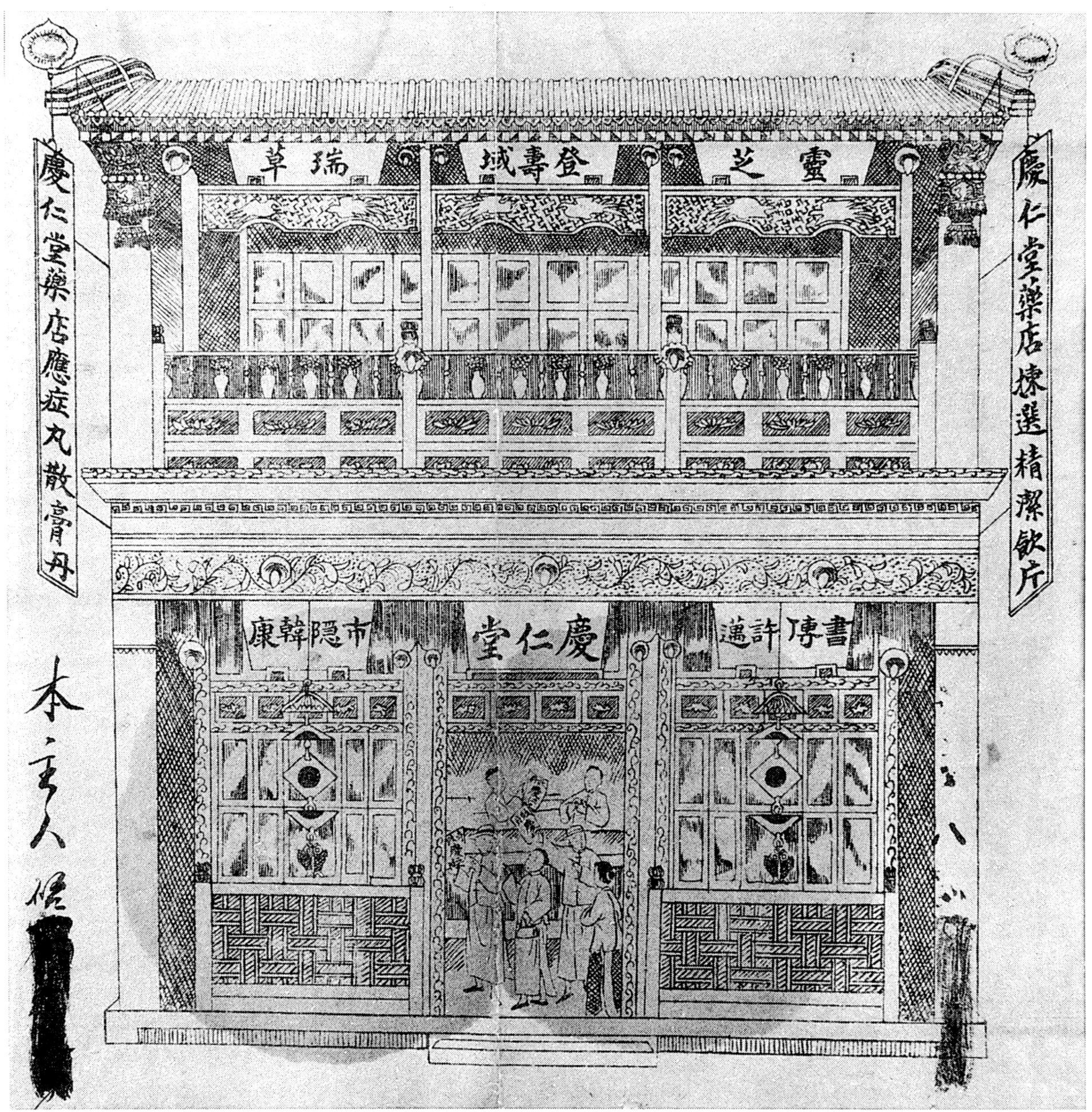


61. Street front of the Qingren Pharmacy. The characters on the signs projecting into the street state: (right), "Qingren Pharmacy. Selected [pressed herbal] tablets of the finest quality for [the preparation of] potable [decoctions]," and (left), "Qingren Pharmacy. Pills, powders, ointments, and boli, effective for conditions of distress." The characters above the second floor railing state (from right to left): *lingzhi* (miraculous Soma mushroom), *dengshouqu* (place where one ascends to longevity), and *shuicao* (Herb of Good Fortune). The three signs above the ground floor windows and door state (from right to left): *shuchuan xumai* ("transmitted in the texts: Xu Mai"; Xu Mai 許邁 is the name of a hermit from Chinese antiquity. He is said to have sacrificed his fortune during an epidemic in order to buy remedies for the sick and to have saved 408 "dead" patients that had been brought to him), *Qingrentang, shiyin hankang* ("unrecognized in the market: Han Kang"; Han Kang 韓康 was a hermit from the Eastern Han dynasty. For decades, he sold medicines on the market without charging inflated prices like the other merchants, which had to be bargained down by the customers). From *Qingrentang yaomu* 慶仁堂藥目 (*Index of Medicines from the Reward for Humaneness Pharmacy*). Unfoldable end-paper. Private print, 1912.

### *1. Form, Inscription, and Decoration of Containers*

Comparable to the gradual emergence of mass-produced preparations and specialties in Germany and several other European countries—but possibly anticipating the European development by six or seven centuries—Chinese pharmacies sold pre-fabricated medicines that were aimed at certain illnesses or syndromes, like the mass-produced drugs of the modern pharmaceutical industry. They also served customers who presented individualized prescriptions based on family knowledge or a doctor's formula.

Because quite a few formulas had consistently proven their effectiveness on the same illnesses, regardless of the relative condition of the patient, they were systematically manufactured and sold with great effort throughout the country. Since one and the same remedy, e.g. the "pills with the eight treasures" or the "elixir for the *sha* disease," were industrially manufactured and marketed by many pharmacies, advertising was as important as it is today.

Song dynasty sources report that pharmacies as well as physicians presented their clients with gifts at the end of the year in order to ensure their continuing loyalty in the coming year. Depictions of the door gods, amulets made out of peach wood (plate 153), and a variety of drugs served this purpose.[52]

Also notable in this context are the form and inscriptions of the containers in which the pharmacies sold their mass-produced drugs. The external design of the medicine containers was aimed at distinguishing them from those of competitors and encouraging potential customers to purchase them. Similar to the way in which a contemporary mustard company in Germany designs its jars so that they can be easily reused as drinking glasses, Chinese pharmacies, during the past two or three centuries, have offered medicinal powders and pills in containers that are attractive in shape and reusable.

In fact, it was a popular custom to put medicines into containers that could later be used as flower vases (plates 105, 121–124). Numerous medicine flacons also resembled snuff bottles and could be refilled as such (plates 89–93). Of similar popularity were small, wide-mouthed jars that could be re-used, for example, as water containers for calligraphy (plate 120). Large containers were occasionally shaped like rectangular tea tins and could later be filled with tea leaves (plate 108).

In order to bind customers to a line of products by a certain manufacturer, some pharmacies designed serial containers, often decorated with scenes from Chinese history and mythology. Customers might be induced to return to the

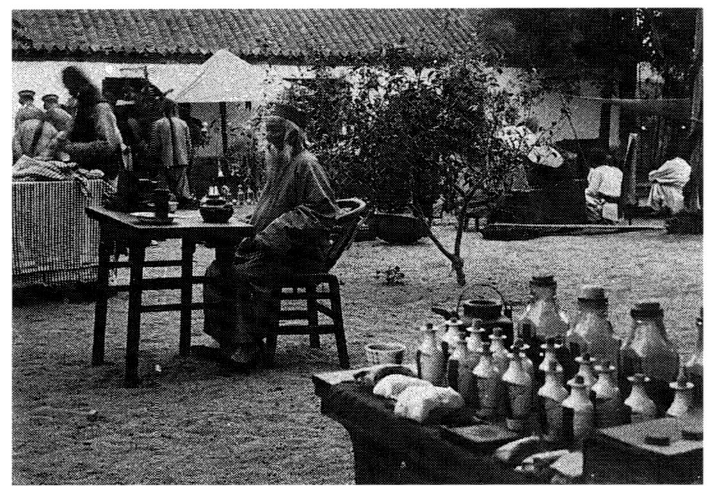

62. Fortune teller and letter writer (seated), and traditional, mass-produced remedies in glass and ceramic containers with plugs and labels. Photograph on the occasion of an industries fair in Litsun, Shandong Province, 1907. Museum für Völkerkunde, Berlin.

same pharmacy, or at least its products, in order to collect an entire series of the eight genies (plates 117, 118), a line of containers with illustrations and biographical descriptions of famous warriors of the past (plate 116), or a line of containers in the shapes of animals (plate 92).

Many medicine containers were also shaped like lucky charms and talismans. Some depicted the circle of the eight trigrams from the *Yijing* 易經 with the yin-yang symbol in the center (plate 94), while others offered encouraging sayings—addressed especially to scholars (plate 103)—such as New Year's greetings or wishes of good luck on forthcoming exams for those in bureaucratic careers. Some containers were inscribed with famous lines from classical poetry and appealed to the customer's level of education (plates 96, 130). The marketing strategies of these pharmacies in general indicates that their clients were primarily from the wealthy and, therefore, formally educated classes of the Imperial and early Republican periods. The itinerant doctors who offered remedies for sale to the common people used their own techniques for increasing sales (plate 76).

When the name of a medicine was not fired under the glaze on the vessel that contained it, it was occasionally written on top of it in ink so that it could be wiped off and the container reused. The same result was reached with a label, usually a red piece of paper, that indicated not only the name of the medicine, but also information regarding its intake.

The name of the medicine might refer to a well-known formula or be very general, (e.g. "eye remedy") and, in this way, indicate a secret recipe. With the addition of a pharmacist's name, a preparation could be elevated from the class of generic drugs to the level of a pharmacy specialty. The *Desheng tang* pharmacy, for example, marketed its version of the Elixir [with the Strength] of a Sleeping Dragon, distributed around the country through countless manufacturers, as *Zhushi wolongdan* 朱氏卧龍丹 (Mr. Zhu's Elixir [with the Strength] of a Sleeping Dragon). The *Baozitang* pharmacy in Canton chose a different path. It marketed *Zhuge xingjunsan* 諸葛行軍散 (Zhuge's Powder that Causes Soldiers to Run), one of the most popular massproduced drugs towards the end of the Imperial period, under the name *Jiuweibabao honglingdan* 救危八寶紅靈丹 (Divine Red Elixir of Eight Precious [Ingredients] for Rescue from Danger), thereby setting itself apart from the competition with a name that could not be found in any formulary dictionary (plate 37).

Since the eighteenth or nineteenth centuries at the latest, we also find erotic scenes on medicine bottles, not only as decoration, but as an indication of their contents. The concern for male potency and the incorporation of sexuality into physical hygiene have been important elements of Chinese medicine since the beginning of its written documentation, i.e. since the Mawangdui manuscripts. Chinese pharmacies offered a great number of essential aphrodisiacs. It was fashionable, at least since the beginning of the Qing

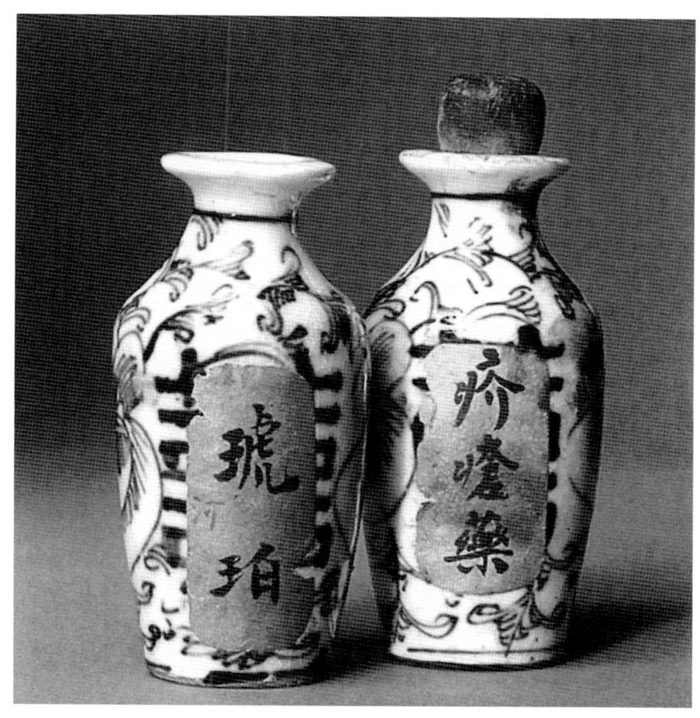

63. Two pharmacy delivery containers in the shape of vases. (left) Red paper label indicating the content 琥珀 "amber." Porcelain, height 10 cm. (right) Red paper label indicating the content 雄黃散 "powder of realgar," arsenic disulphide, and the indication 疥瘡藥 "remedy for scabrous sores."

period, to carry snuff or medicine bottles that were decorated with motifs suited for a visit to a brothel; erotic scenes, moreover, were believed to be talismans for good luck or protection from evil (plates 100, 101).[53]

Also worth mentioning in this context are opium containers. Towards the end of the eighteenth century, brothels in the cities along the coast and the Yangzi River frequently offered their customers a combination of opium and prostitutes. The prostitutes or, in the more upscale houses, special servants were responsible for the tedious task of preparing the pipe and the opium; the customers were also served tea or wine. While the smokers in the opium dens lounged on their sides on narrow divans, in brothels, they rested in wide beds with prostitutes on one, if not both, sides in order to enjoy the narcotic and girls simultaneously.[54] In the second half of the nineteenth century, the poppy-based drug had reached such popularity that the clientele of many brothels, at least in Shanghai, were primarily interested in opium and only secondarily in sexual pleasure.[55]

The accessories for the combination of sexual play and narcotics included, besides an elaborately decorated pipe, a small lamp, opium containers of white brass (plate 97), and several needles for picking up the opium balls. Like the containers for other medicines, those for opium were ornamented in various ways, often with erotic engravings. Commonly, these scenes became visible only after removing an outer casing that was itself engraved with less suggestive motifs or poems such as those of the famous painter Qin Linbing from the Qing dynasty, in order to "provide the sort of literary elegance which appealed to the aesthetic tastes of the users of this form of erotica."[56]

## 2. Advertising: The Example of Topical Ointments

At a time when there were no newspapers or other mass media, in the modern sense, manufacturers of pharmaceutics depended on other techniques to advertise their products. Word of mouth propaganda was highly valued and quite effective, as were the above-mentioned packaging and the inscription techniques, for binding a customer to a pharmacy and its products. These visible efforts to gain the loyalty of customers suggest at least two things. First, that the pressures of competition had been experienced in Chinese cities centuries ago by pharmacies who produced their own specialties, forcing them to develop their own strategies in order to survive this kind of situation. Second, that the manufacturers also considered it useful to repeatedly draw attention to their own existence and that of their products. This fact illustrates both the high degree of mobility among the population and pharmacies' attempts to reach a clientele living outside of smaller neighborhoods with local pharmacies. Posters and hand-outs, which the manufacturing pharmacies used to advertise their products, were particularly useful in reaching these customers.

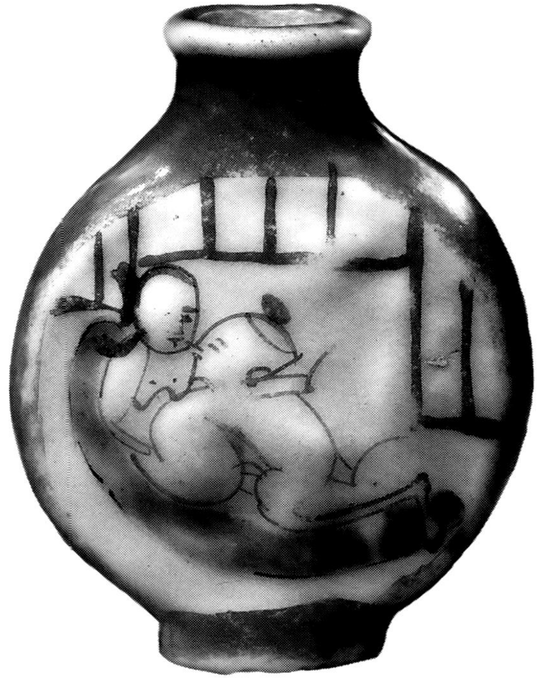

64. Porcelain pharmacy delivery container with figures in relief depicting a love scene.

The mass-produced medicines sold by Chinese pharmacies that were supposedly able to cure a large number of ailments, regardless of a patient's individual condition, can be classified into two groups. The first category, according to the lists of indications in the formularies or on the labels, contained drugs that were able to cure any number of health problems without the patient having to modify the form or location of the remedy's application. Medicines in the second category were also said to cure several different ailments but required specific ways of taking or applying them, depending on each condition.

It seems to have been widely assumed that a formula could be directed to various locations in the body to cure specific problems if the patient simultaneously ingested different conduction agents that guided the medicine through the body (see below pp. 81–82).

Equally popular was the concept that applying one and the same remedy at different, but clearly defined body parts, facilitated the entry to specific conduits inside the body. Therefore a certain ointment was able to produce different effects depending on the types of application.

Two documents illustrate this concept (figures 66, 67). These are advertising texts for ointments that were manufactured and sold by two different Chinese pharmacies under different names, but with partially overlapping indications. Neither of the texts is clearly dateable, but their design and condition suggest that they originated in the late nineteenth or early twentieth century. Chinese pharmacies of the late Imperial period used such flyers to advertise, among other products, topical ointments. Such ointments were applied to specific points on the body for different therapeutic results.

Generally, these points on the body were identical with known acupuncture openings (*xue* 穴) of certain conduits. According to the theory of acupuncture, the individual conduits in which the qi flows are connected to certain functional centers in the body. Therefore, manipulating a specific conduit with a needle is aimed primarily at influencing related functions. The application of topical ointments is based on the same theoretical principle.

The names of the ointments advertised by the texts referred to the manufacturer's specializations, not to the standard formulas whose composition was documented in the relevant literature. Thus, the potential buyer of these preparations did not know which drugs had been used in the recipes and was unable to establish a potential connection between their individual components and his or her ailments. Their persuasiveness, therefore, was based solely on the significance of the conduit openings to which the ointment was to be applied.

When these body points were associated with widely accepted indications from acupuncture or moxibustion, the advertisements for the ointments were able to convince customers, even though they did not know out of which drugs the ointment had been produced. In fact, a comparison of the indications mentioned in these advertisements

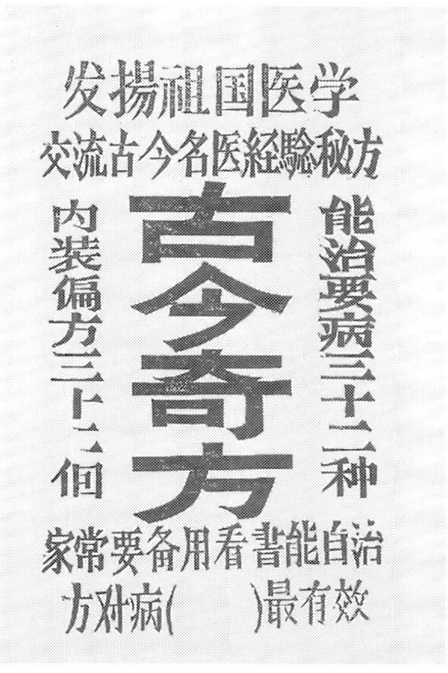


65. Advertising slip for a formula collection, ca. 1955, which states: "old and new extraordinary formulas that make use of the medicine of the motherland and offer contributions from the secret experience-based formulas of famous physicians from antiquity and modernity. Thirty-two popular recipes for internal application that are able to cure thirty-two important illnesses. Be prepared to use them in everyday life. Just read them and you will be able to use them yourself. The formulas are extremely effective for the disease [...]."

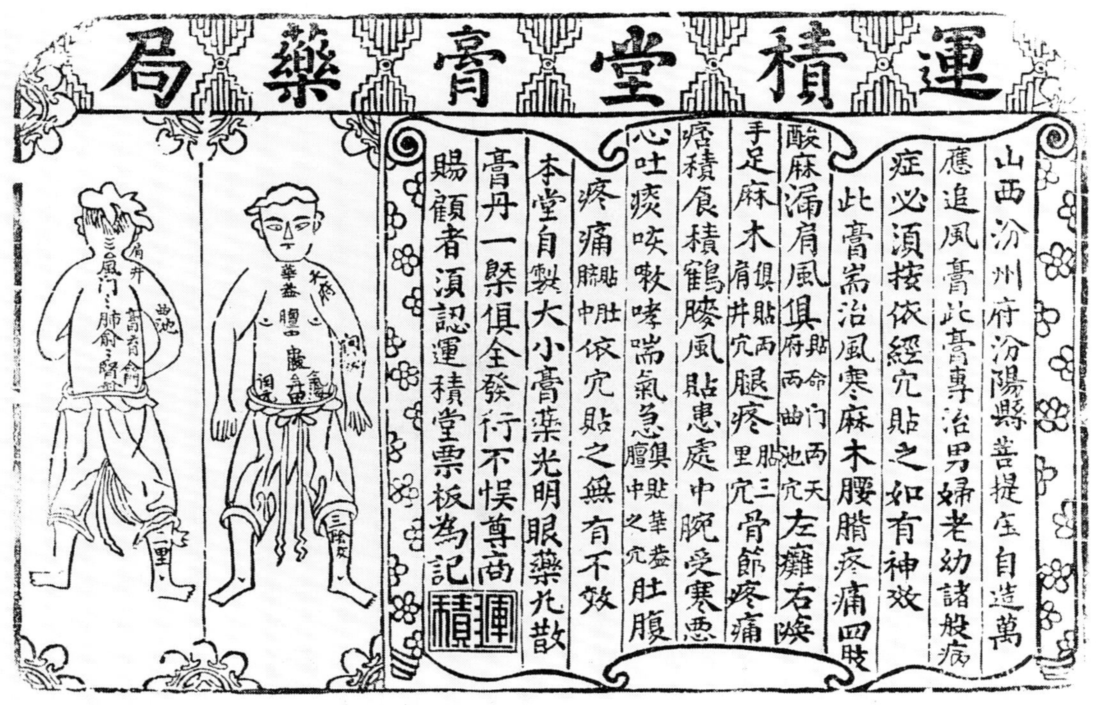





## OINTMENT PHARMACY HALL OF MOVEMENT AND COLLECTION

Shanxi Province, Fenzhou government district, Fenyang county, Puti municipality.

Special preparation: Ointment Which Successfully Dispels Wind One Thousand Times.[57]

This ointment is a special [preparation] for the treatment of all forms of illness on the trunk. It has to be applied to [specific] conduit openings and unfolds its effects as if by the hands of spirits.

This ointment specifically treats:

Numbness [due to] wind coldness, pain in the lumbar and back regions, pain and paralysis of the four limbs, pain in the shoulder joints.[58]
For all these [conditions], [it should] be applied to the openings of the Gate of Life, the two Heavenly Palaces, and the two Flexing Lakes.[59]

Cases of paralysis and numbness of the hands and feet, alternating between the right and left side.
For all these [conditions], [it should] be applied to the two Shoulder Well openings.

Leg pains.
To be applied to the Three Mile opening.

Achy joints, accumulations of blockages, accumulations of food, crane's knee wind.[60]

[It should] be applied to the affected areas.

Receiving cold in the central stomach cavity, unrest in the heart, spitting phlegm, coughing, panting, and pressed breathing.
For all [these conditions], [it should] be applied to the Blossom Canopy and Central Chest openings.

Stomach and abdominal pain.

[It should] be applied to the navel.
If one applies [the ointment] to the appropriate openings, it will always be efficacious.

Our pharmacy prepares large and small [amounts] of ointment medicines and eye remedies in private production and sells any kinds of pills, powders, ointments, and elixirs. We will not treat your valued business [requests] with negligence.

Customers should memorize the company trademark of the Yunji Pharmacy.

58

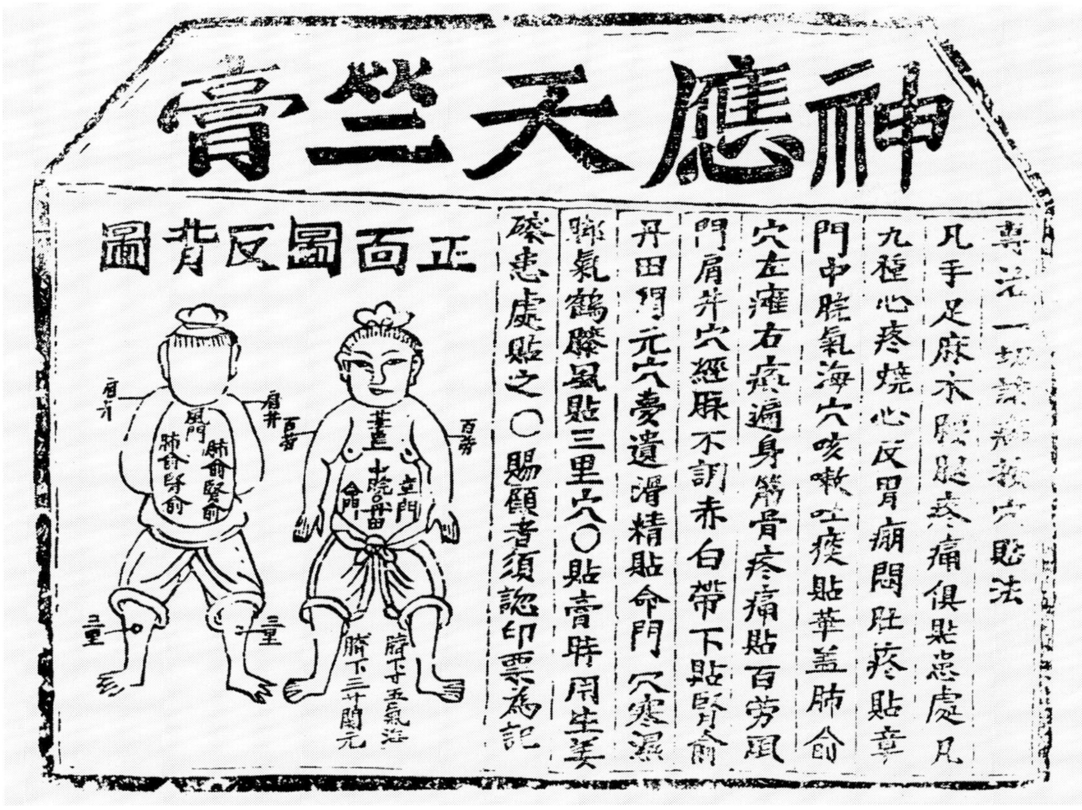



67. Text and illustration on an advertising slip for "Indian [point] ointments of spirit-like efficacy" by a pharmacy of unknown name. Wood-block print, early twentieth century.


## INDIAN OINTMENT OF SPIRIT-LIKE EFFICACY

[Serves] specifically for the treatment of all illnesses depending on the method of application to specific openings.

In any cases of numbness in hands and feet, pain in the lumbal area and legs: [it should] be applied in the affected areas.

In cases of any type of cardiac pain, heartburn, gastric expectoration, hemorrhage, chest pressure, and stomachache: [it should] be applied to the Camphor Gate, Central Gastric Cavity and Qi Lake openings.

In cases of coughing and spitting phlegm: [it should] be applied to the Blossom Canopy and Lung Transport openings.

In cases of paralysis alternating between the left and right sides, pain in the whole body, in the bones, and in the tendons: [it should] be applied to the Hundred Exhaustions, Wind, Gate and Shoulder Well openings.

In cases of irregular [flow in the] conduits and vessels, red and white discharge: [it should] be applied to the Kidneys Transport, Cinnabar Field, and Pass Origin openings.

In cases of ejaculation while dreaming or unintended loss of semen: [it should] be applied to the Life Gate opening.

In cases of cold dampness, beriberi, and crane's knee wind: [it should] be applied to the Three Mile opening.

When applying the ointment, one should first rub the affected region with a slice of fresh ginger.

Customers should memorize the trademark.

for a topical application of the ointments and the indications of the same points in acupuncture does, indeed, reveal a high level of correspondence.[61]

Thus, the manufacturers' brochures of such ointments not only served as advertisements, but also as directions for their use. In both cases, the text to the right of the front and back views of the human body provides the locations of the conduit opening points.

### 3. West-East Product Advertising

When European pharmaceutical companies began to market their products in China in the late nineteenth and early twentieth centuries, they certainly did not encounter an unprepared society. It was simply their methods of advertising that sometimes differed from those that were common in China. Consequently, the importers of aspirin, for example, adopted local customs when they established their distribution network. In order to draw the attention of the Chinese public to the pain killer from the West, they commissioned banners with both Chinese characters and Latin letters; these were designed to leave a lasting impression when carried through the cities, accompanied by orchestras playing Western tunes.[62]

An aspirin poster from 1935 demonstrates the unproblematic connection of this Western drug with traditional Chinese categories of illness. Below the characters *zhuanzhi* 專治 (cures specifically), which also introduce conventional banner advertisements by Chinese physicians for their abilities (plate 177), it lists the seven indications *toutong* 頭痛 (headache), *yatong* 牙痛 (toothache), *shangfeng* 傷風 (wind damage), *hanre* 寒熱 (cold heat [states]), *fengshi* 風濕 (wind dampness), *gutong* 骨痛 (bone pain), and *tongjing* 痛經 (painful menstrual period).

The smooth transition from the advertisements for traditional Chinese mass-produced preparations to modern-day European pharmaceutical products is illustrated even more clearly in Japanese advertising posters from the end of the nineteenth century, the first place where the commercial interests of both traditions found a visible expression in East Asia. The Japanese Meiji government decided in 1869, as part of their comprehensive reforms, to introduce the German variant of Western medicine to Japan and make it the foundation for its scientifically oriented medicine.

Consequently, advertising posters soon appeared in Japanese pharmacies that extolled the virtues of both the mass-produced *kampo* 漢方 (Chinese formula) preparations that were already common in Japan and the newly introduced European remedies, frequently with German terminology.

A good example of this combination of Chinese and European medical culture in Japan is a wooden board from a pharmacy in Nagasawa (plate 44). On the right side is a Chinese advertisement for an ophthalmologic formula called *yifangshui muyao* 一方水目藥 (Japanese: *ipposui megusuri*), while on the left side is an advertisement for a

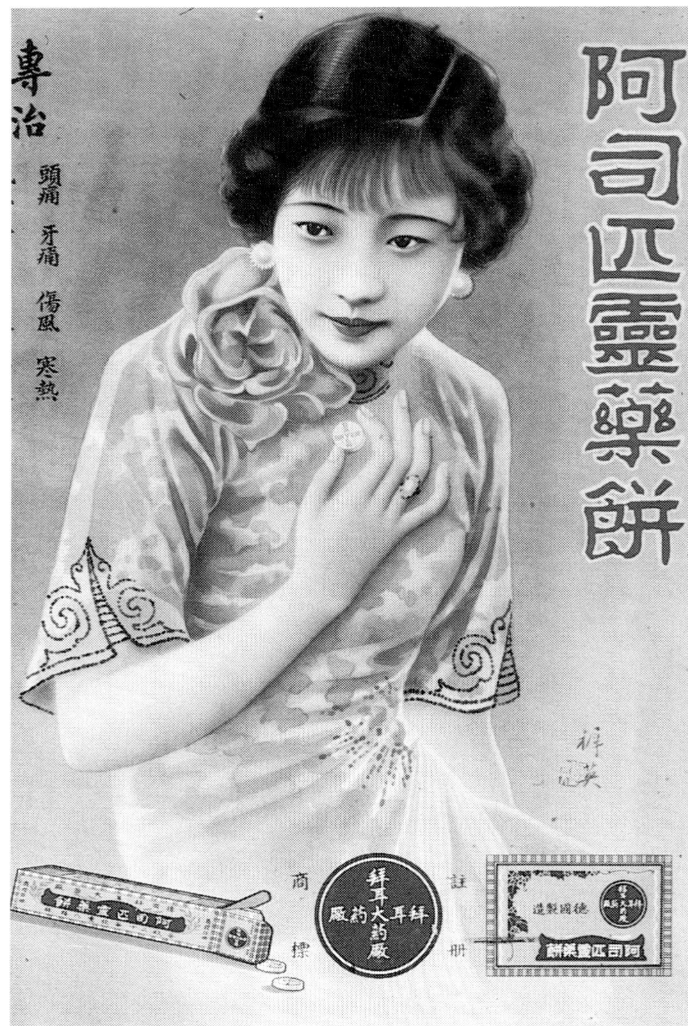


68. Chinese poster advertising aspirin, Bayer Corporation, 1935.

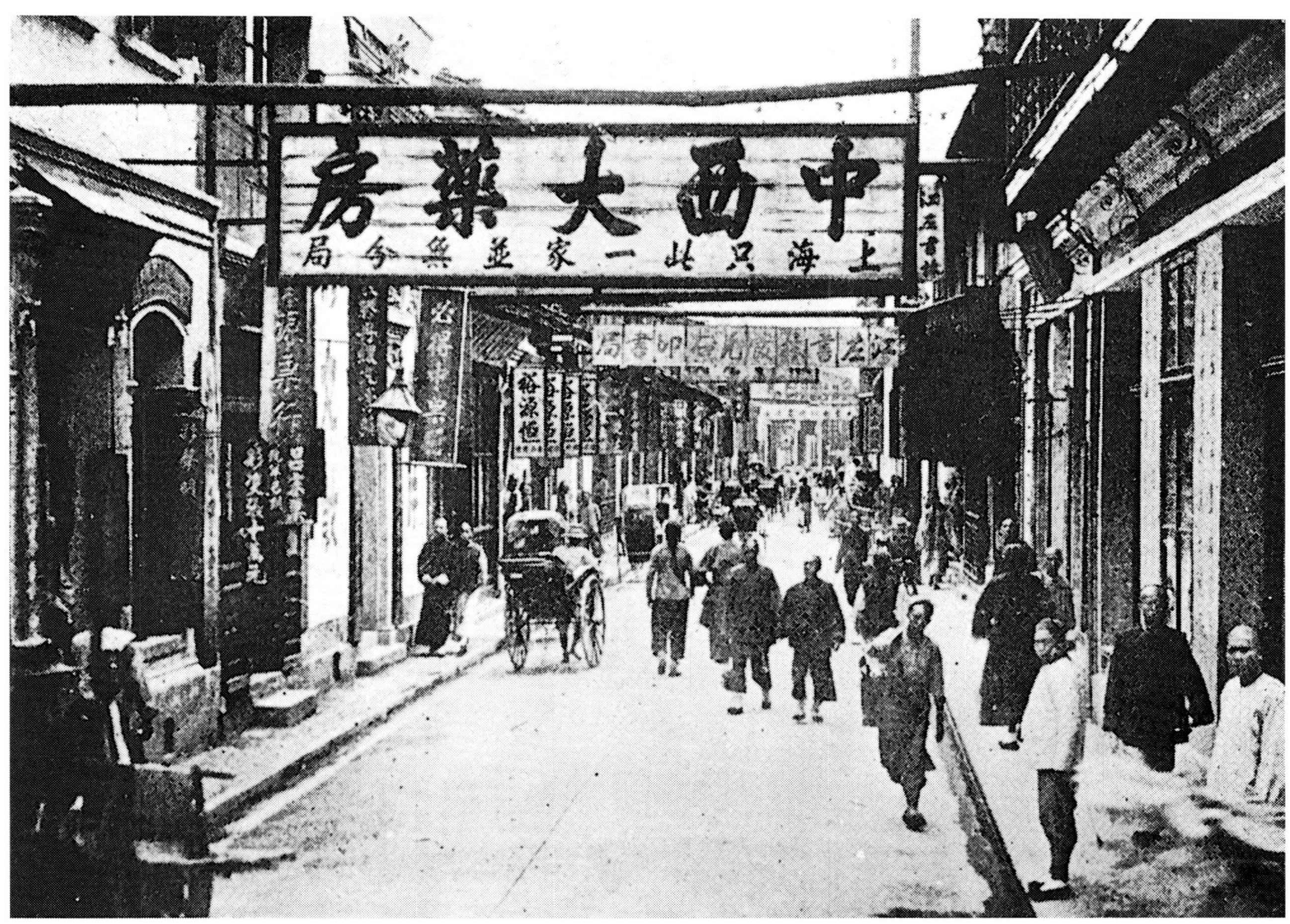



69. Street scene in Shanghai. The advertisement in the foreground states: "Pharmacy for Chinese and Western [medicines]. In Shanghai only this one establishment. No affiliated branches at all!" From W. A. Cornaby, *The Call of Cathay*, London, 1910.

Western gonorrhea remedy produced by Shiseido 資生堂 (Hall of Nurturing Life) in Tokyo. Below the Latin terms *Capsulae Gonor.* are, from right to left, the two Chinese characters *zhilin* 治痲 (Japanese: *chirin*), which mean "heals gonorrhea." The next line-in Katakana writing, used for rendering non-Japanese terms, contains the characters for Gonoru, i.e. "gonorrhea"; below this, finally, is the German word *Innerliche* (internal).[63]

# THE CHINESE PHYSICIAN, HIS PATIENTS AND HIS INSTRUMENTS

## MEDICAL TRAINING AND SOCIAL STANDING OF PHYSICIANS IN CHINA BEFORE THE TWENTIETH CENTURY

The fact that people realize the necessity of medical activity does not automatically guarantee a high social standing or governmental regulation for the medical profession as such. For many centuries, up until the Modern period, individual Chinese and European physicians were able to obtain great fame and extraordinary wealth. But the majority of medical practitioners were not able to regard themselves as members of the upper classes or draw above-average incomes. In China, this situation was caused primarily by Confucian ethics. Medical knowledge was viewed as general knowledge that was obligatory for any responsible person; it allowed the literati to work for the benefit of their own families, but not to earn a living.[64] The ideal patient therefore, was a relative. Confucian texts taught that it was immoral to entrust one's own parents to a stranger who engaged in medicine for financial gain.

Regardless of this basic Confucian attitude, there is evidence of many groups of medical practitioners since the beginnings of Chinese medicine in the Han dynasty. One reason is that the court needed medical experts for its own safety; these may have been trained in special academies or chosen by examination from a large pool of professionally active physicians.[65] It also happened that physicians who had acquired a reputation in the country were called to court in order to treat high-ranking patients on a short-term basis, or to work long-term as court physicians.

There is evidence that many doctors from the elite class applied their medical knowledge not only within the boundaries of their own families, but to strangers either for a charge or for free. The transition from these physicians to those who practiced professionally in the modern sense is fluid. Numerous sources, not least the malpractice legislation since the Tang dynasty [66], prove that, while such doctors might have been treated with contempt by the advocates of Confucian ideology, they were irreplaceable in the provision of medical care for the general population. At the very bottom of the social pyramid were the traveling doctors. In general, they were itinerant medicine

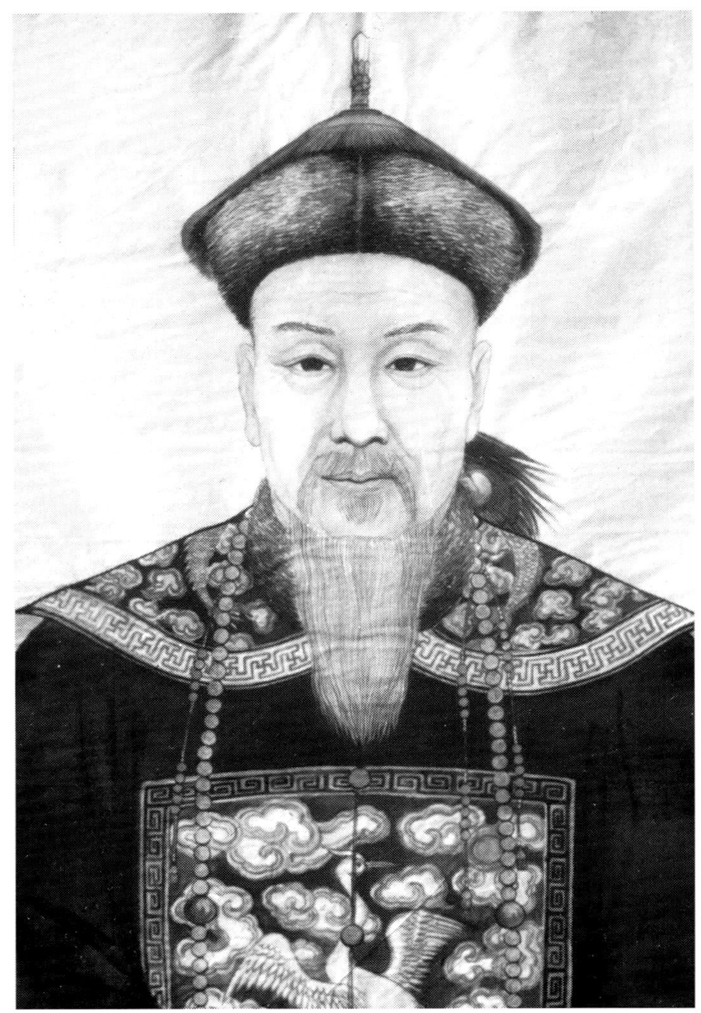

70. The scholar, doctor, and author Xu Dachun 徐大椿 (1693–1771). Drawing after an original in the possession of the Xu family. College for Chinese Medicine, Guangzhou.

sellers who engaged in diagnostic activities in order to recommend and sell the drugs that they carried with them to their clientele.

Since there is no historiography of the development of the medical professions in China comparable to that in Europe, information about all these classes is extremely fragmentary. Current research does, however, permit the following survey.

## MEDICAL OFFICIALS
## AND PALACE PHYSICIANS

Records from the early Han period state that, during the preceding Zhou dynasty, doctors of various specializations and duties worked at the king's court in the status of officials. Among them, the ruler and the general population could choose between dietary physicians (*shiyi* 食醫), physicians for illnesses (*jiyi* 疾醫), physicians for ulcers (*yangyi* 瘍醫), and veterinarians (*shouyi* 獸醫). Their payment, in food, was determined at year's end according to their treatment results: a 100 percent success rate meant inclusion in the highest rank; physicians with a 60 percent success rate were ranked in the fifth and lowest category. The Han records also note that:

> When someone in the country suffers from an illness or ulcers on the head or body and turns to the [palace physicians], the appropriate specialist should treat them. When someone dies prematurely or concludes [their life] in old age, then the cause is recorded and reported to the highest-ranking physician.[67]

Medical experts in the service of the court, or *taiyi* 太醫, were documented continuously for the following centuries of the Imperial period.[68] In the period from the Qin dynasty (second century B.C.E.) to the era of the Northern and Southern Dynasties (sixth century C.E.), there was an Office of the Palace Physician (*taiyiling* 太醫令) with a varying number of doctors. In the Sui and Tang dynasties, an Imperial Department of Medicine (*taiyishu* 太醫暑) primarily responsible for the medical care of the emperor is also documented. After about 605, however, when the Palace Office of Pharmaceutics (*shangyaoju* 尚藥局) that had been founded in the Northern Wei dynasty took over these functions, it became increasingly responsible for training and licensing physicians for government service.

During the Sui dynasty, this office included a director, an assistant, two pharmacists, 200 head physicians, two medicinal herb gardeners, two scholars for general medicine, two scholars for massage, and two scholars for exorcism.

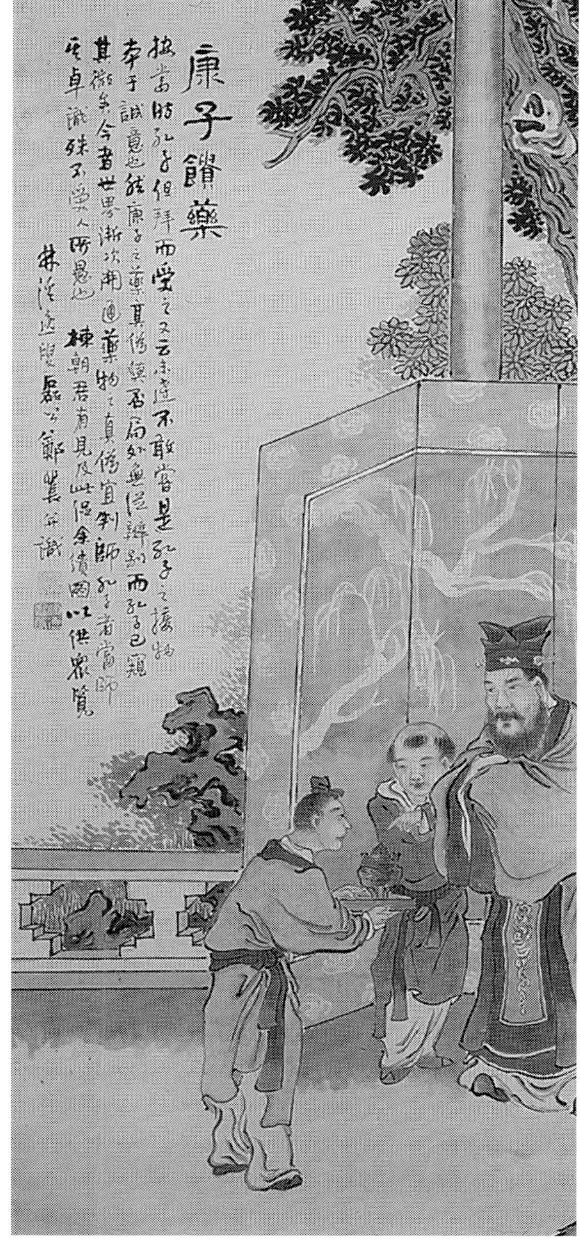

71. "Kangzi offers medicinal drugs [to Confucius]." Scroll drawing by Zheng Chang 鄭萇 from Canton, early twentieth century. The calligraphic text states: "At that time, Confucius merely accepted [the drugs] with a bow and said: 'I don't know anything about it. I dare not take them.' These [words] reflect the straightforward attitude with which Confucius received things. Now, there was basically nobody, except for a pharmacy, who could have distinguished whether Kangzi's drugs were real or fake. Only Confucius had already recognized the proper signs. People of the present are increasingly open towards the world, and it is therefore appropriate for them to distinguish whether drugs are real or fake. Those who take Confucius as their teacher should take his extraordinary knowledge as their model. This makes them insusceptible to the ignorance of the [other] people. [Mister] Dong Chaojun has reached this conclusion. He asked me to leave an [appropriate] painting in order to illustrate this for everyone.  By Zheng Chang, the Old Hermit of the Forest Creek, the Lord of the Rock Pile."

63

Little changed in this composition during the Tang dynasty, with the exception that the office now had two directors and one or several scholars for acupuncture. Teaching activities covered the four subjects of medicine—internal medicine, external medicine, pediatrics, diseases of the ear, nose, throat, and teeth, and cupping—as well as acupuncture, massage, and demonic spell-binding.

During the Sung and Liao dynasties, the Imperial Department of Medicine was renamed the Imperial Office of Medicine (*taiyiju* 太醫局) and, as a department of the central government, was subordinated to the Department of Imperial Sacrifices. Apparently the token of conflicting interests at court, the Imperial Office of Medicine was repeatedly dissolved and then resurrected; after 1102, it was, for a short time, even assigned to the Department of Education.

The Mongols gave a new name to the Imperial Office of Medicine, *taiyiyuan* 太醫院, the Imperial Academy of Medicine. At the same time, they established a subordinate department, the Bureau for the Supervision of Medical Schools (*yixue tijusi* 醫學提舉司), that included among its responsibilities the selection of instructors for the Academy of Imperial Medicine. [69] The Imperial Academy of Medicine remained in existence throughout the Ming dynasty; the subsequent Qing rulers kept court physicians at their disposal until the end of the dynasty. The education of physicians by the Imperial Academy of Medicine ended near the beginning of the Qing dynasty, and in the nineteenth century, this responsibility had been long forgotten.

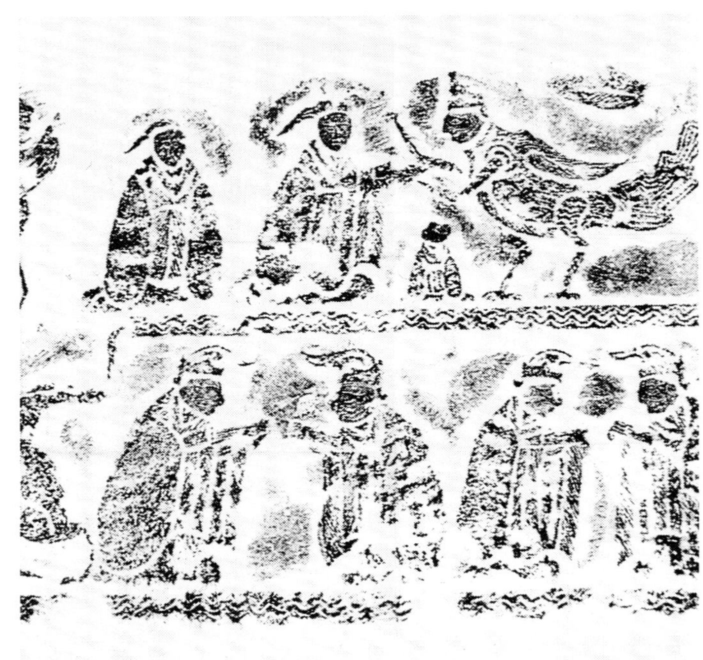

72. Tomb relief from Liang-chengshan 兩城山, later Han dynasty. Bird creature with human head (possibly Bian Que) in front of a person with disheveled hair (possibly a patient).

## MEDICAL SCHOLARS
## AND SCHOLAR PHYSICIANS

Among the doctors of the Imperial Office of Medicine during the past 1300 years are several whose names are still well known today. Chao Yuanfang 巢元方 (ca. 550–630) was the author of the *Zhubing yuanhou lun* 諸病源候論, the first text of Chinese medical literature to specialize in etiology. Zhang Wenzhong 張文仲 (ca. 620–700) worked as palace physician for the Empress Wu (625–705) and compiled a *Collection of all Formulas for the Treatment of Wind and Qi* (*Liaofengqi zhufang* 療風氣諸方) on her orders. Qian Yi (ca. 1032–1113) obtained great fame as a pediatrician and cured the daughter of the Song emperor Shenzong. He published *Straight-forward Instructions for the Treatment of Pediatric Ailments with Drugs* (*Xiaoeryaozheng zhijue* 小兒藥證直訣) and "Rehmannia Pills with Six Components" (*Liuwei dihuangwan* 六味地黃丸), which was marketed until the twentieth century. In the early Ming period, Dai Sigong 戴思恭 (1324–1405) worked as palace physician for

64

thirty years (1368–1398). His book *Essential Instructions for the Therapy of Ailments* (*Zhengzhi yaojue* 證治要訣) in twelve chapters was reprinted in numerous editions, the last one as late as 1959. Gong Tingxian 龔廷賢, finally, was the son of Imperial Palace Physician Gong Xin 龔信. After his spectacular treatment of a concubine named Lu Fan 魯藩, he was employed as Imperial Palace Physician. Later generations remembered him not so much as a creative thinker, but as a hard-working compiler of the thoughts and formulas of earlier authors. Several of his books, in which he covered practically the entire spectrum of medical specializations, have been reprinted until the present. The most famous is the *Wanbing huichun* 萬病回春 (*Return to Spring from All Illnesses*).

The education in the Imperial Office of Medicine was apparently never structured to teach newcomers to the profession. Rather, the system was aimed at refining the skills of individuals who had already created a reputation for themselves outside of court as medical scholars or scholar physicians.

Individuals were referred to as medical scholars when they were knowledgable in medicine, used their skills from time to time outside their family, but never treated patients to make a living. Often their work was committed to posterity through their publications. Scholar physicians were those doctors who used their classical medical education professionally, for the treatment of patients, and who gained fame either as practitioners or as authors.

The first two Chinese biographies of physicians are found in *Records of a Historian* (*Shiji* 史記) by Sima Qian from 90 B.C.E.; they are devoted to a scholar physician called Bian Que 扁鵲 and a medical scholar called Chunyu Yi 淳于意. Since Bian Que died a violent death and Chunyi Yi was sentenced to death, but subsequently pardoned, it is entirely possible that Sima Qian included these biographies in his historical records as warnings not to practice medicine outside the family.

## *1. Bian Que*

Bian Que gained fame as an itinerant doctor; in Zhou dynasty sources, he appears over several centuries at different places so it is impossible to determine the extent to which his biography in the *Shiji* is fictional. The description of the events in his life might not have been entirely true, but may represent a synopsis of real facts based on the observations of several physicians from the early Han dynasty.

In this way, Bian Que's name was related to a substantial body of knowledge. In the small states that he passed through, he practiced pediatrics at one place, gynecology at another, and ear, nose, and throat medicine at yet another place, since he found that the people at the latter paid particular attention to the older generation. He combined the application of medicinal drugs, compresses, and, in one instance, a needle in his therapeutic arsenal. One anecdote

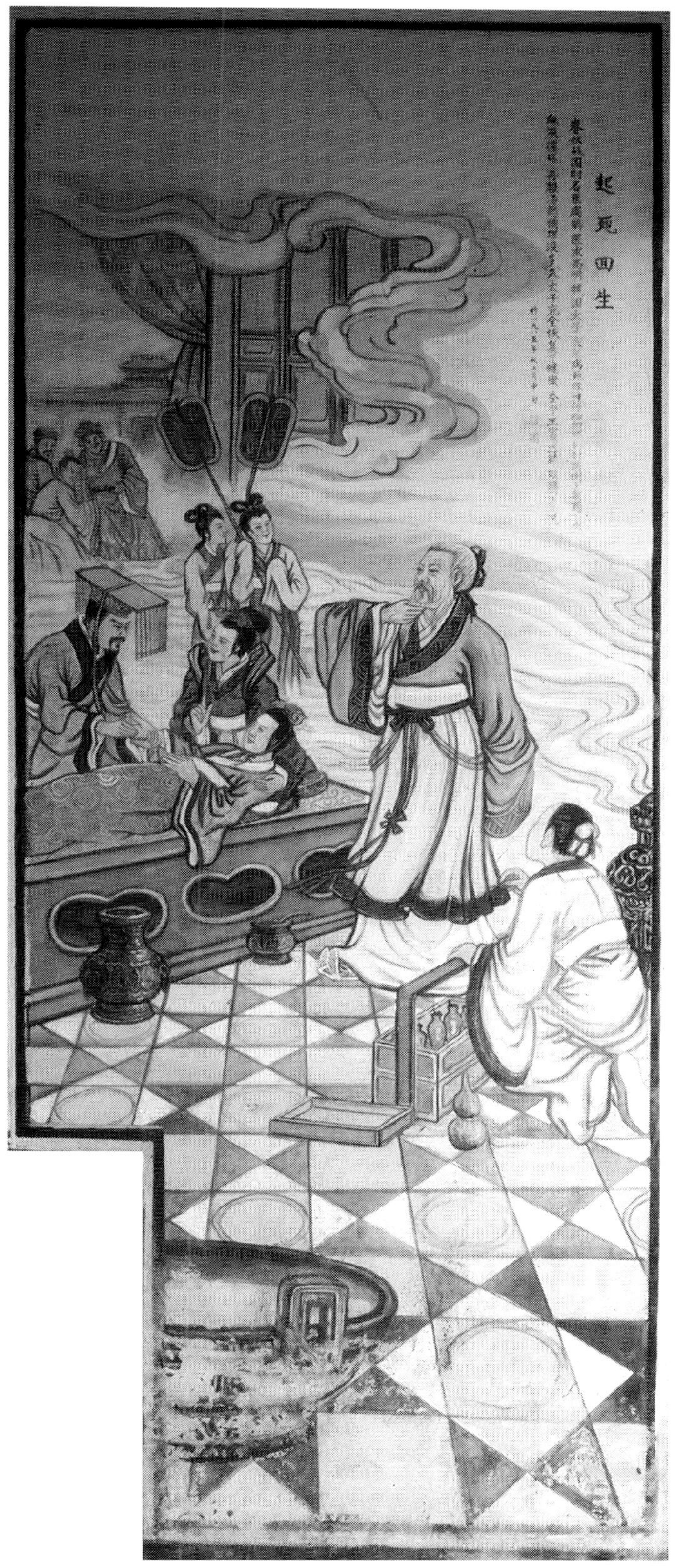


73. "He awakens the dead and brings them back to life." Event from Bian Que's life, *Shiji* 史記 (90 B.C.E.): Bian Que awakens the crown prince of Guo. Temple mural from Anguo near Peking.

even suggests that Bian Que is the originator of acupuncture, but his resuscitation of a "dead" prince in this story, by puncturing the back of his head with a needle, can hardly be regarded as a component of later acupuncture (ill. 73). A jealous palace physician finally arranged Bian Que's execution.[70]

### 2. Chunyu Yi

Chunyu Yi (ca. 215–150 B.C.E.) was not an itinerant healer but the manager of a grain depot in the state of Qi. Among his instructors in medicine was a physician called Cheng Yangqing 乘陽慶, from whom he received several scriptures, among them a *Treatise About Medicines*. For now obscure reasons, Chunyu Yi was sentenced to death and then pardoned, possibly due to the intervention of his daughter who wanted to sacrifice herself as a palace slave. In the course of his trial, Chunyu Yi wrote a report about the medical treatment of 25 patients, thereby providing the oldest collection of case histories in China. Particularly remarkable is the high level to which pulse diagnosis was developed; Chunyu Yi's case histories contain specific terms for more than twenty different pulse states. Apparently, his diagnoses and therapies already reflect the theory of vessel contents as indices for the nature of an illness.[71]

### 3. Zhang Ji 張機

Whereas Bian Que and Chunyu Yi are remembered only as historical figures whose medical knowledge was of no significance in later times, a physician named Zhang Ji who lived roughly 300 years later, was the first author known by name to exert a lasting influence in his profession until the present. Zhang Ji (ca. 150–219 C.E.) studied medicine under a physician named Zhang Bozu 張伯祖 and built a reputation for himself as clinician; he remains famous as the author of the *Shanghan zabing lun* 傷寒雜病論, a text on *Cold Damages and Various [Other] Illnesses* which preceded its time by one thousand years.

Zhang Ji was the first Chinese author to apply yin-yang theories to the use of medicinal drugs and to pay particular attention to the individual condition of each patient.[72] There were no successors to his approach until the thirteenth century. However, the numerous formulary texts that appeared in the ten centuries between Zhang Ji's work and the late Song period contain quite pragmatic formulas for recurring ailments. Thus, it was only logical that the *Shanghan zabing lun* was divided into two texts after Zhang Ji's death. The first of these, the *Shanghan lun* 傷寒論, contains 113 formulas exclusively for the treatment of cold-related damages and stresses the theory of a yin-yang division of the conduits and their problems. The second text, the *Jingui yaolüe* 金匱要略, summarizes 262 regulations against various other illnesses (see also p. 24f.).

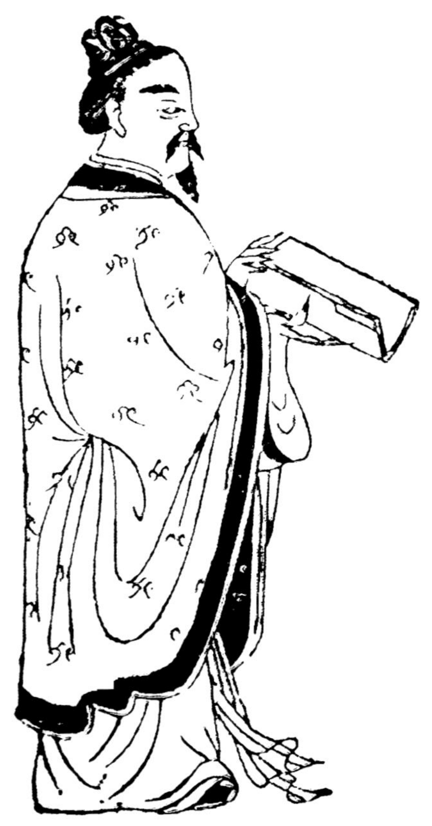

74. Drawing of the medical sage Zhang Zhongjing (Zhang Ji). From *Tuxiang bencao mengquan* 圖像本草蒙筌 (*Removal of Misinformation in Materia Medica, [Expanded with] Diagrams and Figure Drawings*), 1628.

# 4. Teacher–Student Tradition and Medical Schools

Bian Que, Chunyu Yi, Zhang Ji and all of the other physicians whose biographies are documented at least in rough outlines acquired their skills in teacher-student relationships. The first attempt to establish a teaching facility for medicine occurred in 443, due to a request from the Director of the Imperial Department of Medicine, Qin Chengzu 秦承祖, but it did not result in a permanent institution.[73]

In 629, an emperor of the Tang dynasty issued an edict to establish medical teaching facilities, with medical professorships in each, in all important provincial cities. Finally, in 739, the order was given to train twenty medical students per provincial city of 100,000 families or more and twelve medical students per city of 100,000 families or less. As further edicts show, however, these efforts to train a nationwide pool of future medical officials never progressed beyond the initial stages.[74] It is not clear whether these orders actually led to the founding of medical schools and, if so, where the graduates later practiced their profession.

From the Song period on, several attempts were made to raise the standards of doctors in independent practice. An imperial edict of 1188 ordered doctors of the provincial level to pass an examination covering the medical classics, pulse diagnosis, and other related skills. Whether and to what extent these examinations were actually carried out—and in what capacity the successful graduates were employed afterwards—is, unfortunately, not available.[75]

The government-sponsored training of doctors of traditional Chinese medicine has remained questionable until the late twentieth century. Entering a teacher-student relationship has always been regarded as the proven way to acquire the knowledge of a famous physician.[76] Medical knowledge in China has never abstracted from its practitioners to such an extent that it could have been taught in public institutions. For this reason, officials in the PRC failed in their efforts to convince the most recognized physicians to instruct at least two students from those that had been assigned to them; they preferred to select one student as the heir of their knowledge and skills.[77]

Under the Yuan dynasty, professors at the medical schools were ordered to prevent medical students from clinical activities during their training. At the same time, the regularly occurring household census filed the *ruyi* 儒醫 (scholar physicians) as a separate category. Since 1285, all doctors registered as *ruyi* were required to send the supervisory office yearly reports of the patients that they had treated. Examinations were supposed to ensure that doctors were proficient in at least one of the thirteen specializations.

Malpractice legislation from the Tang and Song dynasties mentioned physicians in general; the laws of the Yuan, Ming, and Qing dynasties referred only to the offences and crimes of the common physicians (*yongyi* 庸醫). The term "common physicians" applied to all non-registered, professionally practicing physicians, but the distinction to the

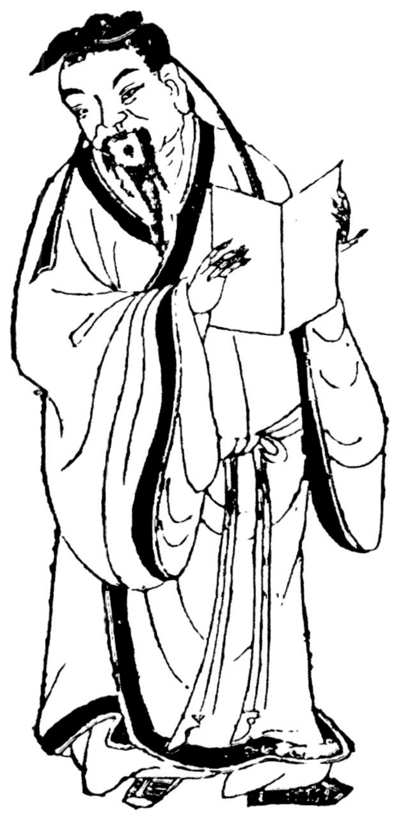

75. Drawing of the Good Physician Hua Tuo. From *Tuxiang bencao mengquan* 圖像本草蒙筌 (*Removal of Misinformation in Materia Medica, [Expanded with] Diagrams and Figure Drawings*), 1628.

"scholar physicians" remained unclear. The title *ruyi* was now claimed by large circles of medically active individuals, since, theoretically, they were exempt from prosecution in malpractice cases.

In China, there was never a strict separation between physician and pharmacist, so these two fields often overlapped. In fact, it was quite profitable to be able to disclose illnesses to patients and then be able to sell them the medications that would supposedly cure their afflictions.

There were always reasons to complain about the lack of qualifications in the medical profession, as seen in the following report from 1268:

> Among the people who open pharmacies, there are those who do not abide by the universally valid laws. Often, they carelessly sell medical drugs with strong toxicity to their clients, such as aconite, croton, or arsenic. This refers to representatives of all social classes. Some of them purposely disobey the laws and cause harm to the lives of their clients, while others merely suffer from a lack of practice in the medical profession. These persons do not understand the medical literature, have no idea about the properties of medicines, and thus deceive the common people. They falsely call themselves physicians, and yet only strive for material profits. They apply needles and medical drugs recklessly and commit assaults against human life. [78]

The phrase "and yet only strive for material profits" expresses only one of the reservations—and, coincidentally, the oldest—that the guardians of the Confucian order had about professionally practicing physicians. In Bian Que's biography, for example, an itinerant healer explains to Duke Huan of Qi that he is ill and should undergo treatment—advice the duke does not accept. After Bian Que leaves, Huan notes sarcastically to his court that "doctors love profit; therefore they love to demonstrate their success on healthy clients!" [79]

## CRITICISM OF PHYSICIANS AND ETHICAL MAXIMS

In China, as in Europe, the criticism of physicians from antiquity to the present has been leveled because of three basic concerns: lack of education, greed as the motivation for medical activity, and abuse of medical knowledge (for example, gaining sexual advantages by devious means). Although the author of the Hippocratic oath is not known, he obviously conceived it as an attempt to relieve fears among the population. In China, the Tang physician Sun Simiao 孫思邈 (581–682?) (see pp. 88–95) tried to eliminate the above-mentioned reasons for distrust in medical activity by composing the first code of ethics for Eminent Physicians (*taiyi* 太醫).

Sun Simiao referred to Confucian and Buddhist values, such as compassion (*ci* 慈) and kindness (*ren* 仁), as well as "not to kill life in order to save life", as the foundations for the practice of eminent physicians. In so doing, he attempted to balance medical ethics with those of the dominant world view. By stressing the emotional neutrality of eminent physicians towards earthly temptations, Sun Simiao tried to dispel fears that doctors might abuse their privileged access to the most intimate details of their patients. In order to dispel the notions of "good" and "bad" doctors, he prohibited physicians from making critical remarks about other physicians in front of patients. Sun Simiao also invalidated the theme of greed by pointing out that eminent physicians were rightfully rewarded by their clients for their good deeds, and that offenses were punished by the spirits.[80]

During subsequent centuries, until the end of the Qing dynasty, opponents of the professional practice of medicine published a long list of writings in which they cited examples of medical behavior that challenged the claims of Sun Simiao and later authors. The accusations were based on reports of physicians who shamelessly cheated their patients out of their money, who took advantage of their patients sexually, or who practiced medicine without any real education. Professional doctors had no recourse but to conceive of ever new suggestions how a good doctor should behave, and point out that only professionally practicing physicians had gained the necessary experience and sufficient skills to counteract all illnesses with success.

Chinese doctors never managed to gain general acceptance of medicine as a professional trade, unlike their European colleagues who succeeded in this from the second half of the nineteenth century on. The European development was partly due to the fact that most doctors agreed upon a single ideology and enacted rigorous trade policies to maintain a professional reputation and unified appearance to outsiders. In China, some progress can be recognized in the 1200 years between the writing of Sun Simiao's deontology and the end of the Qing dynasty.

The evaluation of the practice of medicine began to change during the course of the Yuan dynasty in the thirteenth and fourteenth centuries. This is indicated by the fact that sons of the educated elite increasingly ventured to study medicine and work as official or privately practicing physicians, if they were unable to obtain their ideal careers as government bureaucrats. This change in attitude was accompanied by numerous debates about the high moral value of medical activity. One crucial factor must have been that candidates from upper-class families who failed the examination had fewer opportunities in the Yuan period to engage in teaching as a socially acceptable alternative.[81]

At the beginning of the eighteenth century, professional physicians finally were considered a matter of course. The questions that remained were whether or not there were good doctors among them and how they could be recognized. Xu Yanzuo 徐延祚 (fl. ca. 1875), a physician and author of several texts, composed a few "admonitions addressed to doctors and

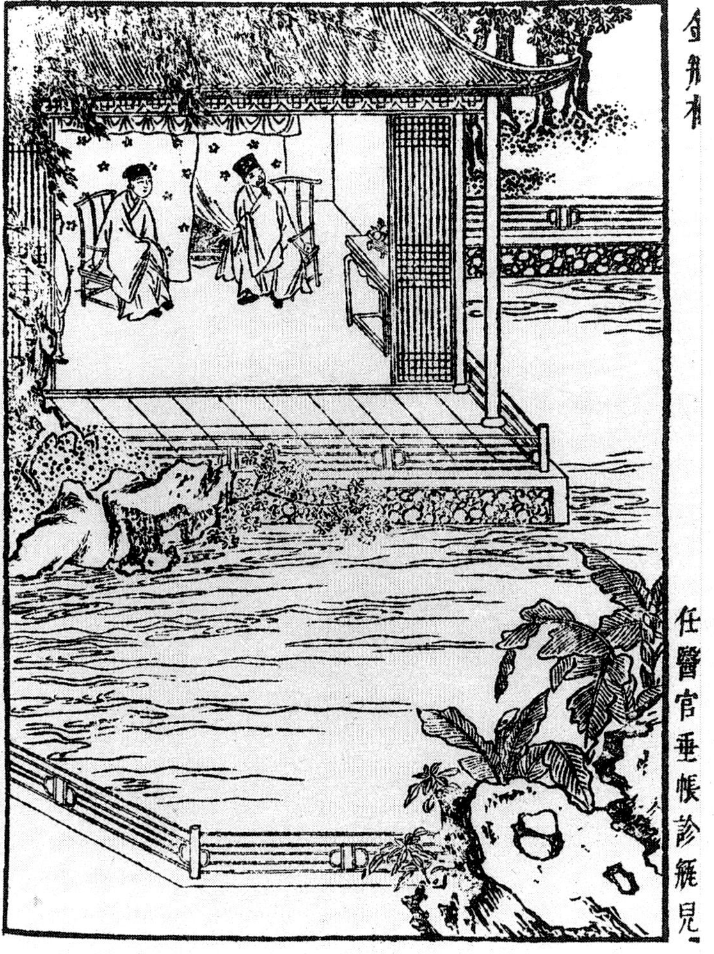


76. "The medical official Ren performs a [pulse] diagnosis with lowered curtain." Illustration from the erotic novel *Jinpingmei* 金瓶梅. Undated edition of the *Jinpingmei*, first half of the seventeenth century. Staatsbibliothek, Berlin.

their patients." They illustrate the status of the ethical debate and corresponding aspects of the doctor-patient relationship at a time when Western medicine and, therefore, new standards were introduced into China:

The intentions of the medical profession are twofold. One is to preserve human life. The other is to make a profit. Does one not need to be careful in the light of these opposing tendencies?

One cannot become a medical practitioner without a superior attitude. And how could one possibly help the world, if one lacks thoughtfulness? A superior attitude allows the principles [of life] to reveal themselves, and thoughtfulness prevents one from striving for fame. If one can combine both elements, one truly does not need to be ashamed, to be a student of Huang Di and Qibo![82] But if one considers eloquence an asset, how could one have a superior attitude? And if one regards success as a matter of luck, how can thoughtfulness be present?

Patients hope for a doctor like an immortal or the Buddha. Doctors save their patients like rain that still comes in time after a long drought. This [relationship] has to be contained in rules. If a doctor is willing to come early [to a patient], the family may not criticize him for that ... A doctor must never intentionally delay his visit. Otherwise, the entire family [of the patient] will be in mourning and fear and will await him sighing on the bed mats. This can only cause the greatest sympathy.

When one places one's faith in a medical practitioner, one should [develop] this trust over a long period of time, but not short-term. I am able to choose and recognize those whom I trust over a long time, under calm circumstances, as if uninvolved and with cool rationality. But doubts and confusion arise towards those in whom I place my trust only short-term [in a crisis], because I act in haste and in a rush, am engaged in the situation, and can no longer remain objective.

Among people, there are those who are wealthy and well respected and those who are poor and looked down upon. Among patients, however, there are neither these nor those, near nor far. A doctor has to treat them all equally and must never stray from an attitude of all-inclusive service. I have encountered those [doctors] who regarded the rich and well respected as important and shook in fear [when they faced them]. Then again I have met those who despised the poor and looked-down-upon and even behaved arrogantly towards them. Were they to come in the morning, the early time of the day did not please them; when one called them in the evening, then they were outraged by how late it was. They responded to unprofitable calls only reluctantly. They lacked in the intent to help people. Both of these types of behavior are not only deficient in every aspect, but one also has to question the conscience of these people. In the Buddhist classics it is said that "all humans are created equal." Medical practitioners should act according to this view.

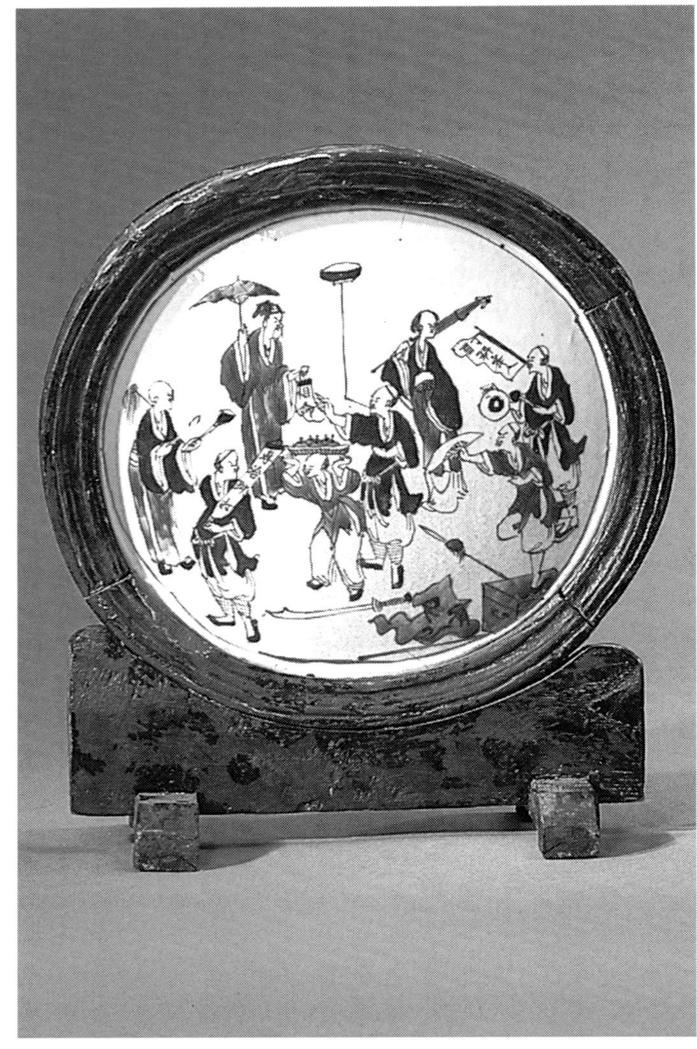

77. Porcelain disk with the depiction of a market scene (mirror image of figure 78). See plate 177.

If a rich person falls ill for a year, he can afford to continue treatment generously for the year and is willing to endure a one-year waiting period. But if a poor person falls ill even for a single day, his work place is threatened within one day and his debts will increase every day. Medical practitioners who only pay attention to those who live in luxury and do not extend their concern to those who live in scarcity can hardly be regarded as serving humanity. They are in fact unscrupulous.[83]

One aspect of the medical profession in China that has differed greatly, until the present, from that in the Western world is that the division between doctor and pharmacist has never been recognized as meaningful. From the above-mentioned Han-era quote, it can be deduced that the pharmacist also diagnosed illnesses and therefore practiced medicine. This situation remained fundamentally the same in subsequent centuries.

At least since the Ming period, many pharmacists also practiced as physicians and physicians sold their own remedies in pharmacies. It is common to this day that pharmacies for traditional Chinese medicines hire physicians as their employees. It remains to be seen to what extent these physicians let patients go without medication. On the other hand, in Taiwanese medical clinics that are affiliated with a pharmacy, medical practitioners are required to prescribe a certain number of medicines every day in order to reach a particular sales objective, instead of taking the conditions of the patients as determining factors.[84]

### 1. Physicians' Advertising and Explicit Ethics

In the PRC, where the government-controlled press does not print any private medical or pharmaceutical advertisements, the use of privately printed flyers to attract customers is still widespread. Doctors or self-defined experts paste such announcements on house walls in the vicinity of their practice to alert the public to their special skills in the treatment of illnesses—nowadays, these are frequently sexually transmitted ones. This is the continuation of a tradition whose beginnings are obscure, but for which there are examples from the late Imperial period.

One such example is the following "self-description" of a doctor who was employed by, or perhaps owned, a pharmacy called Hall for the Preservation of Life:

I was born to the Liu family in Yüyi. In my youth, I educated myself in Confucian scholarship; as an adult, I concentrated for more than twenty years on the study of [the classics of] Qi [Bo] and Huang [Di]. My efforts are not motivated by greed, and I am not like any ordinary doctors. My mind is set solely on helping humanity; my hope is to preserve human life. In my treatment of smallpox and measles, for example, I replenish and drain, regulate the original [qi] and act in

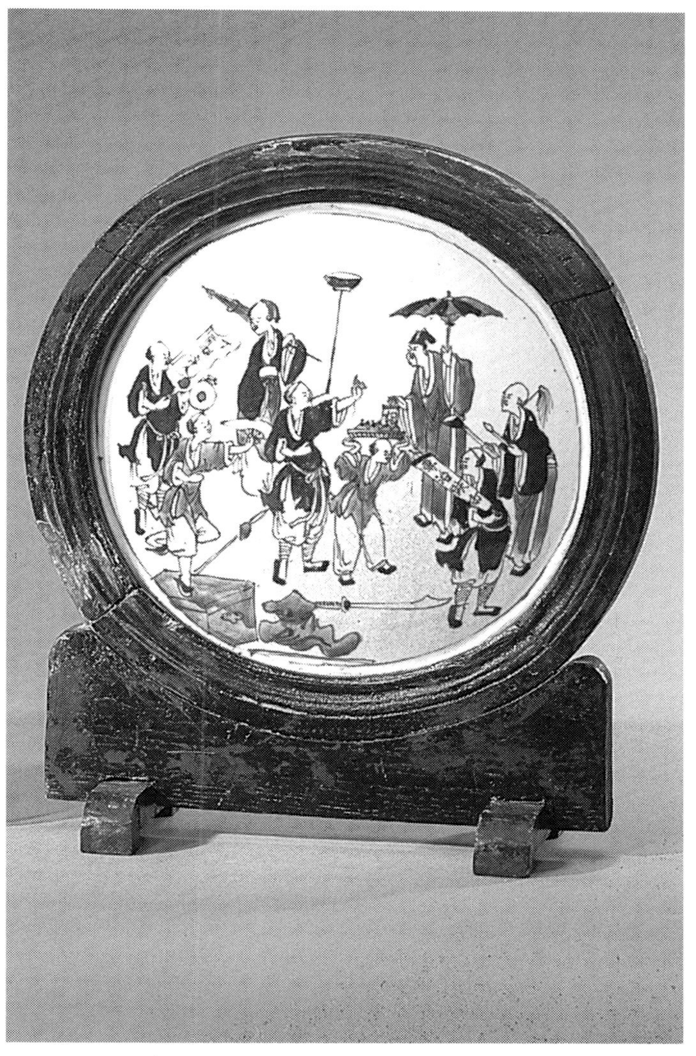

78. Porcelain disk with the depiction of a market scene (mirror image of figure 77). See plate 177.

honest concern and constant fear that I might cause unfortunate harm. Also, when I deal with cholera, acute *sha* disorder[85], or any other ailments, I investigate the build and appearance [of my patients], feel the structure of their vessel [movements][86], and take the seasonal conditions into consideration. Whether rich or poor, [all patients] can receive treatment and will be cured instantly. Further, I am afraid to endanger the invisible rewards that I will receive for my good deeds. Therefore I would never dare to ask for money in the case of an unsuccessful treatment. If someone wants to express their gratitude with a payment, I will not decline it if the illness is cured. (ill. 79)

This is a typical example of a physician's advertisement in the form of explicitly stated ethics, which assisted one physician to win the trust of the population. Such blatantly expressed ethics cannot be equated with the ethical standards which this physician actually followed in his practice. The text contains substantial parts that are characteristic of an incomplete professionalization. That the doctor seeks customer confidence does not serve as an ethical code of a professional trade group per se, but serves his need to set himself apart from other ordinary doctors.

The advertisement also serves to refute the two most prevalent criticisms of doctors and the public's general distrust in professionally practicing physicians. First, the fear that the doctor might not be educated sufficiently is countered by the reference to the fact that he studied medicine for more than twenty years and even engaged in Confucian scholarship as a youth. Second, two remarks are woven into the text with the obvious goal of eliminating the possibility of greed as a motivation. In the manner of Sun Simiao, the doctor here refers to his Buddhist ties and the advantages that good deeds will bring to the metaphysical order. At the same time he indicates that he is aware of the punishments that await those who act sinfully. Mining a similar vein, he also asserts that he will treat the rich and the poor equally. Such a declaration shows that this kind of equal treatment could not be taken for granted in medical practice.

The elaborations on the functional therapies that the advertising physician claims to apply even in the cases of such critical and acute diseases as smallpox and cholera are interesting in terms of a history of medical ideas. This approach was prevalent in scholastic medicine during the Qing dynasty and corresponded, as Xu Dachun 徐大椿 reports, to the population's fear of drastic therapies.[87] As could be expected, the elaborations in the doctor's advertisement reflect the prevailing spirit of the times.

保生堂醫家自叙
余本玉邑劉氏幼習儒業壯學岐黃專心
致志廿餘載非圖射利不與庸醫相等心
純濟世志在活人如醫痘疹補瀉調元深
加微惕恐害魚薰看癰乱急痧一切等
症察其形容切其脈理體乎時令不論貧
富可治便醫又懼敗陰隲未痊不敢支錢
倘有謝儀病愈不卻

79. "Self description of a physician." Wood-block print, late-nineteenth or early twentieth century.

## *1. Early References*

Among all of the doctors in China, the itinerant doctors—
also known as *lingyi* 鈴醫 (bell doctors), *caozeyi* 草澤醫
(country doctors), *zou fang yi* 走方醫 (wandering doctors),
or *jianghuyi* 江湖醫 (doctors [who pass] over rivers and
lakes)—have received the least amount of scholarly attention. This is despite the fact that well into the twentieth
century they constituted the majority of healers for the
general population. It should not be forgotten that the
medicine of the scholar physicians was that of a minority;
the bulk of the population had no access to the theoretical
foundations and clinical applications of the medicine of
systematic correspondence.

Most of the population was forced to trust the skills of
itinerant doctors passing through the countryside when
prayers to deities and spirit exorcisms were of no avail.
From the few sources that are available about this class of
medical practitioners, it can be deduced that their treatments were based on therapeutic concepts which do not fit
into any of the conceptual systems known from literature
(see pp. 36–38).

Official reports about itinerant doctors who exhibited
their skills in market fairs date from as early as the thirteenth century. Representatives of the formally educated
class responded with a complete lack of understanding to
these healers whose arts they believed to be based on deceit
and ignorance, as a document from 1265 states:

> In bazaars and other places where many people congregate,
> one can find types of false doctors and medicine sellers who
> do not obey the universally applicable laws. They handle
> snakes and feathered creatures, manipulate figurines, ring
> little bells, read cards, and play the fish-shaped drum [of the
> Buddhists]. In this way, they attract great crowds who they
> convince deceitfully of the miraculous effects of their reme-
> dies. The ignorant, small people believe that the cheap sales
> of these [false doctors] benefit them and therefore purchase
> pills and powders with their money. They then take these
> medicines according to their claims, but cannot escape from
> death, because none of the medicines corresponds to their
> illnesses.[88]

## *2. The Characterization of Itinerant Doctors in the Chuanya*

Further details about itinerant doctors were confided by
Zhao Xuemin 趙學敏 to his readers in a preface to his
*Chuanya* 串雅 (see p. 36) from 1759:

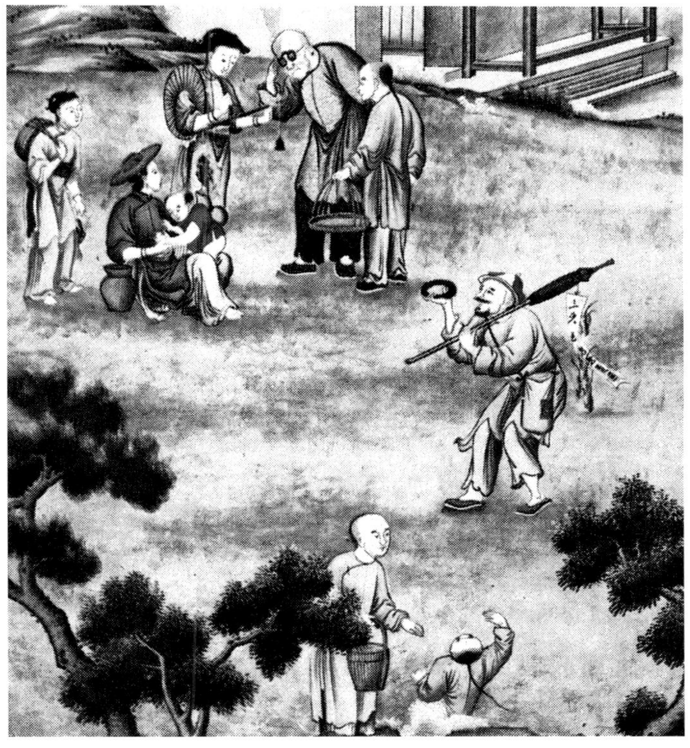

80. Scene of daily street life on Chinese export wallpaper from the eighteenth century, depicting an itinerant doctor with an umbrella and a "tiger sting," a ring-shaped, hollow rattle with which he created the charac-teristic sound for his guild, thereby drawing attention to himself. From *Guang Shi Gao* (*Chinese Wallpaper Book*), n. p., 1957, 26.

In some respects, they stand out because of their behavior. For example, they constantly admonish each other to keep [their knowledge] secret and not to reveal it frivolously in order to keep the circle of practitioners limited. In general, they have a clear idea about what happens [during their activities], but usually not about the reasons why something happens; it is rare that one of them can display a comprehensive understanding [of these contexts].

Mai Sun 邁孫, the editor of the *Chuanya* edition from 1890, apparently knew more details about the practices of itinerant doctors:

Among the common people, those medical practitioners who roam in all four directions with a bag on their backs are called *zoufang* [wandering doctors]. They are always intent on quick results; the complete well-being [of their patients] lies outside of their concern.

They hold an iron implement in their hand which is shaped like a round hollow container. In this otherwise empty container, they swing an iron ball around in a circle. [The implement] has been called a "tiger sting" since the time of Li Cikou 李次口 from the Song period. Cikou was an itinerant doctor. He frequently traveled far into the mountains. Once, he encountered a tiger who had a thorn in his mouth and sought help from Li Cikou. Cikou placed the said implement into the tiger's mouth in order to pull out the thorn. His art later gained fame everywhere. Those who carry on his art all carry this implement as their symbol and call it "tiger's sting."

The medicine bag that they carry is called Wuqie bag, since it is said to have originally been used by Qin Wuqie 秦無且. Their [acupuncture] needle is called "sword-shaped needle". ... Further, they have a small metal tube which they use to pull teeth. It is called *checui* 坼脆 (breaks that which is brittle). Adulterated drugs carry the term *hejian* 何兼 (what is in it?). To offer plant-based drugs for sale in the market is called *jiacao* 夾草 (pinning herbs). ... To dress up as a Daoist or Buddhist priest is called *youfang* 遊方 (traveling the cardinal directions). ... To share payments [with a second doctor] is called *podong* 破洞 (to beat a hole). To collect a fortune from people is called *laozhao* 撈爪 (to fish with clutches). ...

Itinerant doctors follow a maxim of three words. The first word is "cheap." This means, they do not use expensive medicines. The second word is "effect." This means that a drug has to expel the disease in the moment at which it is taken. The third word is "convenient." Those who manage to stick to the principles expressed in these three words in distant mountain or forest regions as well as in urgent cases, assume a superior position among their colleagues.

Itinerant doctors can attribute the trust that they generally receive to four areas of activity, in which their efforts are met with success. These are, first, pulling teeth, second, dabbing skin blemishes, third, removing clouding of the eye, and fourth, expelling worms. In all these four areas, they rely as much on the power of medicines as on manual dexterity.

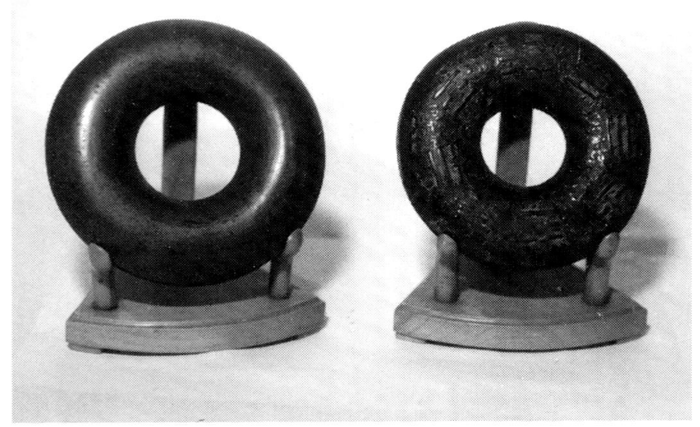

81. Two doctor's rattles, so-called "tiger stings". The one on the right is decorated with the eight trigrams. Academy for Chinese Medicine, Peking.

Itinerant doctors learn their skills far from home. When discussing their theories, one rarely notices a demanding subtlety. They are all experts in one specialty or another and travel around to make a living. When they feel jealous towards each other, they clear each other out of the way. When they work together, they flatter each other. Their communication among each other resembles that of small birds or birds of prey. Now their voices are friendly, then again they argue, without following any regularity.

Among remedies are those which are extremely efficacious. ... Itinerant doctors use these remedies often in order to achieve the most far-reaching results. Every time this happens, people admire their skills with great astonishment. After they have conquered their illnesses, they request further remedies. Then the [itinerant doctors] give them pills which, they claim, are able to remove any further illnesses. [The people], of course, have no idea that these consist of remnants of any roots that were thrown out during the preparation of drugs.

Itinerant doctors know of techniques to transform [a healthy condition] internally or externally into an illness. For example, they use *mugua* dew 木瓜露 in *lepi* pills 樂脾丸 in order to coat the pupils with a film. ... They use mold powder in order to implant ulcers. ... Furthermore, there is *hebiandou* paste 合扁豆膏 in order to induce feverish states. ... Each of these techniques is inhumane. The lower [their social status], the more [they use such techniques]. The reason for such behavior is that they lack in skill, but use these techniques anyway in order to follow their motivation to obtain profits.

Thus, it was not only the theories and practices of itinerant doctors which contradicted the rules and ideals of the higher classes, but also their ethics. It seems that itinerant doctors were primarily wandering medicine sellers who diagnosed real or imaginary illnesses and used clever psychology to incite in their patients a willingness to purchase their remedies (see pp. 76–79).

### 3. Psychology and Strategies of Action Among Itinerant Doctors around the Turn of the Century

The dialogue book of an itinerant doctor from the late nineteenth or early twentieth century in the collection of the Museum für Völkerkunde, Berlin, is the first and, so far, only known document that demonstrates the strategic and professional-therapeutic world of itinerant doctors. The book apparently served as a kind of *vade mecum* for the itinerant doctor who, although able to understand all or most of what potential customers might say to him outside of his home region, was unable to answer in each local dialect. The dialogue book, therefore, contains numerous statements which he could let his audience read or have read out loud by a local person at the appropriate occasions.[89]

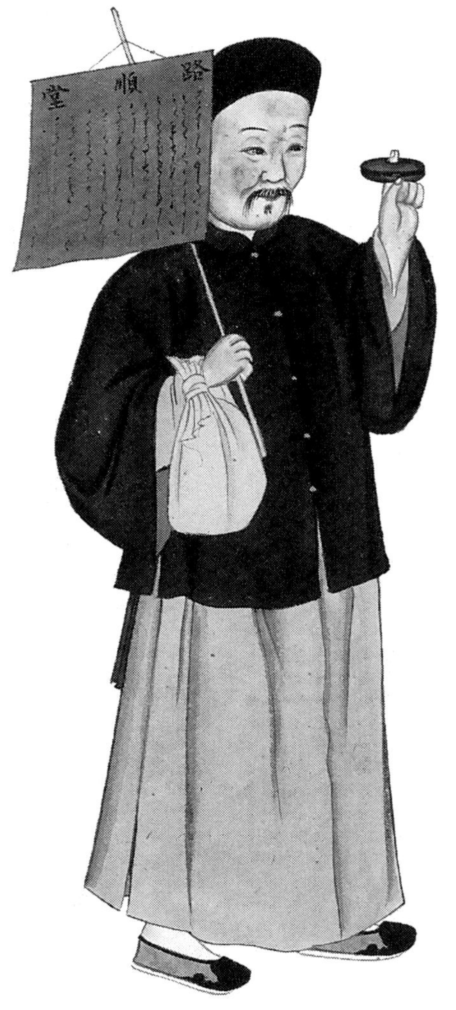

82. An itinerant doctor who holds a stick with a sign indicating the name of his *lushuntang* 路順堂 (Pharmacy for Smooth Traveling), as well as illegible information regarding his remedies and their effects. The bag on his wrist contains the selection of drugs that he is carrying. With his left thumb, he makes the "tiger sting" rattle. From *Beijing minsu baitu* 北京民俗百圖 (*One Hundred Illustrations of Popular Customs in Peking*). Drawing, end of nineteenth century.

The content of the book is unstructured, but from individual answers five thematic units can be isolated which seem to have been paramount in the communication between the itinerant doctor and his clientele. These are: statements concerning the diagnosis and potential danger of illnesses; justifications of the pricing and references to potential discounts in price; explanations about illnesses and their causes; answers to direct questions from the circle of patients and audience; and information regarding the application and prices of the remedies.

It is obvious from several passages that the statements were composed by or for an itinerant doctor who, as usual, carried his remedies on him for sale:

I have come from so far away.
  If I was not concerned with healing [illnesses], why should I have come here?
In any case, your local remedies are certainly no good at all.

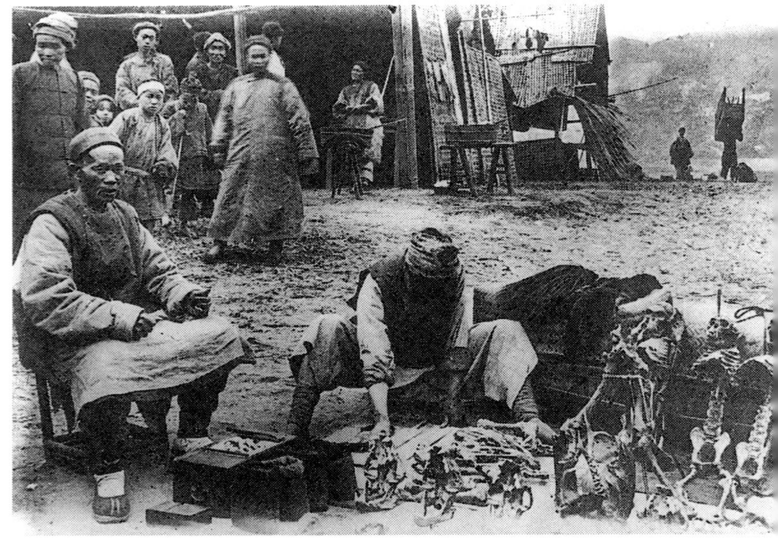

83. An itinerant doctor displays his medicines and waits for customers. Photograph, Sichuan, ca. 1920.

Many of the book's claims served the purpose of convincing patients that they had an illness which was temporarily harmless but could become quite serious in the future:

Sir, you claim that your illness is not serious? What is a serious illness? Wrong. Should an illness only be considered serious after one has died from it?
  It will develop into a terrible problem over the next two or three months. Now it is still easy to treat. [After two or three months, however,] even if you should not die from it, you will still find yourself in a highly critical condition.

Regardless, potential clients seem to have doubted the quality of the remedies and the skills of the itinerant doctor:

You tell me that my remedies are no good? As long as you haven't taken any, you have not tried them. I take into consideration both [the patient's] pulse and [medical] theory at the same time, and say that he is ill. But I can see there are still many ignorant people in this civilized world. You claim to be knowledgeable. As far as I can see, one can never cure an illness if one cannot rely on the good will [of the patient] during the treatment.

The owner of the dialogue book could fall back on numerous formulations in order to point to the origin of an illness or the supposed background of his therapies, thereby giving the appearance of an educated physician:

The reason why you have acquired this illnesses is found in your diet and hygiene. Maybe [your food was] too cold, maybe it was uncooked, maybe [you] drank too much tea/water. This has harmed your appetite. You are taking very little food and drink every day. The illness is worsening day by day. The illness is Coolness of Blood. Later, abdominal distention will develop from this. The fire in the head is flowering. The heart is empty and restless. Sometimes the stomach hurts. Sometimes you don't eat and still are not hungry.

The heart and kidneys are suffering from deficiencies. The Minister Fire is unable to rise and increase the qi of the kidneys. The Minister Fire is moving without regularity. The Fire of the Gate of Life is weak. The Essential Qi can no longer support the Origin. At night, you dream of all those things which men and women crave. If this continues on, you will develop a cough. This comes and goes ceaselessly. This illness is Deficiency due to Exhaustion.

This illness is caused by the fact that poison has invaded the Six Palaces and then escaped from the Palaces. Apply remedies to them, and the [lesions] will be cured soon.

Blood flows like the Yangzi. Places that it does not reach suffer harm.

This illness is a case of Cold Fire. One feels very ill. Coughs. Do not worry if you cough up phlegm. You only have to worry, if you cough up blood.

The owner of the dialogue book was not only prepared for doubts about his professional skills, but also about his ethical motivations:

I don't trust you either! Sir! Humanity! If I was not concerned with healing [illness], why should I have come here? If I don't treat you, I will tell you openly. One who does not plan far ahead will soon suffer. An educated person will rather feed a tiger than an illness. One who is not ill and also does not believe to be ill, will not take any medicines. One who is ill and implores the spirits for assistance cannot be cured of his illness.

Several statements of the dialogue book clearly indicate the problems of the itinerant doctor who was forced to convince his clients in a public place and at the same time defend himself against sometimes derogatory comments of third persons:

Sir, you and I, we don't know each other. This person here [is considering] having his illness treated. This is not a game about money. If he takes medicines, he does not have anything to be afraid of. You must not discourage him. If someone requests a treatment, he will receive a treatment. If his illness worsens, he will accuse you of being bad.[90]

What he says, sounds good to your ears. He says that you should not have your illness treated. I am not angry with you. But it would be better if you let me treat you.

A popular healer was not interested in remaining at one place for long. Therefore he encouraged his clients to make quick decisions:

I did not bring a lot of medicines with me today. I did not come here to make money, but to make a name for myself. I am only treating fifteen patients and am therefore only

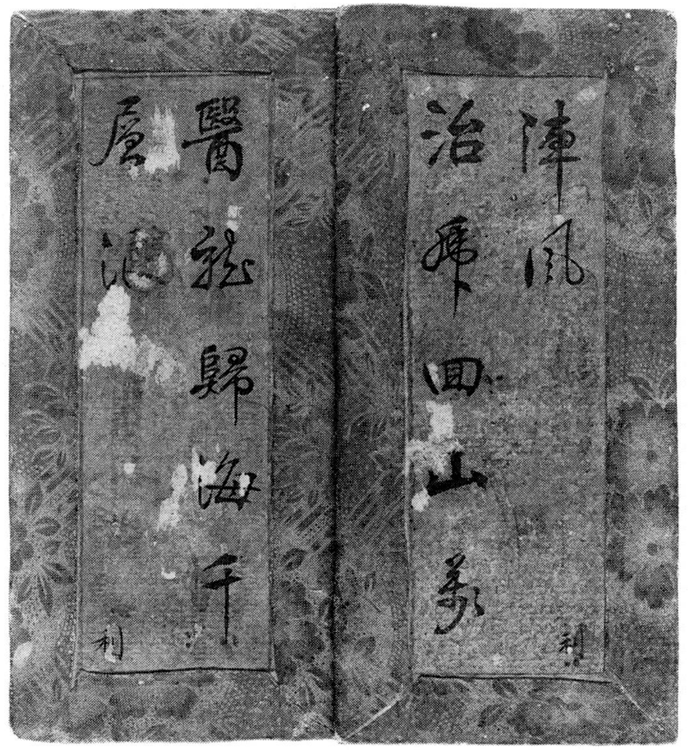

84. Cover of an itinerant doctor's dialogue book, late-nineteenth, early twentieth century, with handwritten maxim: "The healed dragon dives back into the sea [and causes] the waves [to pile up] in a thousand layers. The treated tiger returns to the mountains [and causes] the winds [to roar up] in ten thousand formations."

handing out fifteen numbered tickets. No more. Hurry up. Usually, this remedy costs three dollars; today, an exception for 1.50 dollars!

Many of the above answers to potential questions from clients reflect the wide spread belief nurtured by Confucian writings, that professionally practicing doctors, and particularly itinerant ones, were only interested in making a profit. The following rebuttals may have been directed at patients disputing the costs of treatments and remedies:

I am only concerned with a good reputation. I am not looking for a profit. I am not known for accumulating riches. There are two choices: If [you desire] a treatment, I have the drugs with me. If you trust me, I will treat you. If you would rather keep your money, then there won't be any treatment either.

Where the treatment of illness is concerned, there is no sense in talking about other things. The money is not much.

You are rich because you live. You don't live because you are rich. One can only possess riches as long as one is alive!

Whether you have money or not, that I don't know. But I do know for sure that you have an illness. You should spend [your money]. If you feel bad about the money, then you should not ask for a treatment. If you don't receive treatment, then you won't need to spend money.

Your illness is serious. I think the money [I am asking for] is little. My medicines are exceptionally good, therefore the price is also above average.

The following statements may have been prepared as response to skeptical clients who wished to receive treatment first and pay only after the promised result had materialized:

And if you don't give me the money, should I take you to court? From time immemorial [it has always been the rule:] First the money, then the medicine!

All right, I will reduce the price of my medicine by half for you. As soon as I have cured your illness, examine your conscience again.

Buy one half first. After [you] have taken the medicines, if [you] feel better, then buy the other half. That works, too.

Sometimes, a rougher tone must have certainly been helpful:

Don't talk so much. [I] am treating your illness. [You] pay the money!

You claim that [my] medicines are no good? But you haven't even taken [my] medicines yet? Then how can you know that they are no good? And whose medicines are good? Your local medicines, at least, are certainly no good at all.

Occasionally, the itinerant doctor might have been forced to justify why he had charged different clients different prices. The following statement might have been prepared for such a situation:

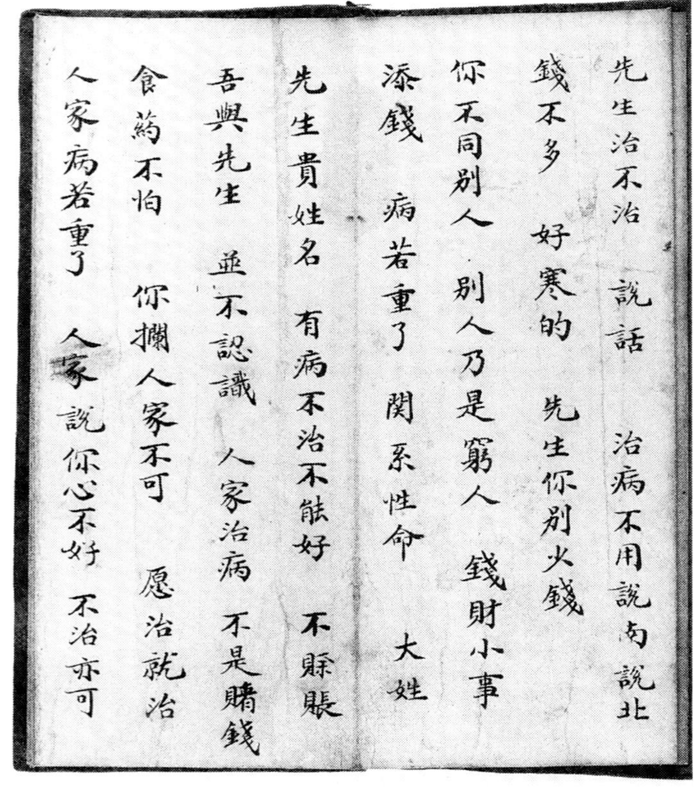



85. Excerpt from an itinerant doctor's dialogue book, late-nineteenth, early twentieth century,: "Sir, now, should I treat you or not? Just say something! Where the treatment of illness is concerned, there is no sense in talking about other things. The money is not too much. How miserly! Sir, you should not give less money. You are not like the other people, are you? The others are poor. Money and riches are unimportant. Add a little more money. If the illness turns more serious, your life will be in danger. Your honorable name, sir, what is it? If you have an illness and don't get it treated, it will not improve. There is no credit. Sir, you and I, we don't know each other. If that person lets himself be treated, it is not a game about money. If he takes medicines, he has nothing to be afraid of. You must not discourage him. If someone requests a treatment, he will receive a treatment. If his illness worsens, he will say that you acted wrongly. If you don't wish to be treated, that is also fine."

Some people are old, some are young. Some illnesses are easy, some are serious. Among medicinal drugs, one distinguishes between those of high and of low quality. Therefore, the prices are also different. The remedies that are used by men and women are also different. People's constitutions and bodies differ. There are differences in the properties of the drugs, since they can be cold or hot, warm or cool or balanced. One does not use the same drugs in spring, summer, and fall.[91]

## 4. Itinerant Doctors in Modern Times

As Mai Sun already mentioned, itinerant doctors used a "dark speech" (*hei hua* 黑話) in order to keep their strategies and skills secret. Later, new insights into the systematic approaches of itinerant doctors were made possible by a *Study of the Internal Secret Language of the Wandering Professions* (*Jianghu neimu heihuakao* 江湖內幕黑話考), published under the pseudonym Xue Mo 雪漠 in 1991.

Xue Mo's contemporary works confirms the claims and reservations against this profession which Zhao Xuemin and Mai Sun had recorded earlier in their prefaces to the *Chuanya* and which were implied by the defensive excerpts cited from the dialogue book.[92]

Even in present-day China, when an itinerant doctor arrives at a place, he first has to win the attention and trust of potential patients. For this purpose, he "glues a circle," *yuan nian zi* 圓黏子. That is, he gathers a circle of curious onlookers around him. He uses two techniques to aid him in this. First, he may "pin a flat one," *dian zhang zi* 點張子. That is, he unrolls a transparency in a suitable location and begins to explain the depicted organs and their illnesses at the top of his voice. A curious audience congregates around him and listens to his explications. Another method is to show the most grotesque things related to the doctor's skills. Thus, he might show exposed brains of a hare in order to call attention to his pills made from them. Nowadays, doctors frequently use spectacular photographs of gruesome illnesses for the same purpose.

Once the itinerant doctor succeeds in finding a listener with an illness, he may feel his patient's pulse, name the origin of the illness, and describe a more or less serious progression of the ailment. The real goal of the conversation is, of course, the sale of medicines.

The itinerant doctor knows many psychologically successful methods to encourage those in his audience, with whom he has established contact in one way or another and for whom he might have already diagnosed an ailment, to purchase his medicines. He might promise potential clients that: "My remedy cures old and new ailments, chronic and acute illnesses. If there is no cure, come back to me and I will refund the purchasing costs and even your traveling expenses. Whoever fails to approach me and demand their money back when the medicines did not help is a coward."[93]

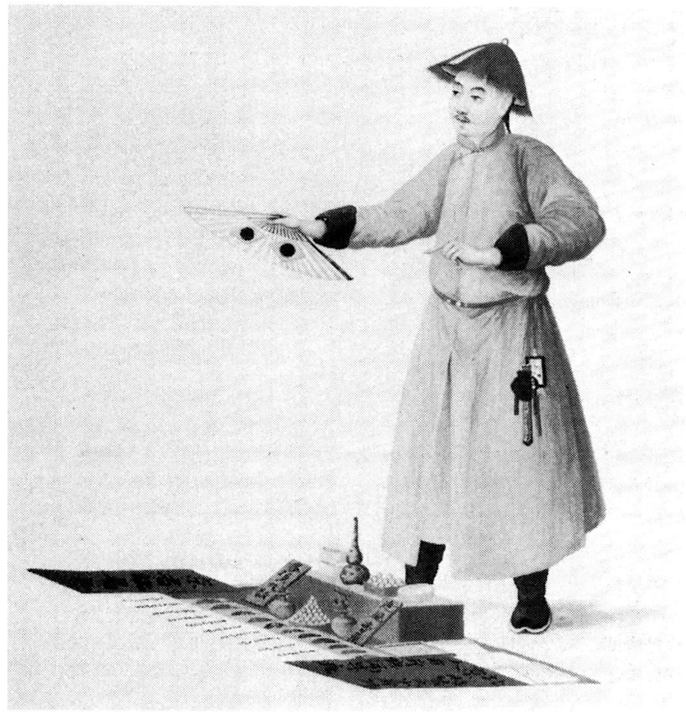

86. A doctor with his selection of medicines. On the fan are the symbols for plaster medicines. Watercolor, China, nineteenth century.

Usually, the itinerant doctor carries the medications that he sells in pre-prepared form. Any efficacious formula contains a basic component on which the result is based. The itinerant doctor might keep two preparations of each of his medications on hand for his customers, one with the active component and one without. The patient first receives one or several pills with the active ingredient as a sample and immediately feels relief. On the basis of this, he or she will decide to purchase more pills, which in reality are a combination of pills with and without the active ingredient. When taken over a longer period of time, the first, active pills cause the patient to feel better, but the last ones have no effect. The patient will not know the reason for this, and if he encounters the doctor again, he might tell him about it. The doctor will answer that there are more and less serious cases of this illness, that his medicine was certainly the correct one since it did show a result, and that the patient will have to purchase more of it, since his/hers is obviously a serious case.

In order to win the trust of still-hesitant patients, the itinerant doctor may make use of the most convincing argument, the oath. This procedure is called *pi lei zi* 劈雷子, literally "to split the thunder," in technical terminology. The oath, in fact, is a seal whose breaking leads to serious consequences in the eyes of the population and in the thinking of the itinerant doctors themselves. In order to escape the consequences, or, in other words, to "split the thunderbolt" that might hit him—i.e. to conduct it to the right and left of his person, and yet be able to swear by the results of his own medicines—the doctor knows two tricks. The first is to make an absurd oath by invoking punishments that are unreal, such as "then cold water shall scald me, a lamp wick stab me, or a pillow strike me dead." The listener pays attention mostly to the words scald, stab, and strike dead and comes to trust the doctor.

A second method is to fall back on ambiguous statements as only the peculiarities of the Chinese language allow. Thus, the itinerant doctor might call out to his clients, "then I will let myself be thrown on a mountain outside [the village, town, etc.], and my dead body will never return home." The oath to forego a funeral in the case of wrongdoing, and to potentially have one's body eaten by dogs or other animals is very impressive. It might convince many hesitant listeners of the honesty of the doctor since he is willing, by these words, to accept one of the worst punishments known to Chinese popular culture. However, if a disappointed customer confronts the doctor and mentions his oath, the doctor would write down the sentence *jiao wo pao shan zai wai, shi bu hui jia* 叫我抛山在外屎不回家, and the cheated client would read: "Let me throw a mountain outside; my excrement will not return home." *Pao shan*, "to throw a mountain," is a colloquial term for bowel movements; *shi* 屎 (excrement) is identical in pronunciation (except for the tone) to *shi* 屍 (dead body).

The itinerant doctor has to be prepared for the possibility that a disappointed patient will blame him, if he later

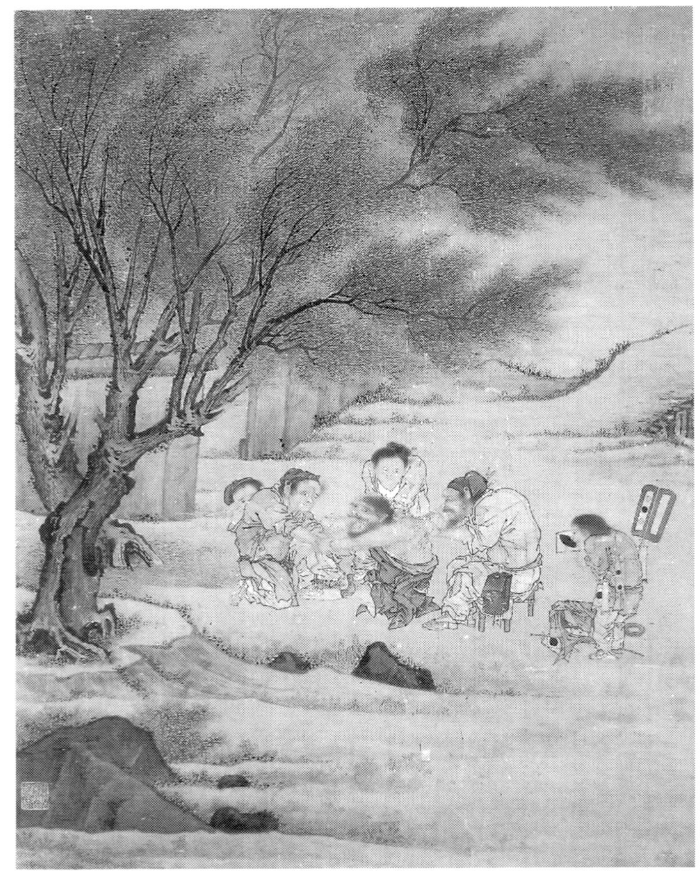

87. "Cauterizing treatment with *moxa.*" While the itinerant doctor works on the back of a patient, his assistant (right) prepares a plaster. Drawing by Li Tang 李唐, Song period.

returns to the same place. The techniques that he uses to exculpate himself in advance for unsuccessful treatments are called, in the secret language of his profession, *chouche kouer* 抽撤口兒 (to pull the way-out), or *la houmen* 拉后門 (to pull shut the back door). After the doctor has praised his medicines and described their effects in highly promising terms, he might add a few words when the patient has paid. He might, for example, tell the patient in parting: "If your illness should still not improve, do not blame me. If you do not get cured, the reason lies not with your illness or my medicines, but with your fate. That is not my fault." Or: "If the illness will not cure itself, it is due to the fact that it is not allowed to be cured." He might also state openly and bluntly: "If my medicines won't work, don't waste your money any further and look for somebody else." As an excuse during a later confrontation with a dissatisfied patient he might also use the comment that the patient had earlier received a discount and could not expect to receive a complete treatment for such a cheap fee.

### *5. Peculiarities of Formulas from the Milieu of the Itinerant Doctors*

Considering how many hundreds of medicinal drugs are known in Chinese pharmaceutics, it was and remains very difficult for an itinerant doctor to carry a full supply of medications and be prepared for all kinds of cases. This problem was addressed by particular formulary rules that are only found in China and are therefore characteristic of traditional Chinese pharmaceuticals.

Chinese medicine has developed a term for "illness conditions" (*zheng* 症). These are conditions which the patient can see or feel himself and which a doctor is able to recognize with the help of his sensory organs. A condition of illness, in Chinese medicine, does not have the same strict correlation to an internal disturbance as a symptom does in Western medicine. In Chinese medical theory, illnesses such as yin deficiency or yang excess has a variety of ways in which they can express themself as an "illness condition."

It is only through the examination of as many illness conditions as possible, in conjunction with any change of movements in the vessels recognized by pulse diagnosis, that a conclusion about the illness in the invisible depths of the organism is reached. This is because either the illness conditions or the movement in the vessels might at first sight point to an illness that is the exact opposite of the actual ailment. "False" heat is, for example, to be differentiated from real heat and "false" cold from real cold.

This method often leads pharmacologists trained in Western, scientifically-oriented medicine to look down on traditional Chinese materia medica. Since one and the same basic disturbance in a given organism has the choice, so to speak, to express itself in any one of a large number of possible illness conditions, likewise, one and the same remedy may be used for a large number of illness conditions. While

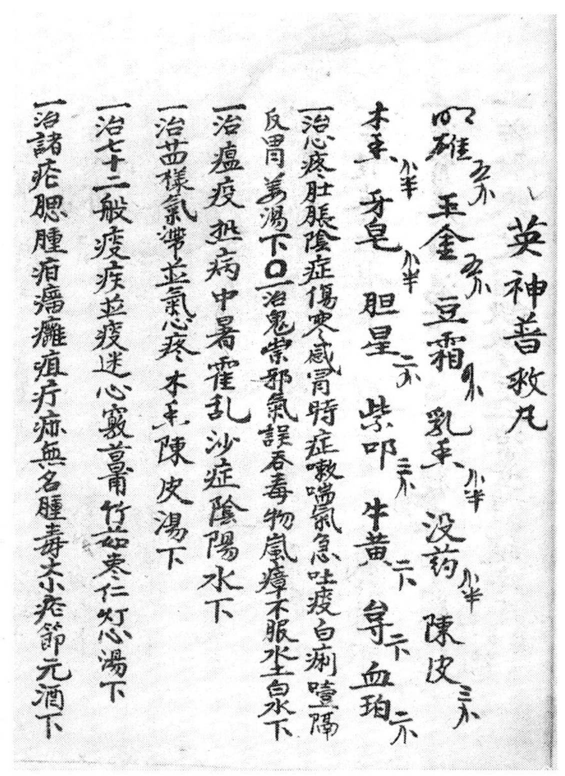


88. "Cure-All Pills Brave Spirit." A list of the thirteen ingredients of a pill formula followed by fifty groups of ailments that can be cured with the same pill when it is ingested with different fluids: *mingxiong* (realgar, AsS), 5 qian; *yugui* (cinnamon bark), 5 qian; *doushuang* (crushed seed of *Croton tiglium L.*), 4 qian; *ruxiang* (rosin of *Boswellia carterii Birdw.*), 0.5 qian; *moyao* (rosin of *Commiphora myrrha Engl.*); *chenpi* (dried peel of *Citrus tangerina Hort.*), 3 qian; *muxiang* (root of *Saussurea lappa Clarke*), 0.5 qian; *yazao* (fruits of *Gleditsia sinensis Lam.*), 0.5 qian; *danxing* (powdered bulb of various kinds of *Arisaema* mixed with cow bile), 2 qian; *zikou* (i.e. *baidoukou* 白豆蔻, seeds of *Amomum kranvanh Pierre ex Gagnep.*), 3 qian; *niuhuang* (cattle bile), 2 spoons; *taicun* (fruits of *Xanthium sibiricum Patr.*), 2 spoons; *xuebo* (amber), 2 qian. —for the treatment of cardiac pain, abdominal swelling, yin ailments, cold-induced damages, influenza, seasonally caused ailments, coughing and gasping, shortness of breath, spitting phlegm, white diarrhea, blocked throat, and vomiting: ingest in a decoction of ginger. —for the treatment of heat-caused epidemics, febrile illnesses, heat stroke, cholera, and sha illnesses: ingest with yin-yang water (a mixture of river and well water). —for the treatment of the twenty-four types of qi blockages, qi accumulations, and cardiac pain: ingest with a decoction of *muxiang* and *chenpi*. —for the treatment of the seventy-two types of phlegm illnesses, phlegm accumulations, and disorientation: ingest with a decoction of *changpu* (rhizome of *Acorus Calamus L.*), *zhuru* (*Phyllostachus nigra* [*Lodd.*] *Munro*), *zaoren* (date stones), and *dingxin* (lamp wick). …" Private medical handbook, undated manuscript.

to the Western eye these might appear to be unrelated, according to traditional theory, they can all be traced back to the same basic illnesses.

The itinerant doctor is, of course, not concerned with these details. Like his clientele, he knows many illness conditions by name and carries around the appropriate remedies, not a complete pharmacy. This is made possible by formulas for multiple indications. For example, in gynecology the basic formula of a remedy with five or six ingredients covers a certain group of illness conditions. The same formula can even treat a variety of additional gynecological problems without modification of its content, if the liquid in which the patient takes it is changed. Because the medicine can be directed against all kinds of ailments by individualizing the way in which it is taken, the itinerant doctor only carries one or two basic premade formulas which may be used to treat an almost unlimited variety of illnesses.

The Leporello manuscript (figure. 89) contains all the applications of a basic gynecological formula. The itinerant doctor can prescribe this formula to several women in whom he has diagnosed different ailments by pointing to different pages in his book which explain: "in case of … take with wine …," "in case of …, take with tea," "in case of …, take with date juice." Altogether, the basic formula can be applied to forty or fifty illness conditions, ranging from tooth aches after birth to bloody stools and swelling of the face and limbs by varying the conducting fluids. In this way, all patients have the impression that they are receiving remedies addressed exactly to their specific ailments.

The fluids which are supposed to guide the basic formula come from the realm of daily life or are easily found and therefore do not have to be brought along by the itinerant doctor. If necessary, he can recommend locally available remedies in addition to his own in order to further increase the width of a formula's indications.

治婦人臨月每服二丸則縮胎易產胎前產後臍腹疼痛婦

米湯砂服即好

治婦人胎前產後胎孕諸病室女經閉男女勞傷童便黃酒送

治婦人胎虛損腹疼寒熱頭眩自嘆少氣不能支持精

羊血少鮮薑少水煎熱服

治婦人血氣血喘下腫或動腹痛艾葉荷湯送下

治室女經閉腹痛不調滾白水送下

治婦人產後胎臍不下落在胎中或難產或死胎不下順數月不

下炒塩湯送下

治婦人臨產前後先腹二九童便黃酒送下能安魂定魄血氣調

順諸病不生養脈調經至效

治婦人產後咳嗽胸膈不利口吐酸水或面目浮腫脅疼痛溫黃酒送下

89. A list of various categories of gynecological problems that may be treated with one and the same formula by ingesting it in different ways. Private medical handbook, undated manuscript.

THE INSTRUMENTS OF
TRADITIONAL CHINESE MEDICINE

The examination of a patient, whether by relatives or a professional doctor, was aimed at diagnosing his or her internal condition via parameters that could be evaluated by external inspection, questioning or feeling. As a rule, these are the illness conditions. Usually it was unnecessary for the patient to undress. The doctor looked at the complexion of the skin, listened to the voice, noticed smells, asked about the daily schedule and physiological changes, and, lastly, felt the patient's wrist pulse.

It has remained uncommon to this day for a doctor of traditional medicine to probe into the private life of his patients, particularly female ones. Even potential psycho-emotional problems are addressed indirectly. While the holistic or psychosomatic nature of Chinese medicine does recognize the interdependency of emotional and physical problems, its diagnostic and therapeutic interest is focused almost exclusively on the somatic conditions. Thus, it tries to influence the emotional state of a patient by influencing the latter.[94]

Traditional Chinese medicine, therefore, does not need any instruments for diagnosis; the doctor's sense organs and fingers suffice to draw conclusions about internal problems within a theoretical framework, from externally recognizable conditions. It is only the recent combination of Western diagnosis with traditional treatment, especially popular in the PRC, which has given doctors of traditional medicine access to a broad spectrum of instruments—no matter how questionable the results may be.

## *1. Acupuncture Needles*

Between the development of surgery in the late Middle Ages and the beginning of the Modern Age, pre-Modern Western medicine developed a variety of therapeutic instruments that preceded technological advances in patient treatment of the mid-twentieth century. This aspect is completely lacking in traditional Chinese medicine. Hence, for treatment, too, few medical instruments are utilized.

Of primary importance are the acupuncture needles which gradually developed from bleeding lancets until they reached their current stage. Most recently, the concern for pain-free treatment has also led to the manufacture of very fine needles in China. Older needles from the first half of the twentieth century, or even earlier, are comparatively crude (plates 140–142). The length and delicacy of the needles depends on the location and purpose of needling.

Probably the earliest enumeration and description of the necessary needles is contained in the *Huang Di neijing lingshu* 黃帝內經靈樞, whose different textual layers were conceived partly before the turn of the Common Era, but primarily in the first centuries C.E.:

The names of the nine needles indicate their different forms. The first one is called "chisel needle"; it is 1.6 inches long. The second one is called "round needle"; it is 1.6 inches long. The third one is called "arrowhead needle"; it is 3.5 inches long. The fourth one is called "spear-head needle"; it is 1.6 inches long. The fifth one is called "sword needle"; it is four inches long. The sixth one is called "round tip needle"; it is 1.6 inches long. The seventh one is called "hair needle"; it is 3.6 inches long. The eighth one is called "long needle"; it is seven inches long. The ninth one is called "large needle"; it is four inches long.

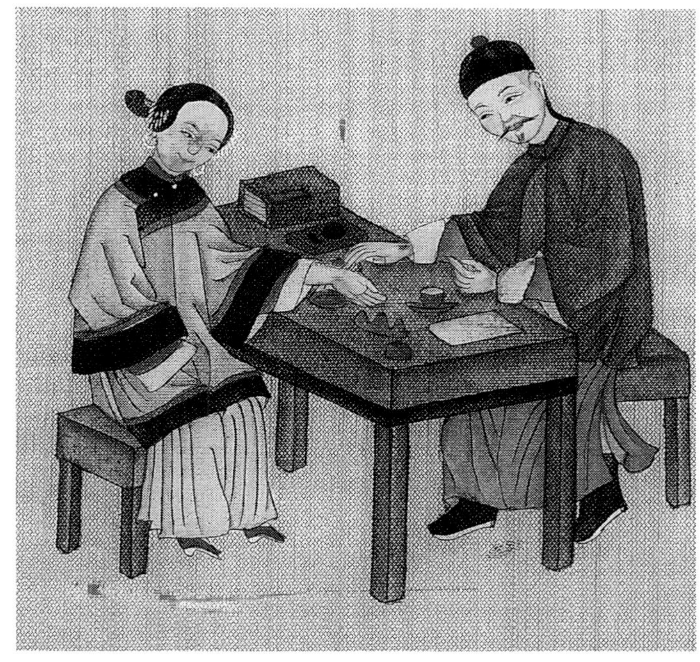

90. "This picture shows a doctor of Chinese medicine examining a patient's pulse and making up a prescription." On the table are a book, an ink stone, a cup of tea, a brush rest, and paper for the prescription. The patient's wrist is resting on a pulse pillow. It is notable that all drawings of this kind depict male doctors with female patients. Gouache, second half of the nineteenth century. Museum für Völkerkunde, Berlin.

The chisel needle has a wide end and a fine tip; it is used to guide yang qi out. The round needle is shaped like an egg [at the front]; one uses it to rub the flesh under the skin. One must not damage the muscles or the [deeper-lying] flesh with it. It is used to remove qi from the area between the hair and the flesh. The tip of the arrowhead needle is shaped like a grain of millet. It is used to exert pressure on the vessels; it is not stabbed into the skin. It causes the pouring in of qi. The spear-head needle is a three-edged sword. It serves to expel chronic illnesses. The end of the sword needle resembles a sword; it is used to remove large amounts of pus. The round tip needle resembles a horse's tail; it has a round shaft and a fine tip. It serves to remove aggressive qi. The hair needle has a tip similar to the proboscis of a mosquito. It may stay [in the skin] until the qi arrives slowly. It is very fine and can remain [in the skin] for a long time. It serves to [nourish] the qi and to remove pain and blockages. The long needle has a sharp point and thin shaft. It is used to remove blockages from distant areas. The large needle has a stick-shaped, slightly rounded tip. It is used to remove water from the joints.

The current shape and function of needles differs from those in this ancient description, as does the modern technique of inserting the needle from the ancient methods. The advice to insert the needle diagonally, for example, in or against the direction of the flow of qi in the vessels, in order to accomplish specific results—and many other modifications in the handling of the needles—was plausible only on the basis of a mechanistic understanding of qi physiology. Nowadays, these techniques do not make sense, especially in Europe and the United States.

## 2. The Pulse Pillow

The history of the support on which a patient placed his wrist while the doctor felt his or her pulse can be traced back about one thousand years. Only ceramic pulse rests from that time are preserved (figure 92, plates 134–136); it can be assumed that "pulse pillows" were also made from softer and possibly cheaper materials in that age, but they are not preserved. Woven and cloth pillows document a variety of shapes only from recent times.

## 3. Acupuncture Models

In 1994, several minor Chinese newspapers reported that an acupuncture figure from the Zhou period had been found in excavations in a small town in west China. The figure is approximately 15 cm long, varnished in black, and painted with red lines which Chinese historians believe to be the conduits of acupuncture theory. The likelihood that this figure is an early acupuncture model is, however, small. Even if detailed tests, which have yet to be performed,

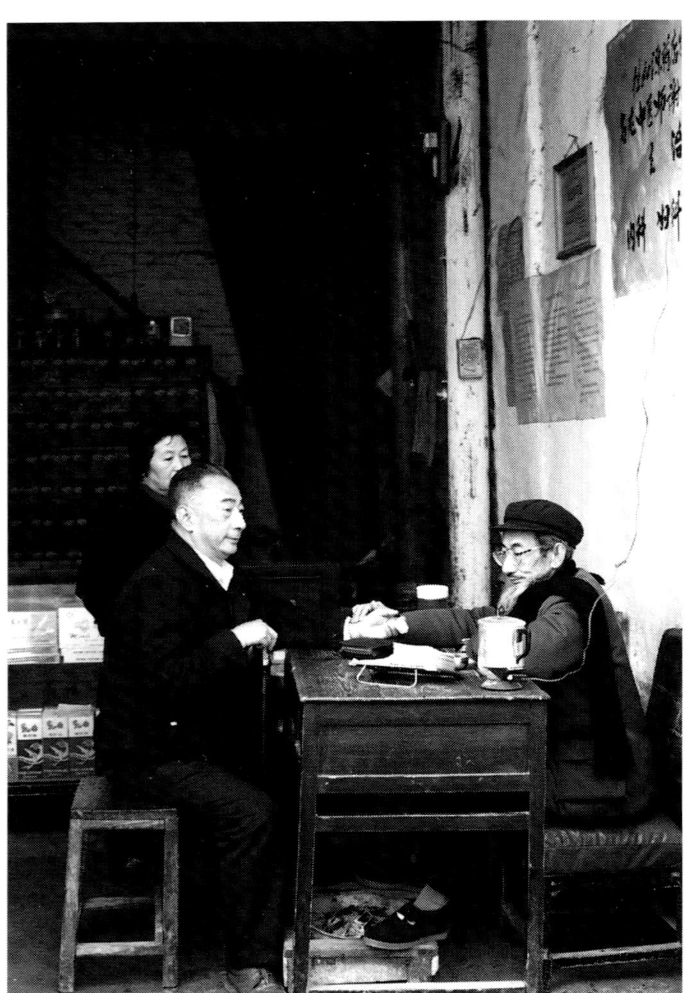

91. A doctor in a drug store for traditional Chinese pharmaceutics feels the pulse of a patient whose wrist rests on a pulse pillow. Photograph, Jiangxi, 1993.

should confirm the age, it is more likely that this is a blood-letting figurine on which red lines have been drawn to indicate the conduits from which blood can be removed; the position of the red lines has no affinity with the conduits of acupuncture that were defined in antiquity. Furthermore, acupuncture is based on the needling of specific points on the conduits. Yet there are no insertion points on the alleged acupuncture model from the Zhou period.

In fact, the earliest manufactured acupuncture model dates from 1027. In 1026, the Imperial Medical Official Wang Weiyi 王惟一 received orders to construct a life-size figure out of bronze on which the conduits and insertion points should be marked for teaching purposes. Wang Weiyi had a figure cast that could be dismantled into front and back halves and which contained organs when closed. The conduits were set into the surface as small grooves.[95]

Since lists with various numbers of insertion openings, the so-called "holes for the transport [of qi]" (*shuxue* 腧 穴), were popular at his time, Wang Weiyi compared relevant sources. He finally decided on 354 insertion openings which he then had poked into the conduits of the figure and marked by name in gold characters.

While neither of the two copies have been preserved, the report of an eyewitness from 1290 still exists. In it, he describes the didactic function of the bronze figures:

> They were used for testing doctors. For this purpose, the holes were coated with wax and the figure was filled with water[96]. Subsequently, the doctors had to measure out [the body to find the insertion openings] according to individually standardized measurements[97] and insert their needles at the openings. When the needle hit the hole exactly, it penetrated, and water ran out.[98]

As a complement to the two bronze figures, Wang Weiyi composed the *Tongren shuxue zhenjiu tujing* 銅人腧穴針灸圖經 (*Illustrated Manual of Acupuncture and Moxibustion with the Transport Holes in the Bronze Figure*). At the government's behest, the text was distributed in all provinces and, at the same time, etched into stone plates.

In the following centuries, similar acupuncture models were repeatedly cast in bronze or carved in wood. However, due to the lack of interest in the morphology of the inside of the body, the reconstruction of the organs in Wang Weiyi's bronze figure remained an option that was soon forgotten.

Today, acupuncture models of the entire body or of individual body parts are made out of plastic or plaster. Since the development of ear acupuncture in France in the 1950's—a contribution to acupuncture that was quickly adopted in China and integrated into specialist literature as ancient Chinese knowledge—plastic ears with insertion points have been particularly widespread as acupuncture models (plate 143).

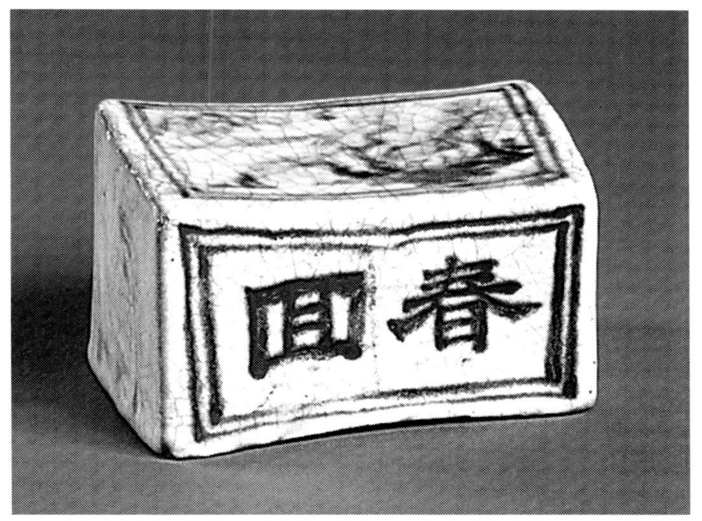

92. Wrist support for feeling the pulse with characters that state: *huichun* 回春 (*Return to Spring*).

## 4. Moxa

Cauterization is mentioned in Chinese sources even earlier than acupuncture. The Mawangdui manuscripts, for example, referred to moxibustion. It is unclear, however, from what point on Chinese mugwort, a type of artemisia, was used exclusively as a cauterizing herb.

Until the Qing period, small mugwort cones were burned directly on the skin—resulting in pain, scarring, and frequent side-effects, especially suppurations, at the cauterized skin parts. Since then, *moxa* has been used as "needles," a term for the cigar-shaped sticks (ca. 15 cm long and 1 cm thick), which are lit at one end and then held close to the skin in order to release their power.

In the 1970s, *moxa* was combined with walnut shell glasses. Based on the idea that the eyes are openings to the body through which qi can enter from the outside, a doctor of traditional Chinese medicine in Peking came up with the idea of replacing the lenses in eyeglasses with walnut shells. He then used a small wire construction to attach glowing pieces of *moxa* sticks, that had been dipped in chrysanthemum water, to the front of the shells. According to his beliefs, the qi of the *moxa* and chrysanthemum flowers would enter the head through the eyes and release its powers by passing through the walnut shells—whose brain-like structure suggested that its qi had a brain-nurturing effect.

There are no procedures in traditional Chinese medicine by which to test or justify such techniques, much less their empirical efficacy, based as they are on generally accepted theoretical premises. Likewise, there is no way of rejecting this or other procedures which claim to be founded in ancient ideological constructs.

## 5. Cupping Implements

Similar to other systems of medicine, the technique of increasing circulation—and perhaps even the technique of breaking the skin to release blood—by creating a vacuum over the skin on non-arterial areas of the body, probably dates back to prehistoric times. "Cupping" is still widely used in traditional Chinese medicine to treat arthritis and several other conditions.

For centuries, the stem of bamboo has been ideally suited for the production of cupping instruments because of its natural division into sections (figure 94; plate 139). Nowadays, cupping glasses are increasingly used since the progress and result of the procedure may be monitored without removing them.

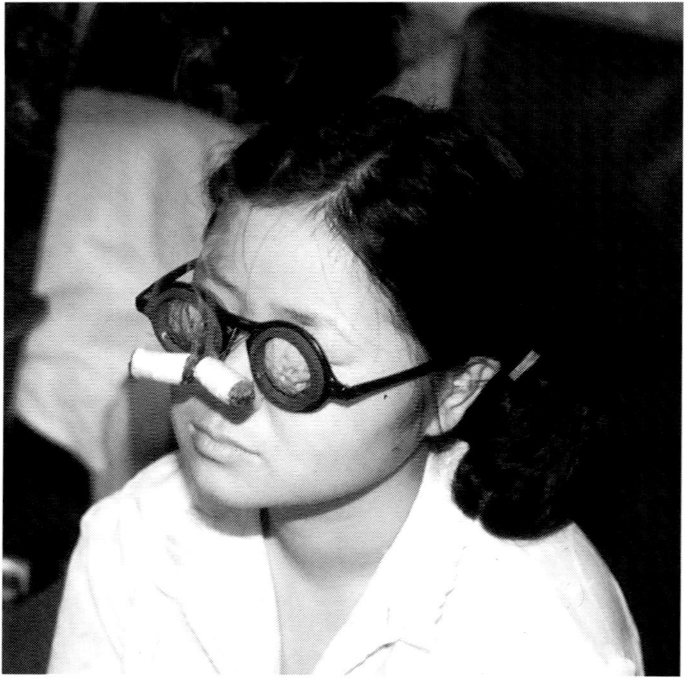

93. Patient with combination *moxa* and walnut shell glasses. Photograph, Peking, 1981.

## 6. Massage and Massage Implements

It is likely that massage, as a therapeutic technique, also dates back to prehistoric times. Traditional Chinese medicine encompasses different types of massage by hand or with mechanical instruments. The different forms of hand massage, especially the *tuina* 推納 technique (pushing and pulling) are regarded as a peculiarity of Chinese medicine—as it has been largely integrated into the theoretical background of scholastic medicine and is described in its own literature. *Tuina* techniques are used primarily in pediatrics.

Massage may also be performed with mechanical aids, such as sticks made out of wood or jade, but it is not known when such aids came into use (plates 146, 147).

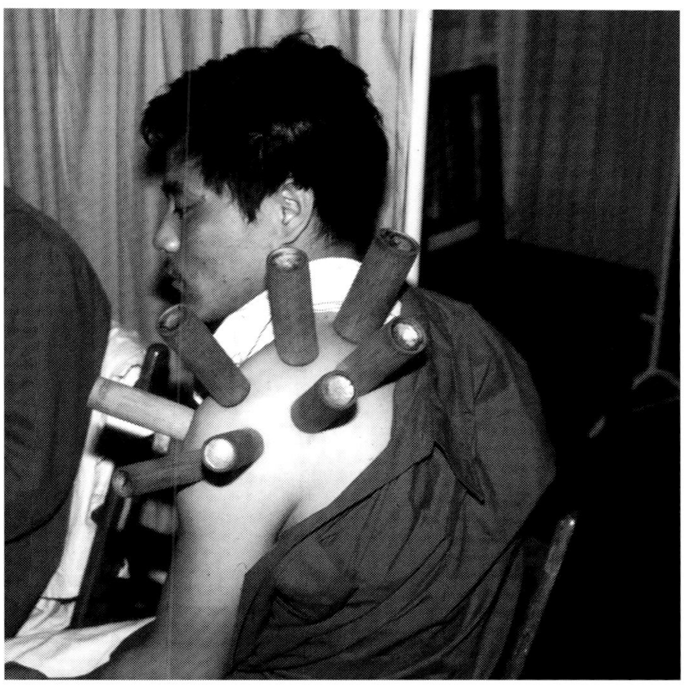

94. Traditional bamboo cupping treatment in a hospital in the PRC. Photograph, Peking, 1981.

## THE TANG PERIOD PHYSICIAN
## SUN SIMIAO: FROM HEALER TO
## MEDICINE GOD

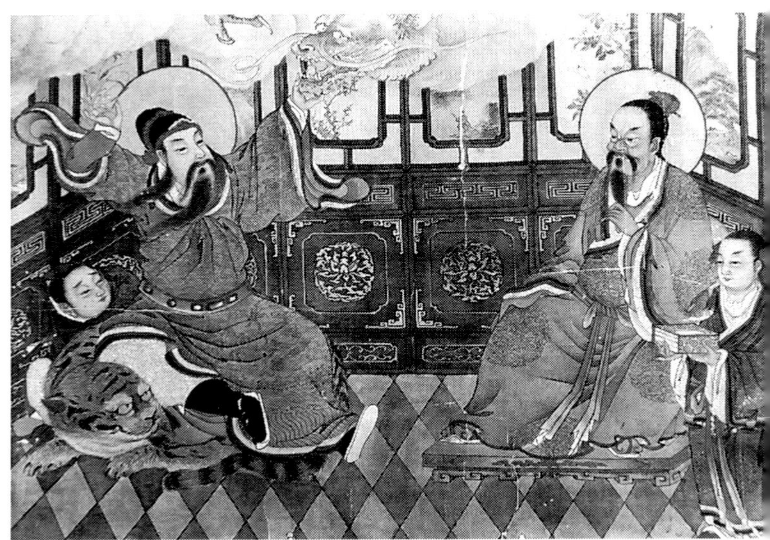

95. Sun Simiao (left), with the characteristic dragon and tiger, in a dialogue with an unidentified figure. Drawing, nineteenth century. Academy for Chinese Medicine, Peking.

### 1. A Survey

Sun Simiao 孫思邈 is one of the most, if not *the* most, interesting figures in the history of Chinese medicine. It is not too difficult to support this judgment, even though biographical details of this Tang physician are only fragmentary. In his lifetime, Sun Simiao was a famous clinician and alchemist; to posterity, he left voluminous formularies that have been influential until the present. In his treatise *Lun taiyi jingcheng* 論太醫精誠 (*Concerning the Absolute Honesty of Great Physicians*), Sun Simiao composed the first explicit medical ethics in China, comparable to the Western Hippocratic oath.

Sun Simiao's fame as a clinician, author, and ethicist caused the posthumous creation of legends about his life and works and finally led to his inclusion in the pantheon of Chinese popular religion. From about the thirteenth or fourteenth centuries on, human Sun Simiao was referred to as the Medicine King, i.e. the quintessential god of drugs. To this day he is venerated by large numbers of the population, and his memory still induces 100,000 pilgrims a year to visit the historical location where he is said to have been born and worked, in order to have their pleas heard. While many doctors in the two thousand year history of Chinese medicine have gained fame as either clinicians, authors, or ethicists, no one has achieved renown for all three areas simultaneously to the same extent as Sun Simiao.

### 2. Sun Simiao's Life and Works

Thanks to a critical analysis of all of the biographical data regarding Sun Simiao by the American historian Nathan Sivin, it is clear how little is really known of the Tang physician.[99] The sources from the Tang period and the following centuries record episodes from Sun's life that cover the period between 537–540 and 860–874. Only a few dates are likely to be more specific. In the final analysis, two or three

biographical facts at best remain. One is that Sun Simiao
may have been born either in 580 or 581 and perhaps died
as late as 682. It also seems fairly certain that he accompanied emperor Taizong to his summer palace in 673.

The question arises as to why, of all doctors around
whom so many legends were woven, it was the biography
of Sun Siamio that was embellished so quickly and exten-
sively. Sun Simiao left an extraordinary impression on his
contemporaries and later biographers that is difficult to
comprehend in detail today. This charisma is today only
reflected in Sun Simiao's writings, and even so it is unclear
whether these are his own words. At least it is known that
the contents of his formulary *Qianjin fang* was modified at
the beginning of the eleventh century by Song period
redactors in the governmental office for the revision of old
medical texts.

Overall, his writings are still quite impressive, and at least
for the most part, authentic. Sun Simiao was a scholar with a
well-rounded education who borrowed those aspects from
any available teachings that appeared to make sense to him.
Apart from his obligatory education for the Chinese bureaucracy, he was also familiar with Buddhism and Daoism, and
aspects of these two world views entered into his writings.

Sun Simiao knew the medicinal drugs of his time and
devoted himself not only to formulary art, for the curing of
illnesses, but also to alchemy for the promotion of longevity. He knew of the existence of male and female spirits
who protected the inner organs of humans, and he recommended a treatment of malaria by magical characters that
were to be pasted to the forehead of a figure of the kitchen
god. He described exorcistic spells in an Indian language
and drew upon astrological calculations in order to use acupuncture to its greatest efficacy. Sun Simiao held the opinion
that the only appropriate goal for medicine was the combined application of drugs, acupuncture, spells, amulets, and
physical exercises.[100]

Thus, chapters one through thirty of the *Qianjin fang* 千
金方 and chapters one through twenty-four of the *Qianjin
yifang* 千金翼方 contain several thousand drug prescriptions arranged in numerous categories of indications,
frequently with detailed instructions regarding the
pharmaceutical processing of individual substances and the
manufacture of the appropriate kinds of medicine. Chapter
twenty-five of the *Qianjin yifang* is devoted to pulse diagnosis; chapters twenty-six through twenty-eight contain a
description of acupuncture and *moxa*. Chapters twenty-
nine and thirty carry the heading *Jinjing* 禁經 (*Classic of
Prohibitions*) and offer a comprehensive list of exorcistic
prohibitions from the realms of demonology and correspondence magic.[101] To alchemy, he devoted a separate
work, his *Danjing yaojue* 丹經要訣 (*Important Oral Explanations to the Classics of Alchemy*).[102]

Sun's ethical teachings for the medical profession in the
*Qianjin yifang* prove his thorough familiarity with its technical, moral, and psychological demands. Certain aspects of
the doctor-patient relationship mentioned there resemble

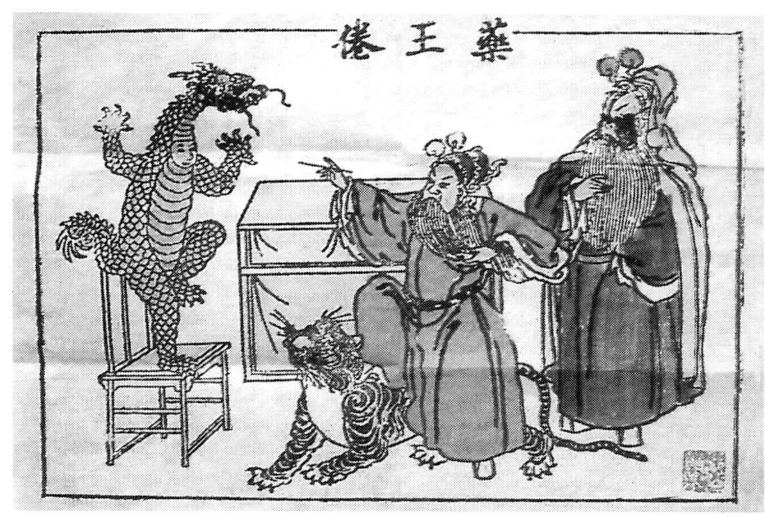


96. Sun Simiao (center), with
tiger, dragon, and an unidentified figure. Colored drawing
by Qian Huaian 錢慧安, Qing
period.

those in the Hippocratic oath in their mixture of ethics
and etiquette. The underlying message in both documents
is that doctors must have the trust of the population in
order to be recognized as helpers. Now and then, this
required proof that a doctor was competent in his profession; that he wanted to serve his patients not because of
greed but because of noble motivations; that he would not
abuse the intimacy of the doctor-patient relationship to the
disadvantage of the patient; and that he was accountable to
a higher, supernatural power, if he failed to live up to these
demands.

Sun's fame led several authors in following centuries to
publish their works under his name. One of the most
famous of these false attributions is the ophthalmological
classic *Yinhai jingwei* 銀海精微 (*Essential Subtleties on the
Silver Sea*) which was probably compiled in its current
condition in the sixteenth century.[103]

### 3. The Creation of Legends around
### Sun Simiao

A legend formed around Sun Simiao which gradually raised
him to the rank of a Medicine King. Pictorial representations of Sun Simiao in his popular religious roles of
Medicine King (*yaowang* 藥王) or Medicine Ruler (*yao-
huang* 藥皇) often show him in the company of a tiger and
a dragon. Also, several themes which had been split among
different doctors in earlier legends of healers coalesced in
Sun Simiao. Stories about an unusual healer who had been
sighted with a black dog or a grateful tiger, and who later
transformed into a dragon, had circulated for centuries.
These stereotypes, in legends, and, later, in the iconography
around Sun Simiao, were gradually embellished with ever
more details.

The efficacy of Sun's formulas required a supernatural
connection, which is why several legends tell of a dragon
king who transmitted numerous formulae to Sun Simiao
in gratitude for saving the life of one of his sons. These
prescriptions proved to be as effective as their metaphysical
donor had promised.

Apparently, these embellishments were still not enough
to raise Sun Simiao above the many famous and venerated
physicians of Chinese medical history. So, from the fourteenth or fifteenth century on, Sun Simiao was identified
with the medicine god from one Buddhist text, albeit the
most important one, the Lotus Sutra. Since then, the doctor and medicine god Sun Simiao has been the predomin-
ant medical figure of contact in the pantheon of Chinese
popular religion whenever humans want to make request
for their earthly well-being.

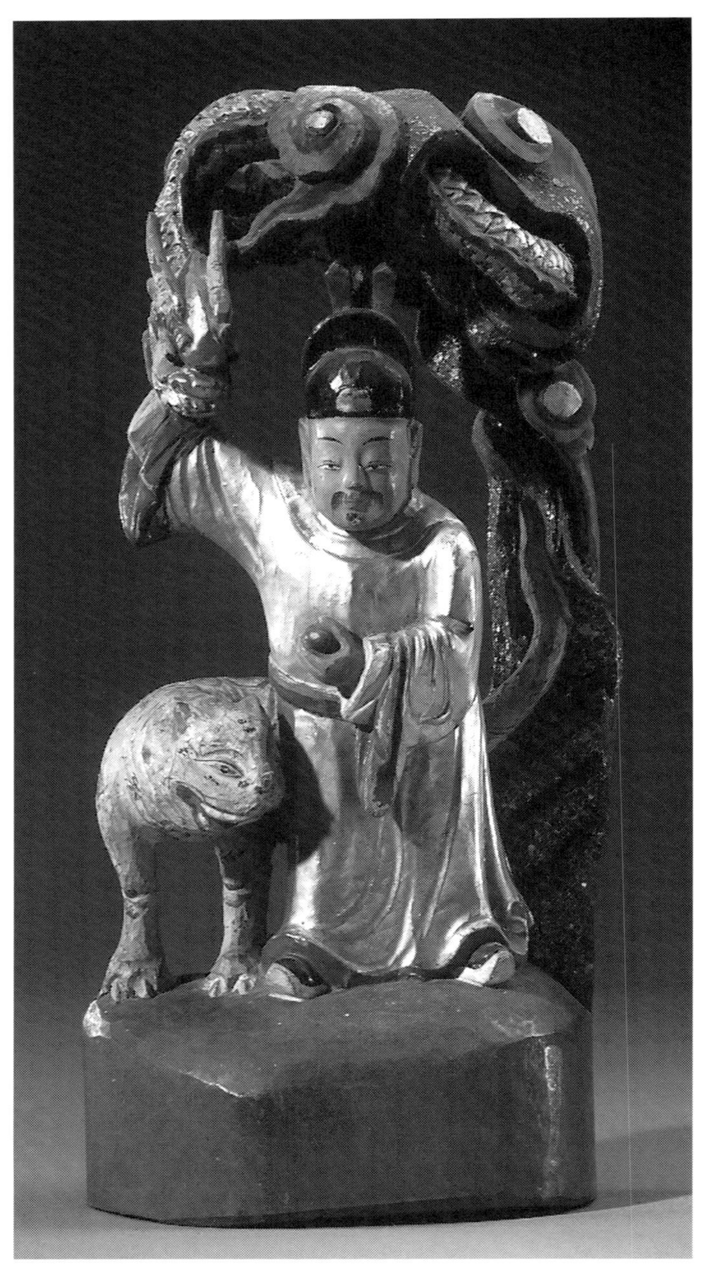

97. Sun Simiao with dragon and
tiger. Wood sculpture, Hunan,
China, nineteenth century.

90

In Shaanxi Province in northwestern China, in the city of
Yaoxian 耀縣, where the historical Sun Simiao had lived,
there is  Medicine King Mountain (*yaowangshan* 藥王山).
In 1954, a group of medical historians from Peking found
a stone sculpture of Sun Simiao there, about three meters
tall and flanked, on either side, by young boys. One held a
medicine bag; the other a medicine container. To the
right, in front of the Medicine King, lay a stone tiger. As
local residents still remember, a wooden screen with a
dragon painted on it stood behind the main figure.[104]
During the Cultural Revolution in the 1960s and 1970s,
the ensemble of sculptures was destroyed,[105] with the
exception of the main figure—found in an inventory from
1981. This figure stood at the entrance to a cave that was,
according to a locally known legend, dug into the rock
and presented to Sun Simiao as a hermitage by a grateful
dragon.[106]

Before the Communist Revolution and again more
recently, the cave was and is the destination of numerous
pilgrims who worship the Medicine King or ask for his
help on the second day of the second month of the lunar
calendar. According to local estimates, approximately
100,000 people have visited this, albeit compared to former
times, increasingly changing landscape since 1990. Indices
of the famous Tang physician are found in a large area,
including a tree under which he is said to have read and a
hill on which he is said to have planted herbs. The center
of the pilgrimages is an area formed by the Northern and
Southern Hills in the immediate proximity of Yaoxian City
and the birthplace a few kilometers away.

On the Northern Hill is the cave, which has been closed
due to the danger of collapse. A larger-than-life-sized,
renovated figure of the Medicine God stands in its entrance
guarded by a concrete tiger to the right; a dragon is attached to the rock wall above. Divine lords stand to Sun
Simiao's right and left, one of them apparently the Dragon
King, recognizable from the formula prescriptions which
he is handing to the Tang physician. In addition to several
steles engraved with prescriptions from Sun Simiao's works,
there is a stone-hewn double basin that points to the
Medicine God on the Northern Hill; where, local legend
has it, he cleaned the raw drugs.

On the Southern Hill, separated from the Northern Hill
by a deep valley, are smaller buildings from the Yuan
period, as well as numerous steles, partly marked with dedi-
cations to the Tang physician. Next to these, modern cura-
tors have reproduced a group of buildings in which Sun
Simiao supposedly lived, held consultations, and stored his
pharmacy. Historical evidence for such an ensemble, however, does not exist.

Similarly, the community in which Sun Simiao's birthplace is located has blurred his actual history. As late as the
1970s, not a trace of his grave could be found there. Now a

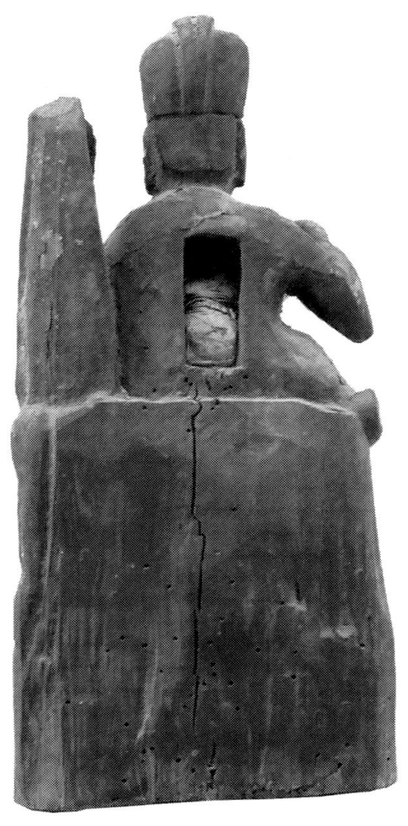

98. Rear view of a wooden
sculpture of Sun Simiao containing various drugs in a cloth
bag. Hunan, China, nineteenth
century.

large park is located in the village center where three dirt hills not only mark the grave of the Tang physician, but those of his parents as well. Furthermore, two nearby "ancestral shrines" to Sun Simiao and his parents also seem to have a different past from what is claimed for them today.[108] The money which the pilgrims bring to Sun Simiao's birthplace, along with the proceeds from a local "Factory for Health-Care Products According to Sun Simiao," permit further construction of the park, in order to increase its attractiveness to visitors.

## 5. Iconography

At least in early centuries, only very few of those who wanted to entrust a wish to the Medicine King were able to travel to Shaanxi for this very purpose. A possibility open to them was to have a wooden figure of the Medicine King carved and donate it to a temple.

These figures follow a characteristic iconographic model with only minor variations. The center of the carving is always formed by Sun Simiao in what was probably the awe-inspiring dress of officials in the Imperial period. The tiger is depicted to Sun Simiao's right, the dragon to his left. Sun Simiao either stands with both feet on the ground next to the tiger (who stands as well), or rests his left foot on the reclining tiger. Occasionally Sun is depicted in a seated position on an uncarved block or on the tiger's back, with his right knee resting on the tiger's head or neck (plate 165.)

The dragon either forms an arch above Sun Simiao or snakes around behind him, in which case the dragon's head is depicted above him or next to his shoulder. Very rare are scenes in which the dragon is depicted as a dog-like creature on the ground to Sun Simiao's left.[107] Often, Sun Simiao's left hand supports the dragon's head or rests on his left thigh. In his right hand Sun holds either the needle with which he healed the dragon—in reference to Ma Shihuang's legend—or holds the Pearl of Happiness.

Some figures of the Medicine King have open palms in Buddha-like fashion, or closed, raised fists, out of which the index and middle fingers are extended. More elaborate figures that depict the Dragon King as well as the Yellow Emperor Huang Di, the Divine Farmer Shennong, the Goddess of Mercy Guanyin—representatives of medical theory, materia medica, and religious healing—in addition to several servants, are more rare. While the figures depicting only the dragon and tiger range from simple to fairly challenging executions, the sculptures that are decorated with the Dragon King and other figures from the pantheon are usually true works of art that were commissioned by wealthy petitioners (plates 170, 172).

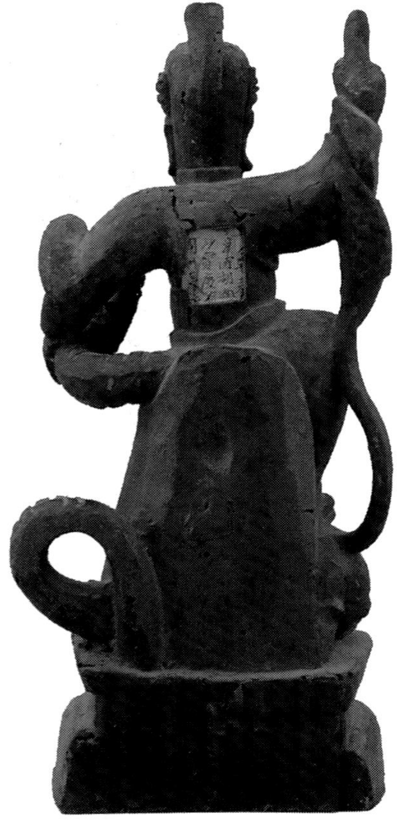

99. Rear view of a wooden sculpture of Sun Simiao in which a donation slip has been inserted. Hunan, China, eighteenth-nineteenth centuries.

## 6. Donation and Petition Slips

The figure of Sun Simiao always has a rectangular cavity carved into its back in which a small cloth bag with different plant, animal, and mineral ingredients was inserted. A folded paper containing the name, residence, and requests of the donor(s) was placed on top of this cloth bag. After the cavity was filled, it was closed with wood shavings and varnish.

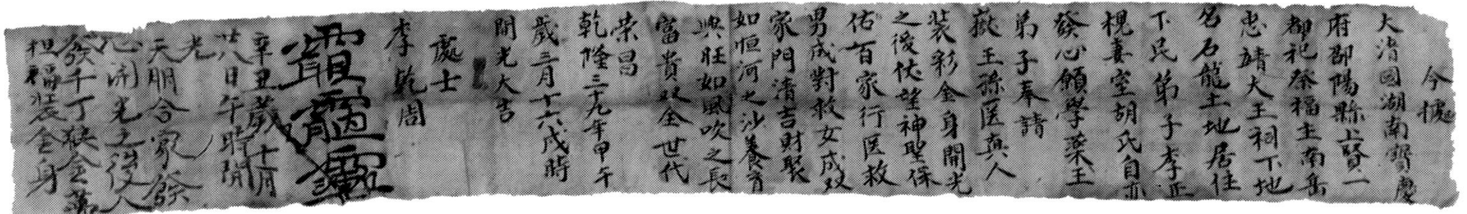

100. Donation slip from the back of a wooden sculpture of Sun Simiao. Hunan, China, 1774.

Such donations were not at all one-sided requests, but brought advantages to both parties. The Medicine King was brought to life in the figure—this is frequently expressed on the donation slips as "opening his eyes,"—and in gratitude, he fulfilled the requests of the donors. The inscription on one such petition slip in the back of a figure from 1774 reads as follows:

In the land of the great Qing, in Hunan, in Bao Qing prefecture, in Shao Yang county, in the First Capital of the Superior Sages,[109] it was sacrificed to the Lord of Charity, the great King of Honesty and Peace-making of the Southern Sacred Summit.

The place where the lowly sacrificers reside is called Stone Dragon.

The adherents from among the common people, Li Zhenghuai and his wife named Hu have made a decision: As followers of the Medicine King, they wish to study his [teachings] and express the following request:

King of the Sacred Summit Sun [Simiao], Physician and Realized Man, after we have provided [you] with a golden body and have opened [your] eyes, we hope very much that [your] Sacred Spirit might support us so that I can practice medicine among the Hundred Families, that I can help men to find a female partner, that I can help women to find a counterpart.

My family shall be pure and encounter good fortune. We shall accumulate riches comparable to the sand of the Ganges. Our descendants shall likewise blossom and flourish without end, as the wind blows.

Prosperity and honor shall double. Each generation shall be famous and glorious.

In the thirty-ninth year of [the reign period] Qianlong, *jiawu* [cycle], third month, sixteenth day, *xu* hour (7–9 o'clock).

The eyes are opened. Very auspicious.

[Written by the] unofficial scholar Li Qianzhou."

On the slip this is followed by three magical characters, as well as—apparently added later by a different hand—a renewed dedication of the same figure by another family. The second date is indicated only as the cyclical date of *xinchou*, which could, in this case, refer to 1781, 1841, or 1901.

In this example, it is of special interest that the petitioner was either already active as a doctor or at least aspired—with the assistance of the Medicine Ruler—to this profession. To be sure, the world views of those who elevated Sun Simiao to the position of a Medicine King were bound to be similar and generally attributed to a particular socio-economic group. However, it is important not to delineate the constellations of medical ideas within Chinese culture—and this also applies for any other complex culture—too sharply from each other or to attempt to attribute them merely on the basis of social class. The donor who had this slip written, for example, may have been an illiterate doctor and therefore without formal education—the phrase "adherent from among the common people" supports this—but he also could have been a formally educated doctor who placed his faith in the hands of the Medicine Ruler for reasons that are incomprehensible today.

Compared to the donation of a wooden figure, printed leaflets that could be purchased in monasteries or from itinerant monks and then pasted to a wall or door were certainly a cheaper option for ensuring the Medicine King's benevolence. One example is represented here (figure 101). In the center is the typical representation of Sun Simiao with the tiger on the ground to his right and the dragon in the air to his left. Translated the caption above the picture reads "Eminent Dao of the Medicine Ruler." Like the picture, the text contains references to the standard iconographic features of Sun Simiao's legendary embellishments:

> Rite for devoting oneself wholeheartedly [to the Medicine Ruler]. The dragon winds around the orange spring;[110] [You, the Medicine Ruler] help the world and bestow on humans the gift of life. The tiger lies in the apricot forest;[111] [You] give back life and raise the dead. Great suffering and great desire [are answered with] great compassion by the great saint. Each request is fulfilled at once. No prayer remains without miraculous response. In the rich region of Jiangxi,[112] [You], famous physician Sun Simiao, realized man, practice medicine in the thirteenth generation and cure illnesses. Great [is your] mercy. Unsurpassed the veneration [that you receive].

In the PRC, depictions of the Tang physician from the past decades rarely take into account the dragon or tiger motifs any more. Historical writings and picture scrolls instead cast Sun Simiao as either the benevolent sage or the popular hero common in Communist China. Likewise, medical figures are often marked with the traditional iconographic element of the gourd, but can be identified as specific historical figures only by newly fashioned iconographic additions such as a text scroll with characters.[113]

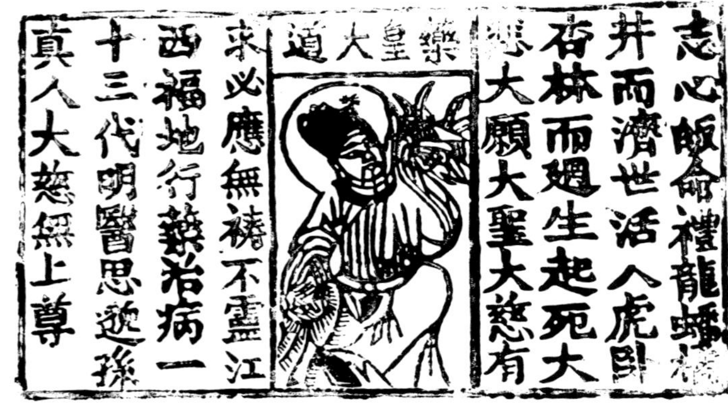

101. "The eminent Dao of the Medicine Ruler." Petition slip with a depiction of the Tang physician Sun Simiao (ca. 581–682), the dragon and tiger, as well as the following text: "Rite for devoting oneself wholeheartedly [to the Medicine Ruler]. The dragon winds itself around the orange well. [You, the Medicine Ruler,] help the world and bestow life upon the people. The tiger lies in the apricot forest. [You] give back life and awaken the dead. Great suffering, great desire [are answered with] great compassion by the great saint. Each request is fulfilled at once. No prayer remains without miraculous response. In the rich region of Jiangxi, [you] famous doctor Sun Simiao, realized man, practice medicine and cure illnesses in the thirteenth generation. Great [is your] mercy. Unsurpassed the veneration [that you receive]."

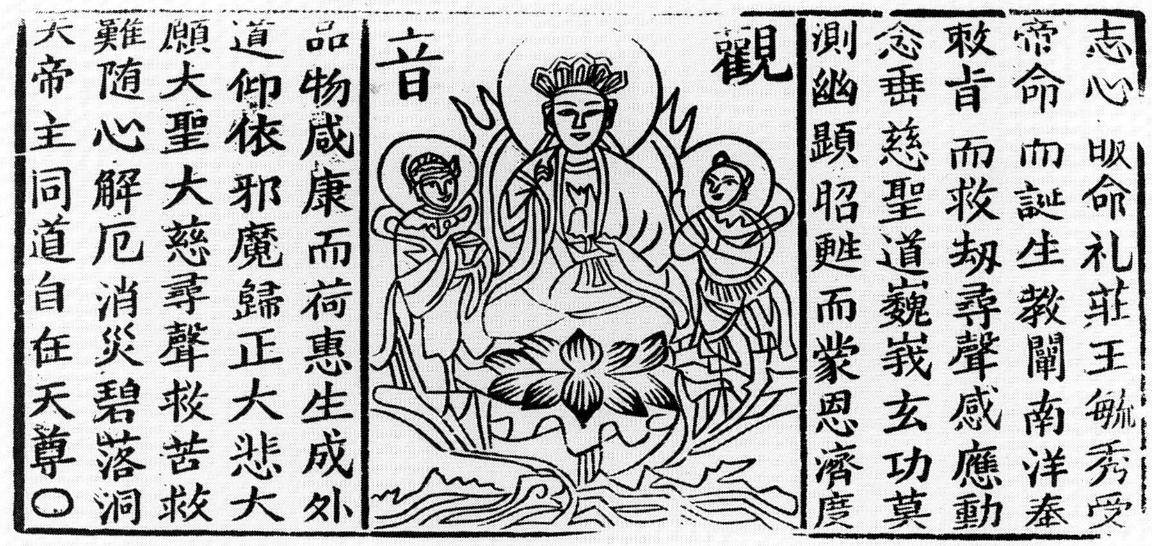


The advertisements by the Factory for Health-Care Products According to Sun Simiao form an exception. They consciously use the traditional iconography to keep the legends of the dragon and the tiger alive.

## OTHER METAPHYSICAL HELPERS AND ACTS OF ASSISTANCE

The pantheon of popular Chinese religion includes, besides Sun Simiao, several non-humans with the power either to keep illnesses away from humans or to drive them out of those who had fallen ill. This transition from scientific to religious healing was fluid, in terms of content and social strata. Therefore, to represent traditional Chinese medicine as purged of its metaphysical aspects would be an artifice. While this might have complied with the ideology of one group of Confucian scholars of the Imperial period that was averse to religious content, it certainly did not correspond to the overall appearance of traditional Chinese medicine in literature and practice.

The close ties between natural knowledge, religion, and magic were often expressed in advertising slips used by pharmacies to market remedies whose names suggested that they were imbued with the power of a benevolent god or goddess. One example are the advertisements of the Zhenyaotang Pharmacy in Peking, which extol the virtues of the "paste with which Guanyin saves from grief," the "elixir with which Guanyin saves from grief," and the "miraculous medicine which imparts the mercy of Guanyin." These "medicines from a trustworthy conscience" that are "able to cure any kind of illness," created a correlation between the

102. Petition slip with a depiction of the Boddhisattva Guanyin (Goddess of Mercy) and the following text: "rite for devoting oneself wholeheartedly [to Guanyin]. Noble seed of King Zhuang, created by orders of the [Heavenly] King in order to teach the [Buddhist] doctrine in the South Sea, in obeisance to imperial orders, [you] save from misfortune. [You] locate the voices [of those seeking help] and respond to them. Moved by the impression [of these voices], you let your mercy descend. The way of the saints is majestic and eminent, the depth of hidden merits measurable by none. When the hidden emerges, there is light and revival, and one receives the mercy to be ferried across [the Sea of Sorrows]. Things of all kinds thrive and receive the favor to develop to perfection. The foreign ways (i.e. non-Buddhist teachings) subordinate themselves, the bad and the devil return to rightness. Great sorrow, great wishes [are answered with] great compassion by the great saint. [You] locate the [pleading] voices and save from suffering, [you] save from misfortune and follow the heart (i.e. the wishes of those pleading). [You] dissolve threats and cause disaster to disappear; autonomous goddess [residing] in the Heaven of the Emerald Cave, having the same way as the imperial ruler!"
(Translated by H. Tessenow)

efficacy of real pharmaceutical substances and the belief in the Buddhist goddess of mercy (figure 102, plate 33).

Furthermore, this transition becomes evident in petition slips whose purchase simultaneously served as an invocation to certain supernatural authorities depicted and addressed on them. To stay with the example of Guanyin, purchasers might implore Guanyin to rescue them from a life of suffering, but primarily to release them from childlessness. Guanyin's 觀音 iconography therefore often relates to the slogan *Guanyin song zi* 觀音送子 (Guanyin Grants a Son). Other gods or goddesses who are often invoked specifically for the release from illness are Leigong 雷公 (plate 157) and the Smallpox Empress (*douzhen niangniang* 豆疹娘娘).

Of purely magic-religious content are printed amulets— still extant in parts of society—that summoned protective demons or spirits for assistance to drive out illness-causing demons or spirits. These amulets are generally designed in a pattern that is closely related to the power structures of the worldly authorities. Written in cryptic symbols—apotropaic characters which differ from ordinary writing—and in everyday script, the amulets announced that the human user was allied with the highest and most powerful authorities and ordered the evil demons and spirits to leave.

Besides such character amulets, that could be written anew at any time, doctors and lay people who were not averse to this kind of world view used other objects for an apotropaic effect. For example, a healer might place a peachwood coin on a painful, or otherwise afflicted, body part. Where real coins are stamped with the period of their minting and value, this coin displays the phrase, "Don't mention feelings. If you want a beating, just come over here!" (plate 153).

After the umbilical cord of a newborn child was cut, the midwife, or whoever was attending the birth, might place a lead medallion on the child's navel to close it from evil invaders (as long as it had not grown shut). The characters *huangtianba* 黃天把 (Yellow Heavenly Rule) informed any unwelcome arrivals of the great power with which they would have to contend if they tried to enter the child (plate 153).

Also very popular in this context were coin swords. The significance of coins as a special symbol of power is obvious. Symbolic swords manufactured from real coins were considered to be especially powerful if the coins carried the reign period of an eminent emperor as their minting date, e.g. in the Qing period that of Qianlong 乾隆 or Kangxi 康熙. Suspended above a house entrance or bed, the coin swords announced that powerful authorities were prepared to fight if an evil spirit should be so inclined (plate 152).

Carved or painted depictions of demons had the same purpose. Their iconography reflects the most influential powers of the universe: the Star of Seven, the characters *taiji* 太極 of the Supreme Pole that holds the world together, the character for king, *wang*, as well as a sword and a menacing grimace intended to induce fear even in demons. Occasionally, small mirrors were inserted since it was believed that demons flee in panic upon looking at themselves (plate 154).

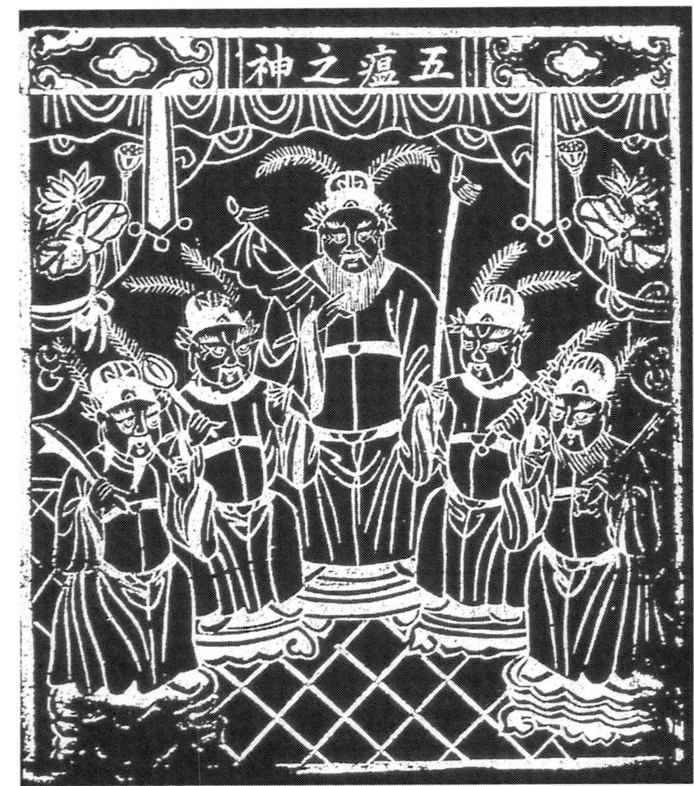

103. "The spirits of the five warmth epidemics." Popular drawing to ensure the benevolence and protection of certain deities.

# CHINESE MEDICINE IN
# ART AND LITERATURE

## MEDICINE AND ART IN EUROPE
## AND CHINA

It would only be a slight exaggeration to claim that every medical historian in Europe could produce a lavishly illus-

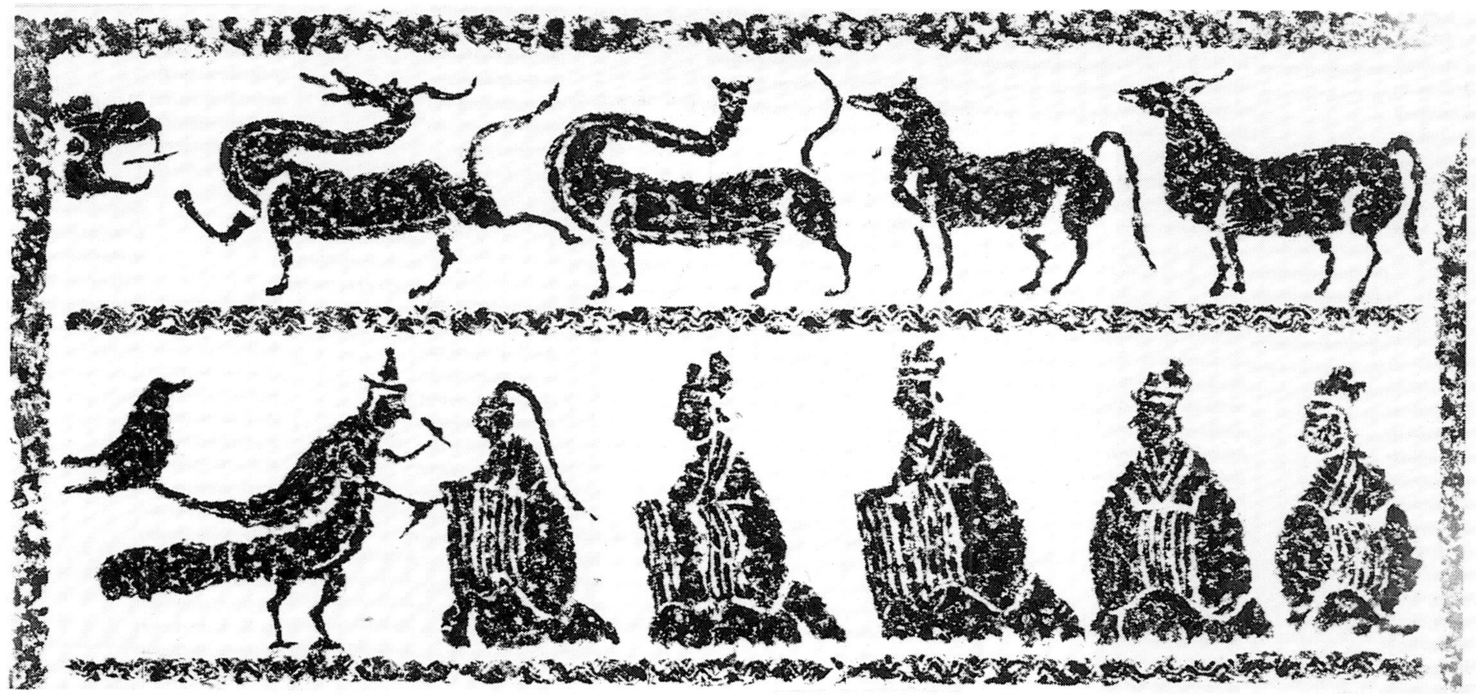

104. Tomb relief from the Han period. Bottom row left: Bird creature with human head (possibly Bian Que) in front of five figures, one of whom has disheveled hair and is apparently a patient.

trated book on the history of Western medicine and therein reproduce a number of illustrations from the arts without duplicating much previously published work by their predecessors.

Medicine in art and literature is a practically inexhaustible subject in Europe; from Greek antiquity, through the Middle Ages to Modern times, artists of every origin have returned to medical topics, whether to depict reality as they saw it or for allegorical purposes—since a multitude of beliefs from both the pre-Christian and the Christian era have been related to the treatment of illness and the figure of the physician, the healer.

Therefore, no aspect of Western medicine has been excluded, whether it was from the lower or higher ranks of the cultural hierarchy of physicians. The autopsy by Dr. Tulp in front of the wealthy citizens of Amsterdam or a surgery by Ernst von Bergmann in the surgical hospital in Berlin were as inspirational for the creation of artistically outstanding oil paintings as were the traveling surgeon in early modern times or the epidemics which Breughel immortalized in his folk scenes. Woodcuts and copperplate engravings, drawings and even sculptures depict innumerable scenes from the field of medicine, in general and specific terms, throughout many centuries. In all their artistic liberty and abstraction they still convey glimpses of a reality which cannot be seen from texts alone.

Chinese culture does not offer a similarly diverse selection of art which illustrates the reality of healing through its mirror. This might partly be due to the fact that no one has yet pursued such evidence systematically. Dispersed in archives and collections, numerous pictures could exist that contain medical motifs. However, the fact remains that medical subjects were usually not deemed worthy of artistic reflection in Chinese art.

The fact that medicine has been ignored by Chinese painters for over two millennia is astonishing. It suggests a homogeneity within Chinese culture that overrides the many examples of social nonconformity which are also known. This facet of Chinese culture cannot be explained by the scornful disdain of medicine as *xiaodao* (small teaching), placing it on the same level as gardening, by the Song philosopher Zhu Xi 朱熹 (1130–1200) and numerous other writers of later centuries.[114] An equal number of writers attempted to raise the status of medicine as an important aspect of culture, claiming it to be an ideal base from which to translate the values of Confucius into concrete action.

To be sure, one could argue that Western medicine, with the procedures of anatomy and surgery, offered far more graphic models. Traditional Chinese medicine does not know of any comparable spectacular interventions. But even the activity of folk healers and midwives, the interior of a pharmacy, or the physiognomy of patients remained for the most part unnoticed in China.

Western artists reacted to issues such as the plague epidemics of the fourteenth century—an incomparable encounter of a civilization with death—with pictorial translations of the Vanitas and *Memento Mori* motifs. China was also familiar with large-scale epidemics and wars, but the reflection on the constant presence of existential threats to mankind—a topic that in Europe was also expressed in artistic discourses on the problematics of healing—found no manifestation in Chinese secular art, and only rarely in religious art.

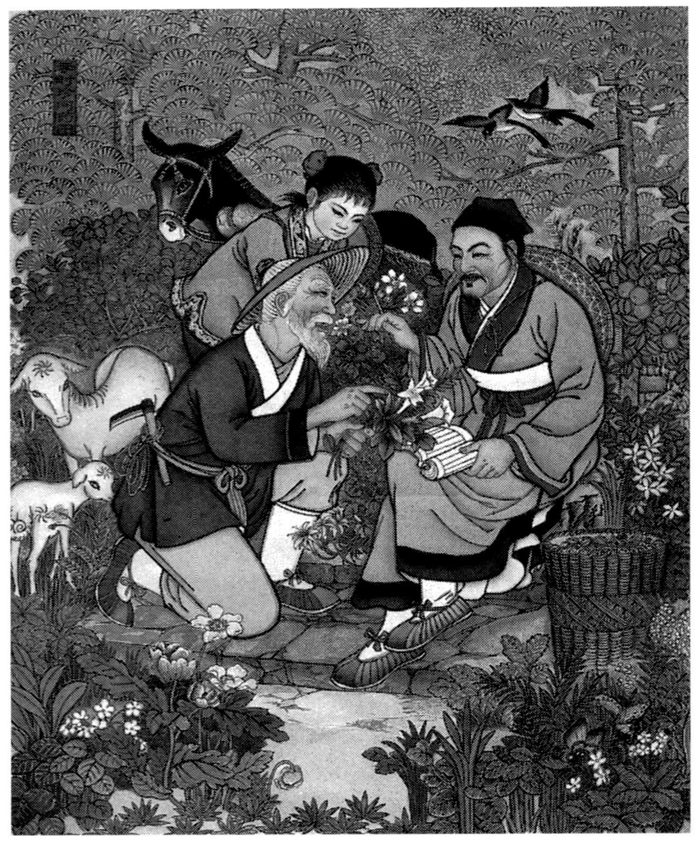

105. "Li Shizhen 李時珍, famous pharmacist and doctor of the Ming dynasty, gathers information about medicinal plants from the common people." Idealized depiction of the author of the encyclopedia of natural history and materia medica *Bencao gang mu* 本草綱目 (1596), on a postcard. Tianjin, 1988.

This is the reason why most portraits, sculptures, and other objects, which can be categorized as art and simultaneously touch on the area of medicine, were not created as an artistic exposition of the human answer to the threat of illness and the possibility of premature death.

It is not known when the demand for representations of famous physicians arose. Four tomb reliefs survive from the Han period which depict the same motif albeit in differing artistic styles. A bird with a human head faces a row of humans who might be identified as patients due to their disheveled hair. The bird-human creature is holding the wrist of the patient in front of him with his right hand while grasping in his left hand an elongated object, possibly sharpened at the tip. Chinese authors have interpreted these murals as depictions of the ancient itinerant physician Bian Que 扁鵲, for two reasons. First, the reliefs come from the province of Shandong, an area which traditional sources also associate with Bian Que. Second, the character for *que* in Bian Que's name includes the two components "old" and "bird", allowing us to assume a connection.[115] Japanese researchers have even speculated that Bian Que was one of the shamans who, in ancient times, traveled throughout Eastern China in bird costumes (figures 72, 104).[116]

Whoever the figure on the Han reliefs might be, it is likely that a medical treatment of patients is depicted. For this reason, these reliefs are unique in the history of Chinese art and medicine. A few rare depictions of Chinese physicians and patients exist from the nineteenth century. The same applies to portraits of physicians which, when they do exist, depict them not in a medical context, but as personalities who could be practicing any profession of an elevated social status.

From the twentieth century several depictions exist, for example, of Li Shizhen 李時珍 that show this author of the *Bencao gang mu* 本草綱目 (*Materia Medica Arranged in Monographs According to Topics*) as a thoughtful scholar (figure 105, plate 173). More recent paintings of the semi-legendary Han physician Hua Tuo 華佗 or of the prototypical barefoot doctor of the early seventies, follow the motif of the proletarian folk hero (plate 163). The line between heroes of Chinese medical history and the Sun Simiao figures of the Medicine God is fluid. Mao Zedong's picture is displayed in many taxis and buses, not because the drivers are supporters of Mao's ideas—most of the time they are not even familiar with them—but because they have heard of him as a ruthless government leader and want to oblige his spirit as an ally in a ruthless environment. Similar notions lie behind the desire to own a painting or statue of Guanyin—to implore the "goddess of mercy" in times of need.

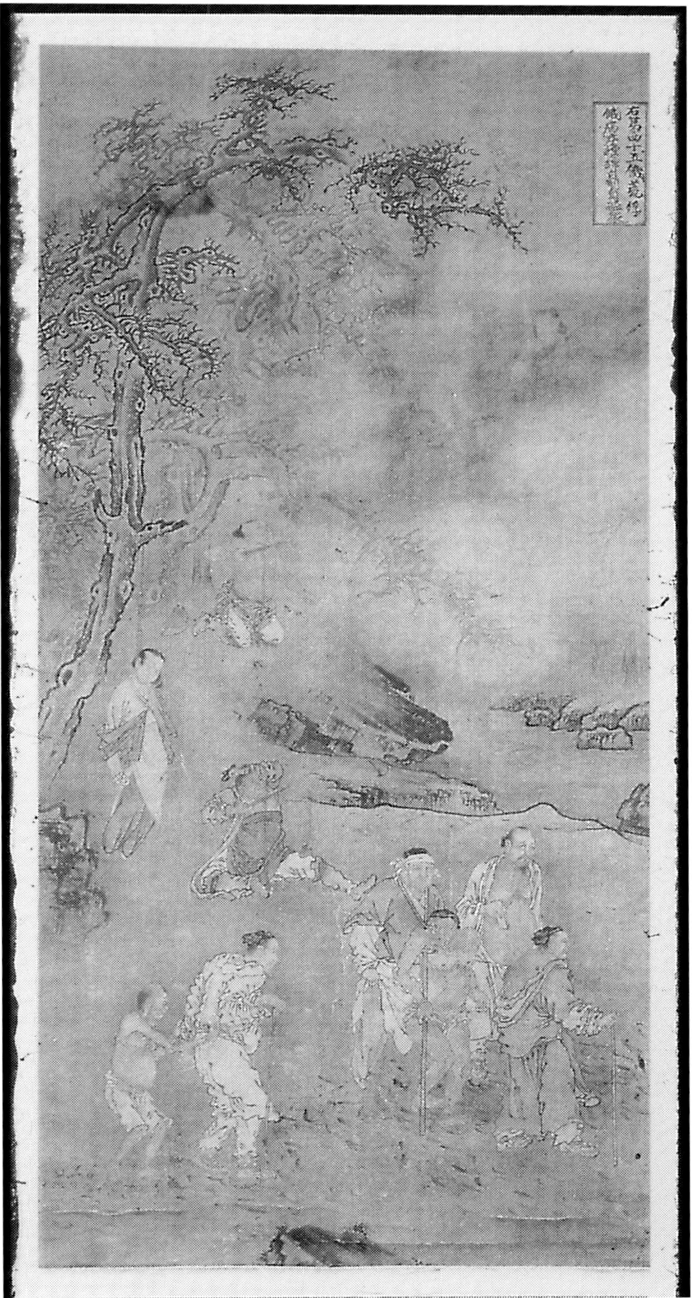

106. "All those who [have died] from hunger and related illnesses as well as from self-inflicted punishment and hanging themselves." Ming period depiction from the context of the Water-and-Land Ritual. From *Provincial Museum Shanxi, Ming Dynasty Shui Lu Paintings At Bao Ning Si*, Peking, 1985.

99

The Ming paintings of the Buddhist Water-and-Land Ritual (*shuiluhui* 水 陸 會) from the Baoning 寶 寧 Temple in the district of Youyu 右 玉, 120 km west of Datong 大 同 in Shanxi Province, also remain in the realm of religious art. These silk paintings (a total of 139), by an anonymous painter do not directly depict medical subjects, but express human pain, the bodies of sick persons, and the agents responsible for such suffering.

According to tradition, the Water-and-Land Ritual was introduced as a festival for poor souls by emperor Wudi (464–549), a ruler of the Liang Dynasty and a devout Buddhist. To this day, it is performed annually according to a ritual which has remained unchanged for centuries. It is intended to shorten the suffering of ancestors who are doing penance in hell for a variety of reasons. For similar reasons, people pray for poor souls who have died from injustice, misfortune, or illness, and are unable to find peace.

The murals in the Baoning Temple and the *shuilu* paintings elsewhere illustrate the realistic context of these prayers for believers. The suffering depicted is quite closely related to metaphysical notions, but it also offers insights into the dark side of the Ming and preceding dynasties which otherwise would not be imaginable. The ghosts of people who have been wrongfully executed are shown clubbing the responsible high officials with their chopped-off heads. This could be interpreted as a criticism of the situation at that time, but might also be a reference to the atrocities performed by the previous, now defunct dynasty.[117]

The *shuilu* paintings depict demons who can cause illness to humans in a symbolic manner that can be only partially interpreted today. Human figures depicted with horse, chicken, crow, tiger, or human heads, holding buckets, fans, daggers, swords, or gourds—the symbol of pharmaceutics—in their hands, signified more to people half a millennium ago than they do to viewers today. Included in this context are rare depictions of the victims of serious illnesses, accidental deaths, suicides, and other events (figures 106, 107). Among the subjects depicted is an itinerant physician receiving a thrashing from the relatives of his patient who is now spitting blood (figure 109).

The background for a series of executions in the city center is the pharmacy of a Mr. He (figure 108). From a Western perspective, it might be assumed that the artist purposefully linked ineffective methods of ending one's life (only entry into Nirvana is the true end of life) with ineffective methods of healing (true liberation from suffering is achieved not by taking drugs, but by turning to the Buddha's teachings), but this is uncertain. Signs of a new beginning are evident in all this suffering: women are washing a newborn baby, while the mother rests in a warm bed on the stove nearby, cared for by the midwife (figure 110). In order to shed light on these and other scenes which are more or less related to healing through secular art, we are limited to coincidental finds. Depictions of market scenes, for example, sometimes include healers, but the known pictures of this type may be counted on one hand.



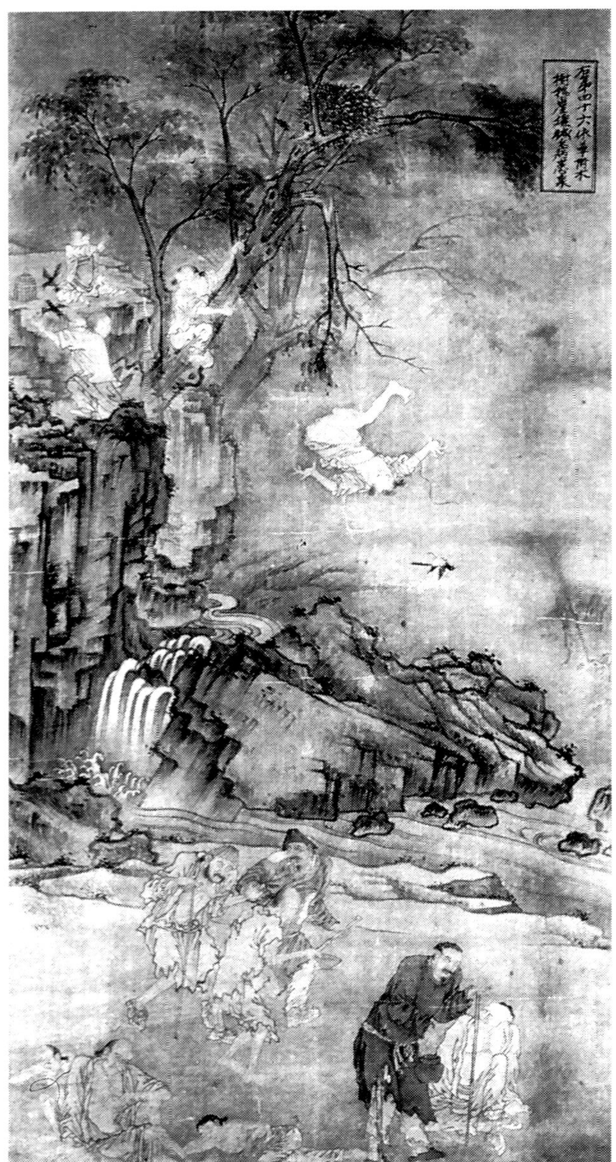

107. "All those who [have died] from broken trees or dropping rock cliffs or from acupuncture and moxibustion, as well as from sickness." Ming period depiction from the context of the Water-and-Land Ritual. From *Provincial Museum Shanxi, Ming Dynasty Shui Lu Paintings At Bao Ning Si*, Peking, 1985.

A good example consists of two round porcelain disks with blue marks on a white base. Besides an artist, a fortune teller, a fruit peddler, and a messenger announcing the results of civil service examinations, we can see an itinerant physician/drug merchant moving through the crowd. His banner announces that he specializes in injuries arising from being struck or falling. (plate 177)

Even rarer than such coincidental depictions of medical subjects is a painting that was created at the beginning of the twentieth century by the Cantonese artist Zheng Chang 鄭萇, who supposedly was able to paint only in a state of intoxication. This might explain the unusual motif of the painting: *Kangzi kuiyao* 康子饋藥 (*Kangzi Offers a Medicine*), a well-known anecdote about Confucius, in which the great philosopher is presented with medicine by Kangzi, one of the few statesmen to be convinced by Confucius' ideas. Confucius accepts the gift, but states, "I am unfamiliar with this; I dare not taste it." [118] (plate 175)

To the left of the figure of Confucius, Zheng Chang wrote a calligraphic inscription explaining that Confucius rejected the drugs because he had immediately recognized that they were inappropriate (adulterated)—a fact that usually only experts in a pharmacy were able to recognize. Nowadays—Zheng Chang is here referring to the time of initial reforms at the end of the Qing period—China had been opened to the world, making it essential that everyone be able to distinguish good from bad, appropriate from inappropriate remedies. One should acquire the outstanding knowledge of Confucius in order to avoid falling victim to the general ignorance. This may have been a reference by Zheng Chang—or whoever inspired him to paint the picture and write the text—to the many "prescriptions" which were supposed to show China a way into the future. Perhaps the message of these lines is the conservative notion that true, appropriate medicine for the future formation of China was to be found only within the frame of Confucianism.

If this interpretation is correct, Zheng Chang's painting is a unique document, since no other painting has used a medical scene—even if there are no physicians and patients present—as a metaphor for a political statement.

## ILLUSTRATIONS IN MEDICAL LITERATURE

Very different from the fine arts is the purpose of pictures in medical literature. Their function is technical and primarily didactic, i.e. for the study of medical and pharmaceutical subjects. However, it would be a mistake to view such illustrations only as technical depictions. The transition from the

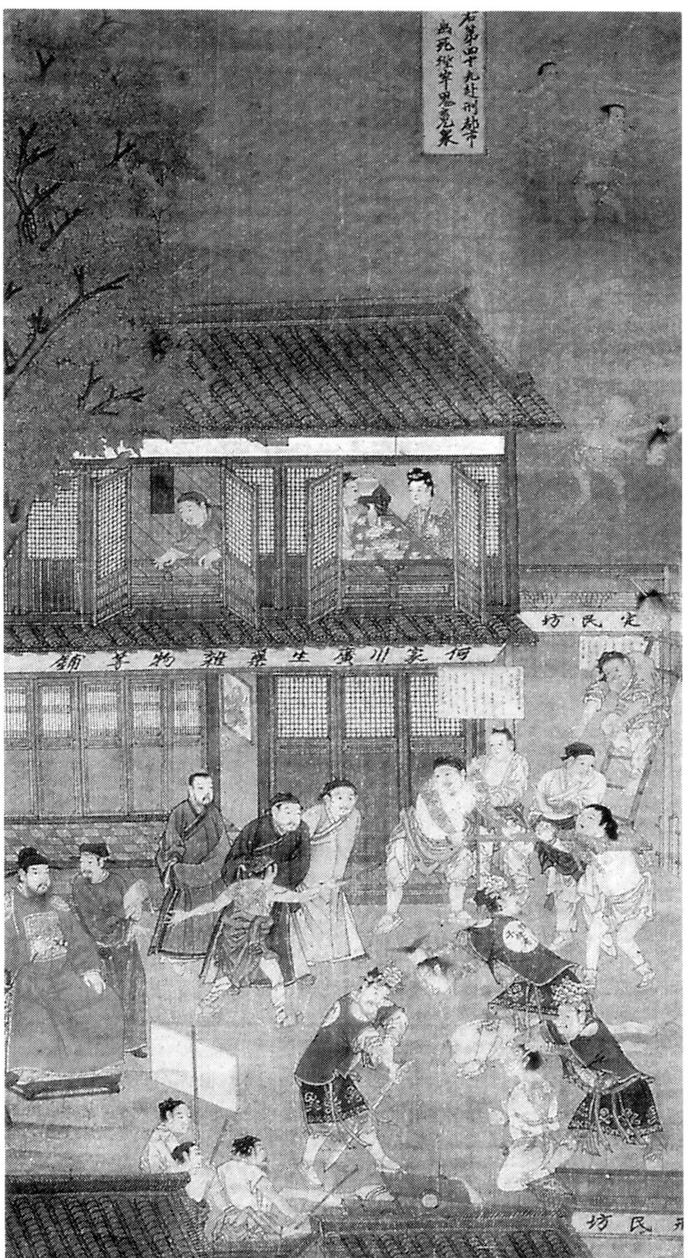

108. View of an execution site in front of a pharmacy that has a tea house on its second floor. The characters above the pharmacy contain the information: "House He. Store for fresh medicinal drugs from [Si]chuan and Guang[dong], as well as various items." Ming period depiction from the context of the Water-and-Land Ritual. From *Provincial Museum Shanxi, Ming Dynasty Shui Lu Paintings At Bao Ning Si*, Peking, 1985.

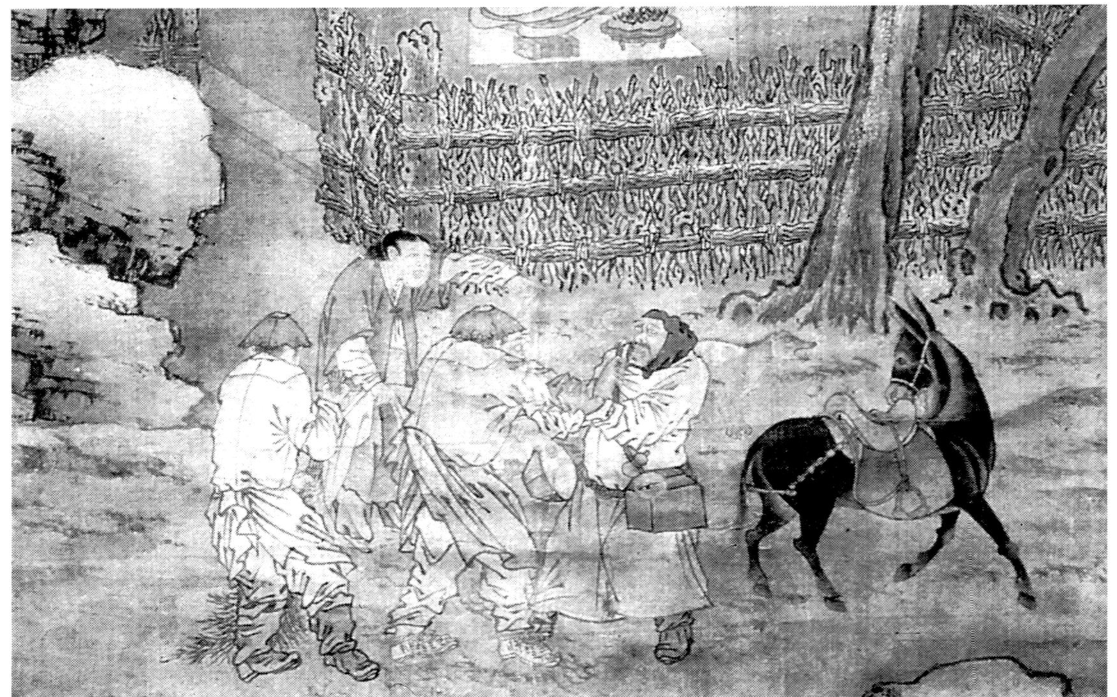

109. Villagers fighting with an itinerant doctor, identified by the gourd at his side. In the house, a patient is spitting blood into a bowl. Ming dynasty depiction from the context of the Water-and-Land Ritual. From *Provincial Museum Shanxi, Ming Dynasty Shui Lu Paintings At Bao Ning Si*, Peking, 1985.

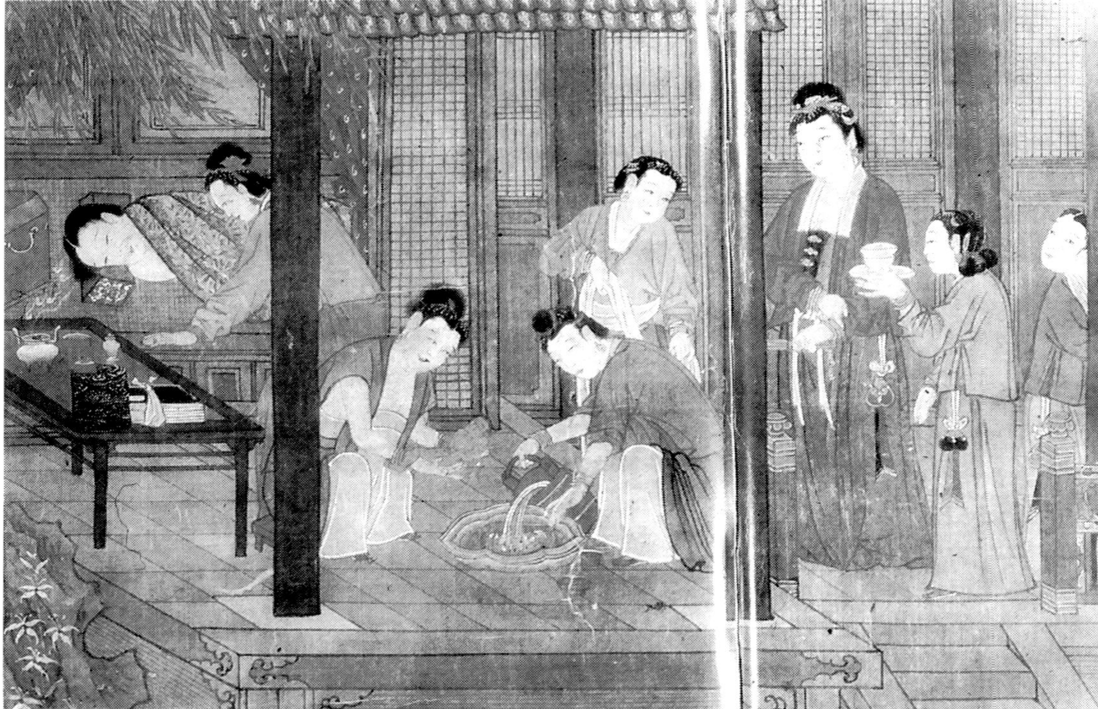

110. Scene after a birth which depicts the mother resting on an oven bed (left), and a woman pouring water into a basin in order to bath the child (center). Relatives and servants are also present (right). Ming dynasty depiction from the context of the Water-and-Land Ritual. From *Provincial Museum Shanxi, Ming Dynasty Shui Lu Paintings At Bao Ning Si*, Peking, 1985.

flat, anatomical images of scholasticism, in the style of woodblock printing, to the perspective drawings by Stefan von Kalkar in the *Fabrica* of Andreas von Wesel (called Vesalius) is not only a part of art history, but also of intellectual history, and marks a completely new view of the world which can only be understood within the changing conditions of Europe at that time.[119]

The difference between the development of medical illustration in Western and Chinese technical literature, however, is apparent, since the significant breaks which molded Europe at regular intervals of a few centuries did not occur in China. The continuity of Chinese medicine from the Han period to the nineteenth century mirrors the continuity of its political environment. All developments within medicine corresponded to developments in its social context. These transformations, however, were much less substantial than the upheavals in Europe. Changes in China between the Han period and the end of the Imperial period were always within the system, never of the system. Therefore it will not be surprising if a history of illustrations in the medical literature of Imperial China, which has yet to be written, fails to yield a multi-faceted, pictorial broadsheet comparable to European development.

In Europe, we can trace the development of certain styles of illustration through late Classical, early Medieval, and Byzantine copies of traditions back to the Hellenistic period—that is, to the time when the Mawangdui tomb in China was closed—without having access to originals from the second century B.C.E.[120] In contrast, the Mawangdui excavations have yielded a series of original illustrations (see above, chapter 2, pp. 19–21) which are followed by a gap of several centuries.

The bibliography in the official history of the Sui dynasty (581–618) offers the first list of books whose titles suggest that they contained illustrations. It is entirely unknown whether illustrated medical or pharmaceutical texts existed in China in the meantime. The Sui dynasty titles suggest primarily anatomical texts and illustrations which indicate the position of insertion points for needle therapy.

Of particular interest among these titles is the still unexplored *Frog Classic of Huang Di* (*Huang Di hamajing* 黃帝蝦蟆經) whose peculiar content has been dated by several Chinese historians to the Han period.[121] At the beginning of this century, Sudhoff called attention to the oldest illustrations of European medical texts, which he dated to the Hellenistic period, the so-called Five Pictures Series of anatomical figures.[122] These figures, drawn in the supine position with straddled thighs and flexed arms, were transmitted in European medical literature until the high Middle Ages. Medical historians have given them different names: "Squatting Pictures" (Sudhoff), "Frog Position" (Garrison) and "Table Pictures" (Herrlinger, who wanted to indicate that these figures assume the typical position of bodies that have been laid out for preparation on an autopsy table).[123]

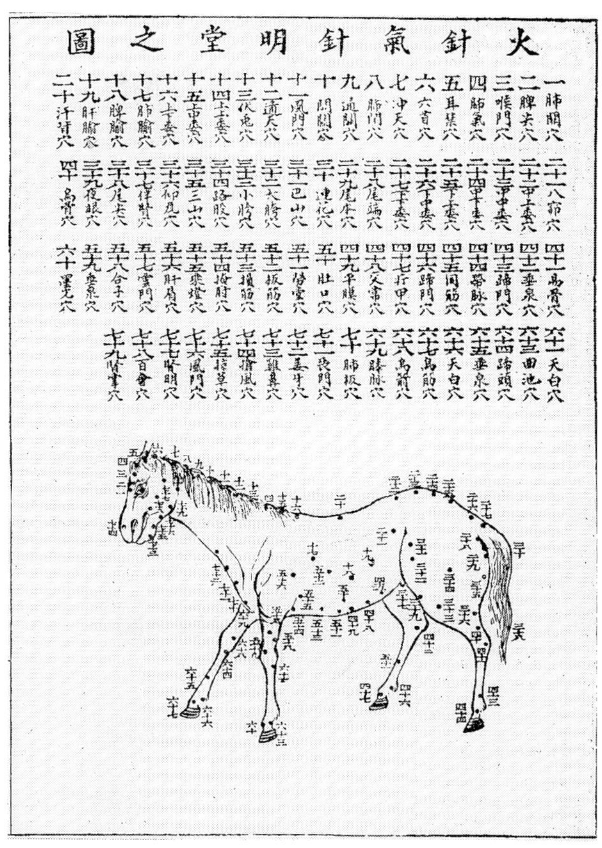


111. List of names and site plan of the insertion points for heated needles ("fire needles") and for ordinary acupuncture needles, in order to influence the qi in a horse. From *Yuan Heng liaomaji* 元亨療馬集 (*Collection of Horse Medicine by [Yu Ben]yuan and [Yu Ben]heng*), 1608. Undated edition, publisher Saoyeshanfang 掃業山房, Shanghai.

Drawings of the human body which are remarkably similar to the Five Pictures Series of European antiquity are found only in a fragmentary manuscript of the "Frog Classic" preserved in Japan.[124] The only significant difference between these two sources is the fact that the arms are flexed inward in the Western frog pictures and outward in most Chinese ones.

The Chinese "Frog Classic" supposedly originated in a legend in which Chang E 嫦娥 stole the drug of immortality and fled to the moon, where she was transformed into a toad.[125] The text contains instructions on the days and times during which cauterization and needling are counter-indicated and thereby mirrors classical Egyptian and Babylonian concepts about the relationship between astrology and blood-letting, which also influenced European texts on blood-letting until the Renaissance.[126]

Fragments of a Tang dynasty manuscript, which is now part of the Stein collection in the British Museum in London, are also concerned with cauterization. The text deals with the use of moxibustion to treat various diseases and is interspersed with simple contour drawings of the human body on which the points for cauterization are marked.[127] This manuscript was found in the early twentieth century at Dunhuang, and it remains to be seen whether it forms a link to the numerous cauterization texts of Hippocratic medicine in late antiquity which were illustrated in a similar fashion.

References to the first-known illustrated drug work in China also date from the Tang period. Based on a governmental edict, all parts of the country were ordered to send in drawings of known medicinal drugs so that an editorial staff could revise the materia medica. The work was published after two years in 659; besides general descriptions of drugs in twenty chapters, it contained twenty-five chapters of illustrations and seven chapters of explanations to these illustrations.[128] Unfortunately, all the illustrations, have since been lost.

The oldest existing illustrations in Chinese pharmaceutical texts stem from the *Daguan bencao* 大觀本草 from the year 1108. How much they are based on earlier models is only guesswork. Since these illustrations are found in printed works, they conform, by necessity, to a type of schematic woodblock prints. Plants, plant parts, minerals, the instruments used for their preparation, and animal and human medicinal drugs are still frequently and recognizably depicted, indicating that they have been created for didactic purposes.

To be sure, manuscripts from this time, with accompanying illustrations, offer a completely different level of quality. They express a direct translation of close botanical observation and knowledge into colored illustrations, allowing for a positive identification of certain plants up to the present day. One example is the *Lü chanyan bencao* 履巉巖本草 (*Materia Medica of the Mountain Cliff Wanderer*) from 1220, which exists in a Ming period copy.[129] The author Wang Jie 王介 was a high-ranking government official who also became famous for his landscape and plant paintings (figures 17, 18).

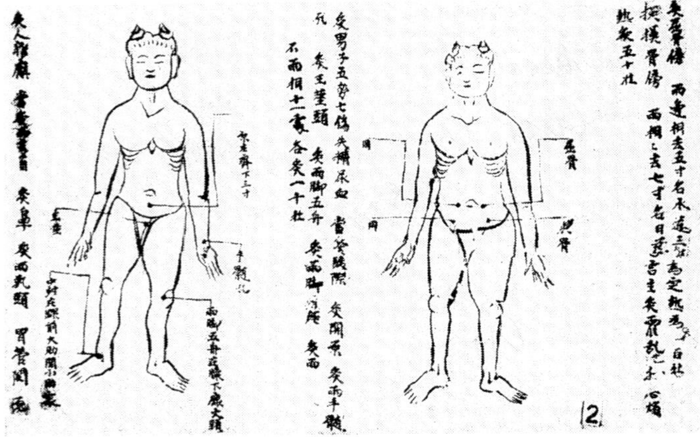

112. Han period (?) drawings of either dissected human bodies or human bodies in frog poses in an almanac of favorable times for cauterization. From *Huang Di hamajing* 黃地蝦蟆經 (*Frog Classic of Huang Di*).

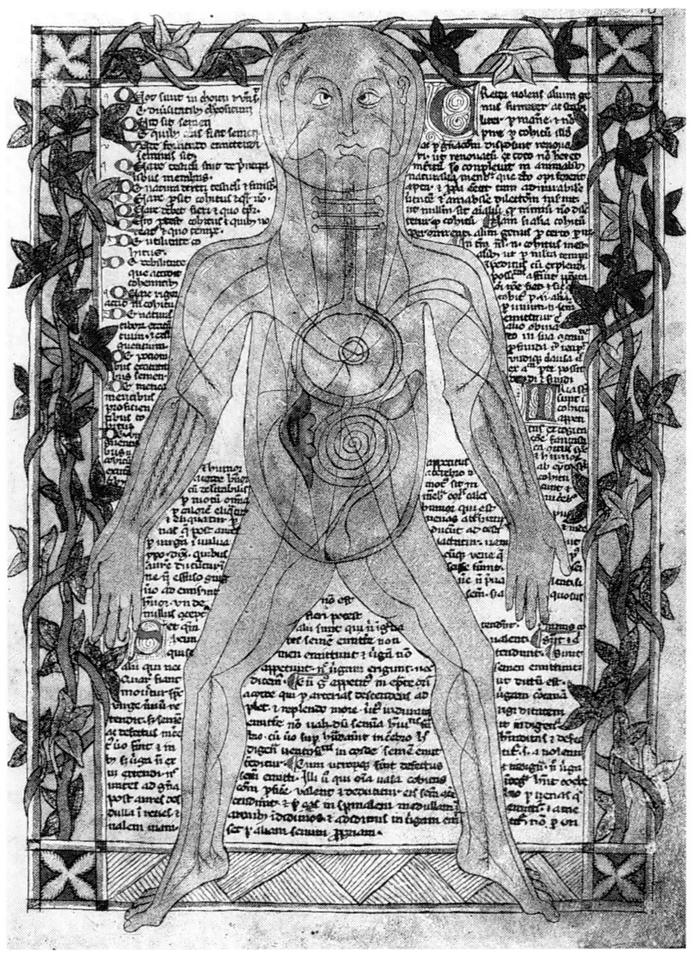

113. A way of depicting the body in dissection or frog pose, dating to the Hellenistic period (?). Series of five pictures in the Codex Ashmole 399. Bodleian Library, Oxford.

Due to the lack of research on this topic it is difficult to say how illustrations in Chinese pharmaceutical works developed in the following centuries. At first sight, a continuous development is not recognizable. The texts which were printed from woodblocks until the nineteenth century vary greatly in the quality of their illustrations. The first observable leap to a new level occurred in 1848 with the *Zhiwu mingshitu kao* 植 物 名 實 圖 考 (*Study of the Names, Facts, and Illustrations of Plants*), whose depictions of plants could still be used in similar literature today.

Since practically all known pharmaceutical books from the Sung period forward are found in printed form, manuscripts such as the *Lü chanyan bencao* constitute an exception, as does the *Yuzhi bencao pinhui jingyao* 御製本 草品彙精要 (*Materia Medica Written on Imperial Orders, Containing the Essential and Important in Classified Order*) from 1505.[130] This encyclopedia contains 1,358 colored illustrations in impressive arrangements. The artist was not content to depict only medicinal drugs, their plant sources and other primary materials. Implements for the production of minerals, for example, convey an image of the production of the drug "iron chips." A plant-based prescription imported from abroad appears in the hands of a foreigner (figures 42, 43, plate 2). In order to illustrate the prescription "Herbs from a Swallow's Nest," the artist painted swallows flying back and forth above a Chinese house where several men on a ladder are busily cleaning out their nests.

To be sure, illustrations are not only found in pharmaceutical literature. Theoretical and clinical books used pictures to supplement the text. But for this genre, the same holds true for pharmaceutical illustrations. Due to a lack of research, no development can be recognized since the Ming period, from which stem the earliest depictions of such subjects as the course of vessels on the body, the position of organs within the body, or patients suffering from certain diseases. The technology of woodblock printing and the willingness of a publisher to invest capital determine the quality of illustrations in a book. Occasionally, a considerable amount of negligence can barely be ignored. For example, a comparison of the illustrations of horses to the directions about the location of insertion points suitable for horse acupuncture indicates that the images could have been used only symbolically; no editor seems to have ever tested the accuracy of the information contained in the pictures (figure 111). Another example of a purely symbolic illustration that contains no factual information whatsoever is found in the depictions of eyes in the ophthalmological literature of the Imperial Age. It was not until the late nineteenth century that the influence of available texts from Western medicine led to considerable changes.

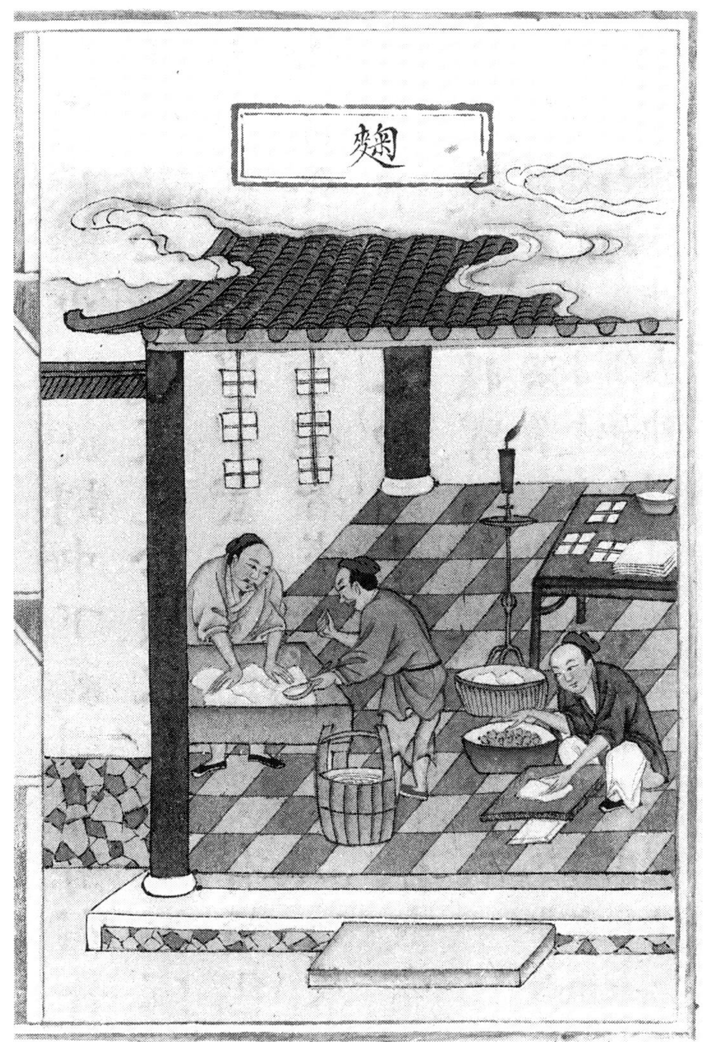

114. The manufacture of yeast. From *Yuzhi bencao pinhui jingyao* 御製本草品彙經要 (*Materia Medica Written on Imperial Orders, Containing the Essential and Important in Classified Order*), 1505. Identical copy of the original, nineteenth century or earlier. Staatsbibliothek, Berlin.

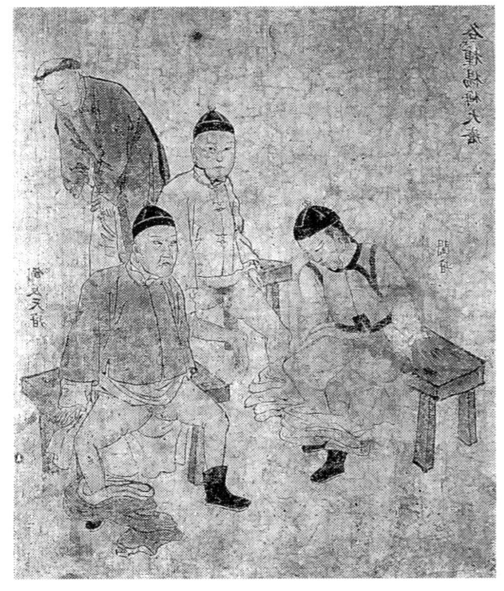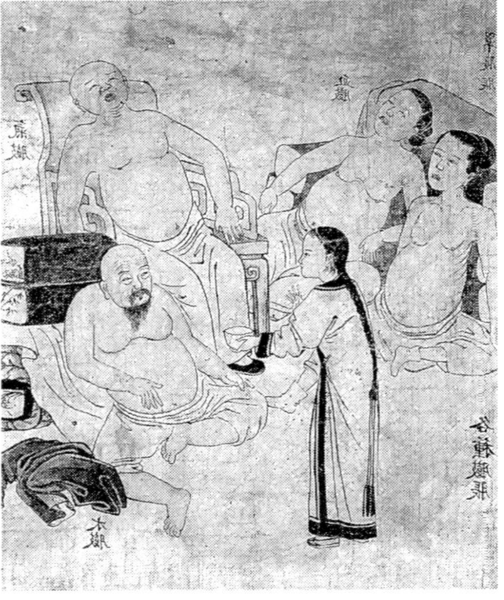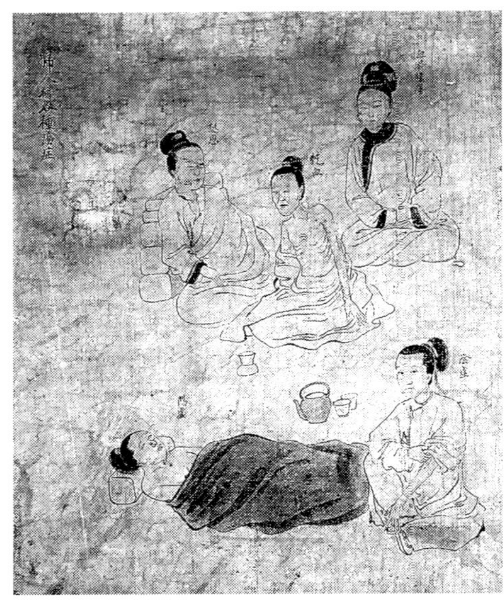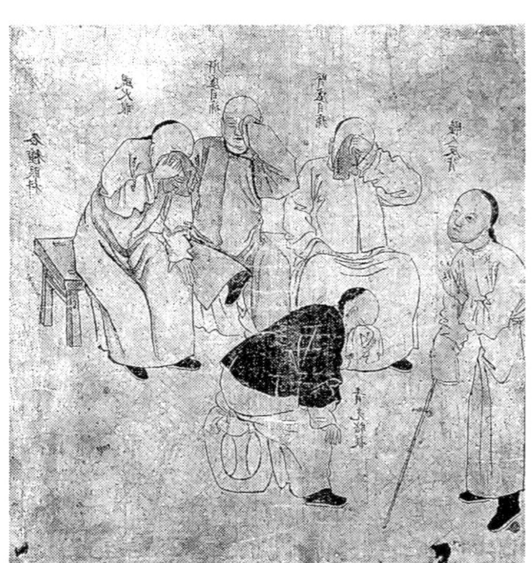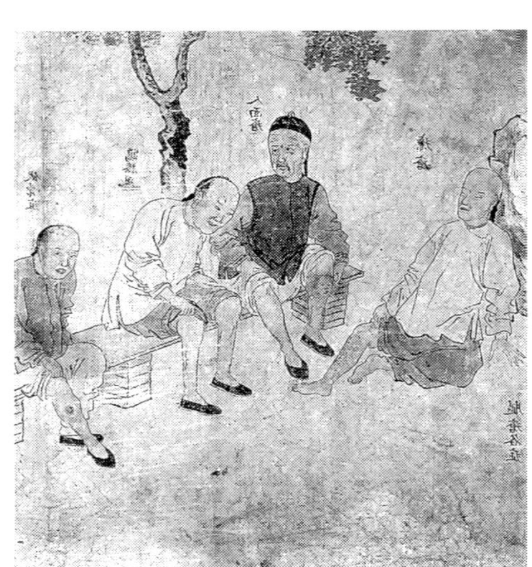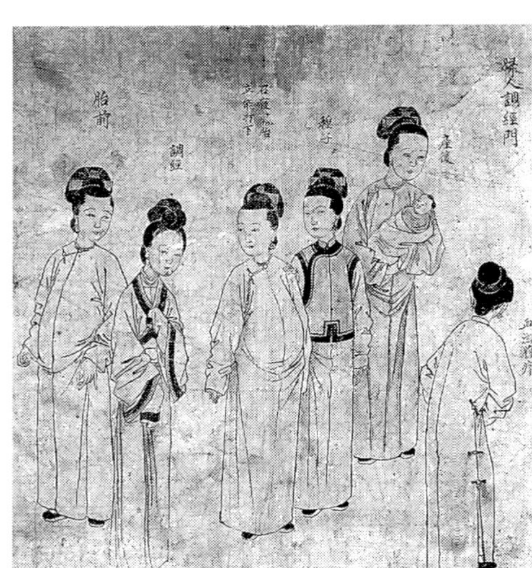

115.

1. "All kinds of large syphilitic sores."
2. "All kinds of abdominal distensions."
3. "Section gynecology. All kinds of conditions of fatigue in women."
4. "All kinds of [problems] from ophthalmology."
5. Depiction of various sores on the legs and in the face.
6. "Section: gynecology, regularizing menstruation"; from right to left: "blood stasis (血游 instead of 血瘀) and abdominal pain," "after delivery," "fertility [problems]," "stone-like indurations and false pregnancy," "regularizing menstruation," "pregnancy." Drawings in an undated manuscript. Wellcome Institute Library, London.

The small number of serious historians concerned with the history of Chinese medicine in Europe and the United States helps to explain the lack of well-founded information about the significance of medical motifs in the *belles lettres* of the Imperial Age as well as the Modern age and the present.

Lu Xun 魯迅 is the most prominent example from the twentieth century of an assimilator of medical themes in Modern literature. Like Sun Yatsen 孫中山, and other reformers and revolutionaries of the last decades of the Qing dynasty, Lu Xun was keenly aware of the ignorance and incompetence of the physicians rooted in the various traditions of Chinese medicine; he saw Chinese medicine as an allegory for a doomed China. Therefore, he decided to go to Japan in order to study medicine and, upon his return, to treat patients, "at the same time strengthening my countrymen's faith in reformation."[131]

When Lu Xun became aware of the real extent of China's precarious situation in Japan, however, it seemed more important for him to adapt the minds of his compatriots to the new age; he believed that he could heal the "illness" of his people much more effectively as a writer. But this did not change his contempt for traditional Chinese medicine and his admiration of the natural sciences and medicine of the West.

Besides scathing statements about Chinese medicine in several of his writings, the short stories "Medicine" and "Tomorrow" from 1919 offer particularly lucid insights into Lu Xun's attitudes. In "Medicine," he drew a detailed picture of the "disgusting, superstitious old medical practices, heightened by the tragedy of a child's death and his mother's grief."[132] In "Tomorrow," Lu Xun describes a traditional physician at work, an "ignorant and callous [man] brushing off the anxious queries of a widowed mother with empty phrases about 'obstruction of the digestive tract' and 'fire overpowering metal,' in order to pocket his fee and get rid of her. After taking his prescription, the woman's son dies."[133]

This medicine, which is so deeply rooted in the old system, stands in Lu Xun's literature for the situation of the Empire in general. Just as the children of Chinese mothers die when they entrust themselves to the doctors of Chinese medicine, China's future is endangered if new political prescriptions are not implemented. The evaluation of traditional Chinese medicine as "backward, inhuman, and disgusting"[134] is expressed even more drastically in 1926 in Lu Xun's story "Father's Illness," which is based on events from his own family.

The widely read author Ba Jin 巴金 was moved by similar experiences to enumerate in his autobiographical novel, *Family*, a long list of "ignorant physicians, priests, and sorcerers" who try their useless skills on the ailing

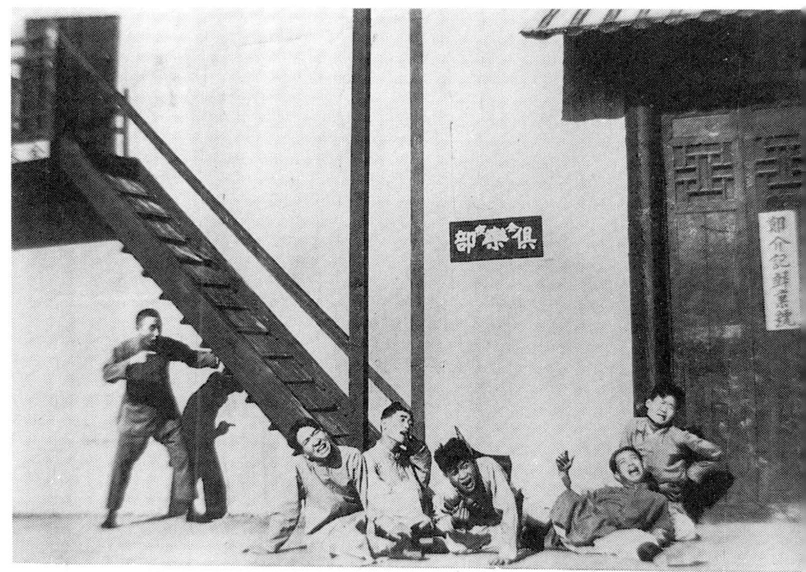

116. Still from Zhang Shichuang's movie, *A Laborer's Love*, 1922. The fruit vendor achieves success with his mechanism that causes guests leaving the second-floor nightclub at dawn to slide down the stairs and land in front of the doctor's door.

family patriarch. This very different document shows just how scornful the attitude was among large circles of the general population and intellectuals of the 1920's, not only towards the theoretical contents, but also the practices and ethics of traditional Chinese medicine. In 1922, Zhang Shichuang shot the silent film *A Laborer's Love*, the story of a fruit peddler who falls in love with a young woman assisting her father, a traditional physician, across the street from his fruit stand. When the fruit peddler asks for the daughter's hand, the father responds that he could only accept him as son-in-law if the fruit peddler could do something to stimulate the physician's business. He could, after all, not even afford the rent for his stall on the street. In his despair, the fruit peddler conceives of a device to transform the stairs leading to a night club above his apartment into a slide. The numerous nightly victims of this infamous device limp and hobble on the next day to the doctor, who makes a big business out of highly questionable treatments and is only too happy to accept the fruit peddler as his son-in-law.

Lu Xun, Ba Jin, Zhang Shichuang and many others agreed that traditional medicine was not only useless, but even extremely harmful.[135] Such an attitude is, of course, related to expectations linked to the development of Western medicine. As long as Western medicine was still unknown in China, traditional medicine was justified in its own right. The premises of its theoretical superstructure—and this was recognized by Lu Xun and others—were identical to those of the general Chinese sociology from which no one was able to escape before the encounter with Western culture. This does not mean that there are no critiques of physicians in Chinese dramas and literature before the end of the Imperial Age. A striking example is the fifteenth-century musical drama *Jiang sangzhen Cai Shun fengmu* 降 桑 椹 蔡 順 奉 母 (*The Mulberry Tree Is Brought Down: Cai Shun Takes Care of his Mother*).

In the musical drama, Cai Shun's mother falls ill and two doctors appear—making fun of their own incompetence in a dialogue and speaking about the tricks by which they are going to clean out the patient's family.[136] One of them is identified as *taiyi* 太 醫 (outstanding physician), while the other likens himself—in the epitome of impertinence—to the Medicine King, Sun Simiao. Moreover, he points out that his family has been practicing medicine for three generations, thereby questioning the validity of the Chinese saying, "If a physician does not yet practice in the third generation, beware of his drugs."[137]

The two healers are characterized by deficient education, recklessness in their dealings with the life of the patient, and greed (in order to share the case, one of them feels the pulse on the patient's left hand, the other the one on the right). While one doctor arrives at the conclusion of a cold disease, the other one supposes a heat disease. As if in a persiflage on the widespread Chinese "both this and that" culture, the two decide that each should treat his half of the patient according to his own diagnostic results. When Cai Shun orders them to end this foolishness and to decide

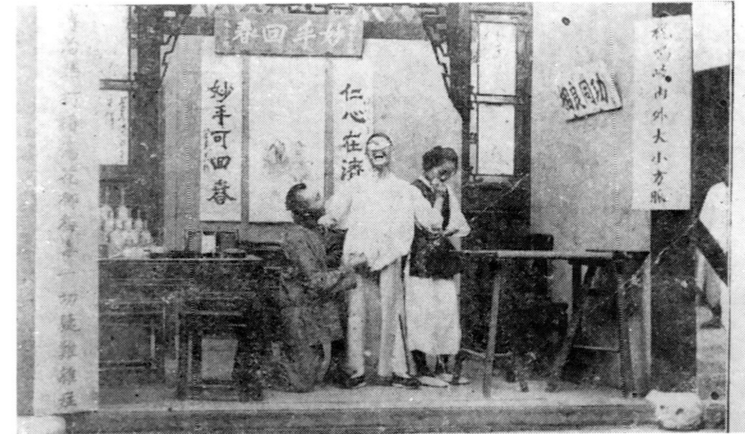

117. Still from Zhang Shichuang's movie, *A Laborer's Love*, 1922. The doctor (center) rejoices at the helpful fruit vendor and gives him the hand of his daughter. In the background are typical calligraphies of a traditional doctor's clinic. The scroll on the left states that "An expert made possible a return to spring," while the center scroll (partly covered by the doctor) notes that "A humane attitude stresses assistance."

which one will treat the patient, the scene concludes with a contest in which the two doctors take turns trying to outdo each other with the most audacious statements about their medical competence. Ultimately, they are chased out of the house. In this play, medical theory appears ridiculous, not because the author—in the manner of Lu Xun, Ba Jin, and others at the beginning of the twentieth century—would have known of a better alternative, but simply because the two physicians have not mastered it.

Until the present, only two examples of a literary treatment of motifs from the environs of medicine in a time prior to the encounter with Western medicine have been researched in detail: the novels *Jinpingmei* 金瓶梅 from the late sixteenth century[138] and *Xingshi yinyuan zhuan* 醒世姻緣傳 from the seventeenth century.[139]

The *Jinpingmei* (*Plum Blossoms in a Golden Vase*) is the most famous erotic novel of the Chinese Imperial Age by an unknown writer; it is set in the twelfth century of the Song period, but an obvious mirror of society in late Ming times. It describes the life of a wealthy family in all details, including numerous episodes of sickness and recourses to medical experts. Unlike the Modern authors Lu Xun, Ba Jin, and Lao She, who purposefully placed reflections on medicine in the center of their stories and wanted to make a statement about its role, the author of the *Jinpingmei* referred to medicine in all its variations as an accessory of daily life which was as self-evident as the various types of housing in which people lived. The treatment of medicine in the novel is a representation which is as true to life as the other components of the environment in which the author has located the story of the bon vivant Ximen Qing.

The great number of medical practitioners consulted by the members of Ximen Qing's household corresponds to the spectrum of groups also known to us from other sources. The so-called *taiyi* 太醫 (eminent physicians) to whom Sun Simiao's ethics of duty were addressed form the top of the hierarchy. They come from a family tradition or have gained their knowledge at a medical school; they hesitate to accept a reward, but then allow themselves to be persuaded. Here a subtle social stratification can be recognized; the beneficiary of medical services is not willing to accept them without prompt compensation since they would have to be reciprocated somehow with later services, as was customary with people of his standing.[140] Even the *taiyi* is a merchant; he earns a living on the medicines he has prescribed and sets up his own pharmacy when his means allow him to do so.

Acupuncture and moxibustion are not employed by the educated physicians; these therapies are reserved for the lower practitioners who gain access to Ximen Qing's home in various ways. The transition between explanatory models is fluid; metaphysical concepts are doubtless of great importance. When all else fails, knowledge about the causation of illness by the gods gains validity. One and the same healer might thus cure ulcers, apply needle therapy, and also attempt to question and appease the gods.[141]

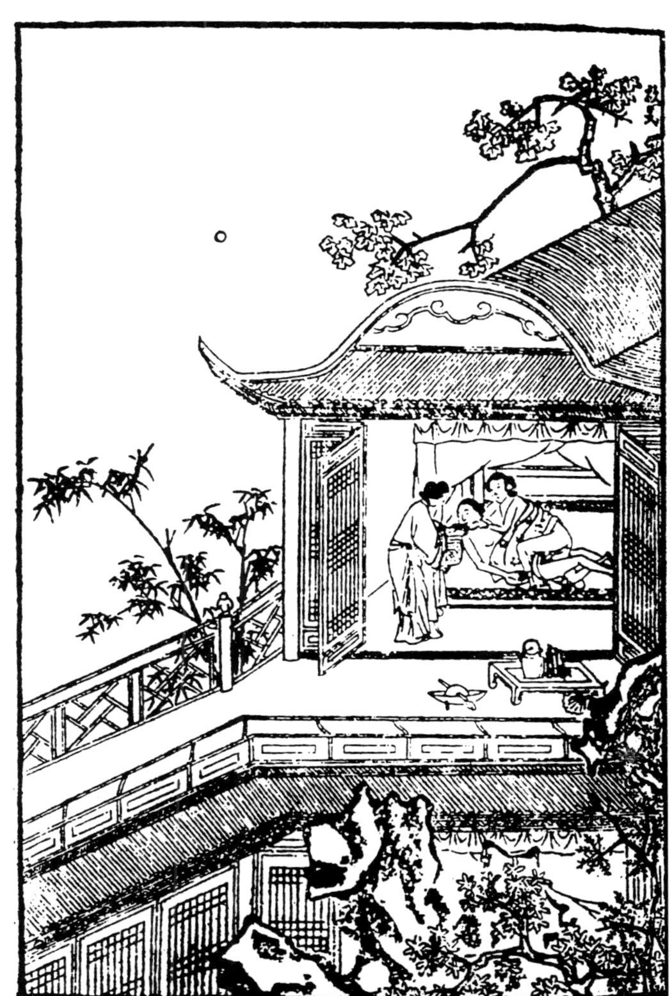

118. "Golden Lotus dispenses an overdose of an aphrodisiac to Ximen Qing." Illustration from the erotic novel *Jinpingmei* 金瓶梅 (*Plum Blossoms in a Golden Vase*). The pharmaceutical context is suggested by the drug boat to the left of the table on the balcony. Undated edition of the *Jinpingmei*, first half of the seventeenth century. Staatsbibliothek, Berlin.

The *Xingshi yinyuan zhuan* (*Record of Marriages that Shake Up the World*) is the longest novel in the history of Chinese literature. Similar to its famous precursor *Jinpingmei*, this epic was written by an unknown author—this time in the fifteenth century—and tells of the dark sides of social life and moral decay in those times. From a medical viewpoint, the more than two dozen practitioners who care for the numerous ailments of main and side characters of the novel are significant. It is noteworthy that the normal hierarchies, as we find them in the *Jinpingmei* and in other sources, are reversed here. Daria Berg, who was the first to discuss this story in detail, was able to show that the eminent physicians, the *taiyi* 太醫, turn out to be charlatans. The itinerant "bell doctors," or *lingyi* 鈴醫, on the other hand, are represented as well educated, effective in their treatments, and moderate in their financial demands. For someone familiar with the social conditions in China, however, this anti-utopian nightmare, as Berg called it, only reconfirmed a century-old assessment.[142]

There is still a great need for further studies of medical statements in Chinese novel literature. It is obvious that this field has remained largely untouched. In 1977, the Dutch sinologist Wilt Idema disclosed a great number of literary works from the Chinese Imperial Age whose contents were of medical interest, but he was compelled to speak only of a "highly provisional" list.[143] The large wall separating ordinary sinology from studies of Chinese medicine has contributed to the fact that Idema's hint has so far remained without effect.


## CHINESE MEDICINE THROUGH EUROPEAN EYES


It is striking that sinology has distanced itself from a study of any cultural areas related to the natural sciences and medicine, considering that the reaction of a foreign culture to illness and premature death is central to any attempt to understanding it. Scholarship and religion, philosophy and language, social conditions, economic constraints, and other aspects also coalesce at this point. Contacts between the West and China, moreover, were already quite active in the eighteenth and nineteenth centuries. Numerous books were published in Europe that familiarized readers with the particularities of Chinese culture. Leibniz and many others were impressed by China. The exotic and foreign motifs were adopted by arts and crafts, leading to the creation of the chinoiser-style, from the kitchen tiles in the Amalienburg in Nymphenburg Park to the porcelain decors from Meissen, from snuff bottles to the wallpaper in elegant salons. This was how knowledge about Chinese medicine arrived in Europe. The first wave of enthusiasm for acupuncture had already sunk into charlatanism before sinology established a serious scientific discourse about China at the beginning of the twentieth century. A second wave of enthusiasm arose in the mid-1970s, but it took until the 1990s for sinologists to discuss the cultural and intellectual background of this phenomenon.

As deficient as the intellectual discussion of Chinese medicine is, so, too, is the pictorial documentation of past decades and centuries in this area of Chinese culture. Only a few depictions of Chinese medical practitioners have been transmitted to the West, but some familiar examples are immediately recognizable as early witnesses to a way of life whose substance is being transformed only now, at the end of the twentieth century.

Pharmacies in the Song period painting *Qingming shang-hetu* 清明上河圖 (*Up River [to the Capital] after the Spring Festival*) resembled pharmacies in China until recently (figures 24-26, 53, 54). In the same way, the depictions of itinerant doctors and drug peddlers, or of a charlatan advertising his drugs made with snake products in dramatic gestures and speeches, correspond to sights which have only begun to disappear from streets of China.

It is unfortunate that so few travelers to China retained their impression of local medical practices in drawings for transmission to Europe. The documentation presented here is therefore stimulated by the goal to secure material testi-monies from the history of Chinese medicine and to make them available for future research. The large majority of objects are items which are found by the thousands in the everyday culture of their country of origin. Everyday culture, however, is neither recognized nor valued as such in China; and it is therefore subject to almost constant change without notice. Thus, it is to be expected that these documented material remains of everyday culture will also disappear silently and irreversibly if they do not receive the attention they deserve.

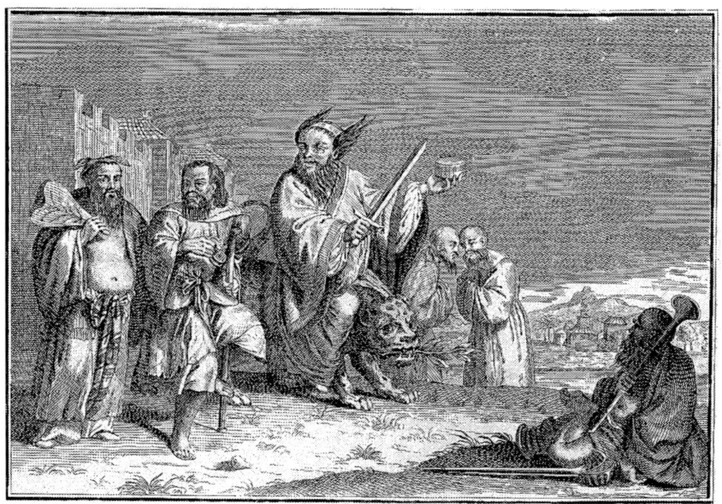

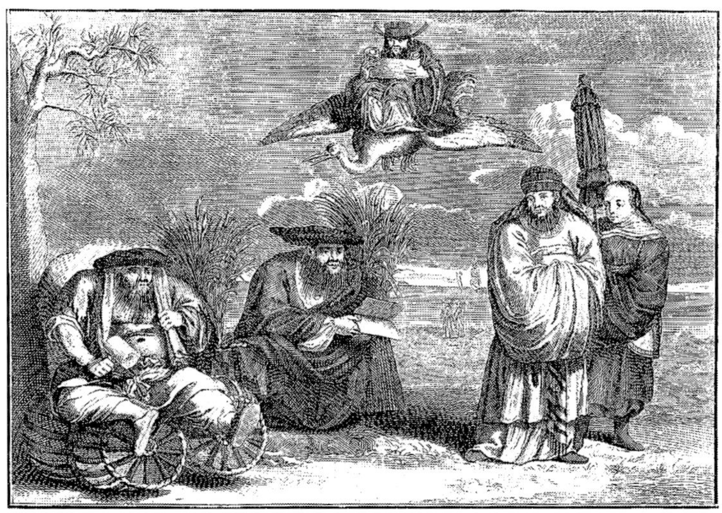

119. *Charlatans, parading around on tamed tigers*. French engraving, nineteenth century.

120. *Charlatans in China, selling the wind*. French engraving, nineteenth century.

121. *The Chinese quack*, an itinerant medicine vendor with spectacular displays. From *China, historisch, romantisch, malerisch*, Karlsruhe, nineteenth century.

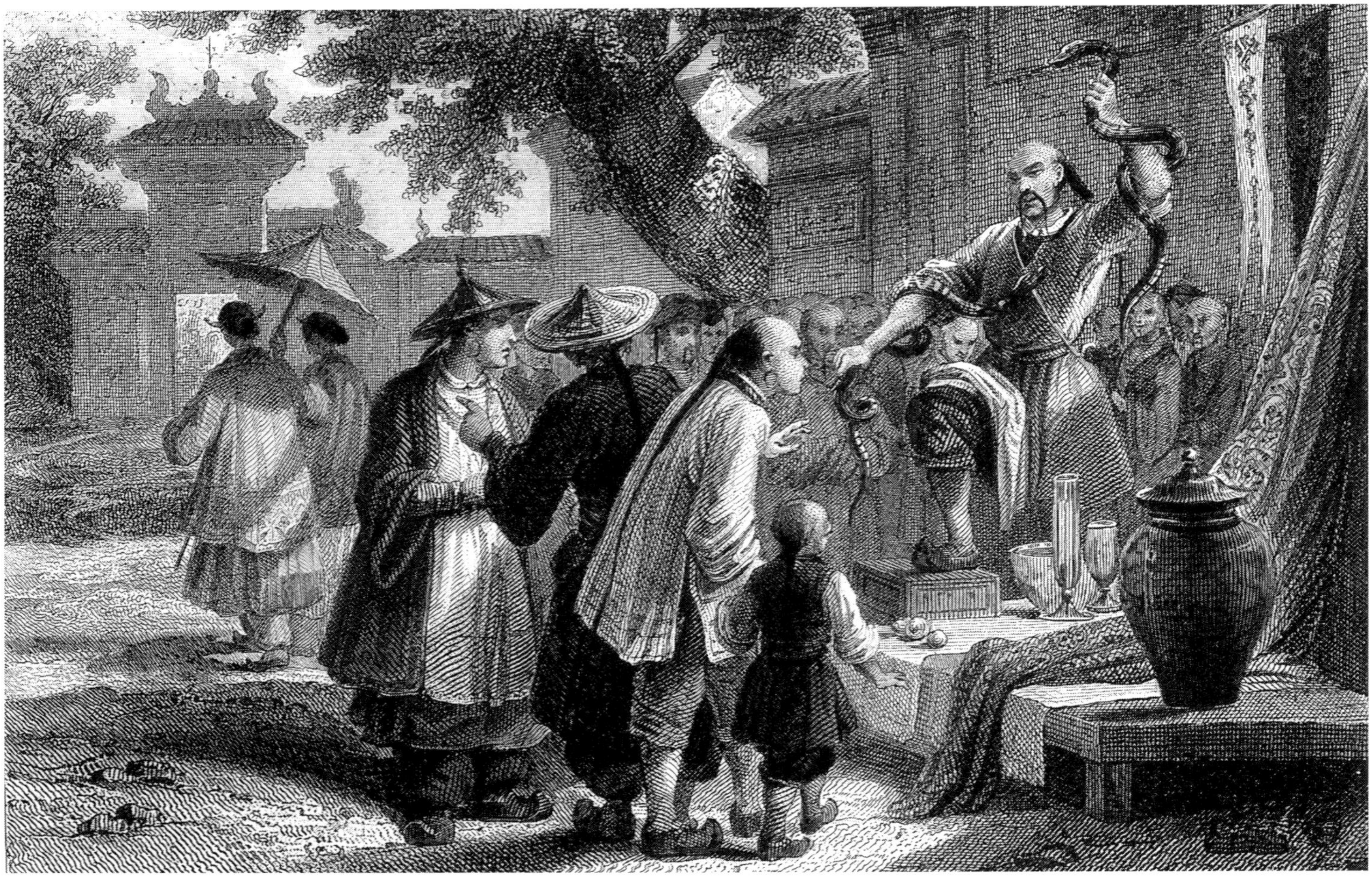

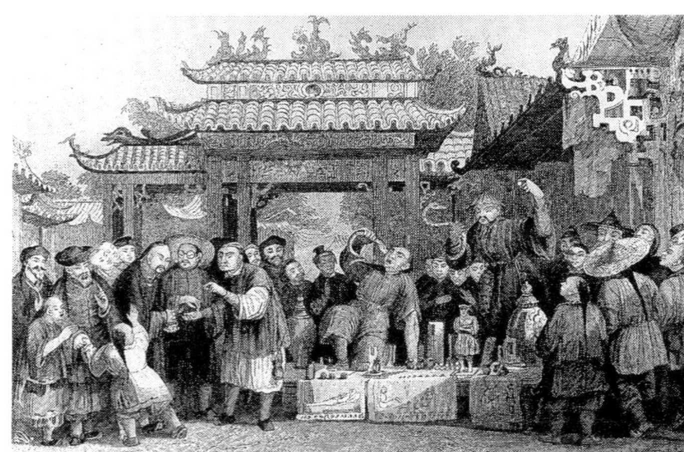

122. *China: artists and itinerant doctors*. Colored French engraving, nineteenth century.

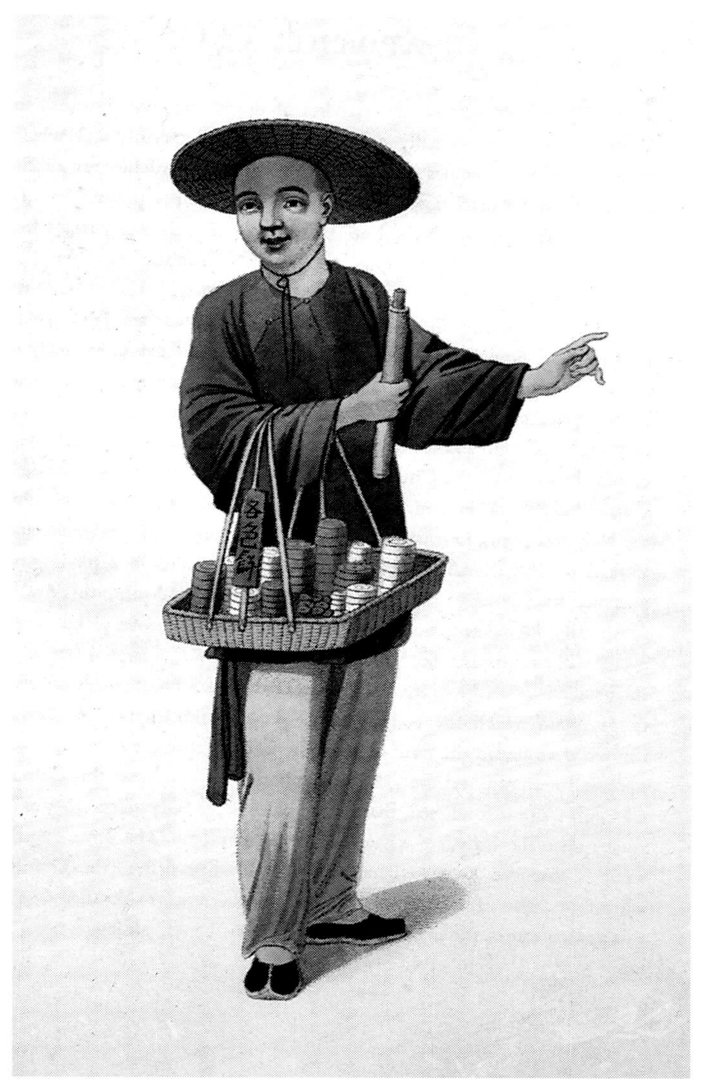

123. Drawing of a cake peddler
inadvertently identified as "An
Apothecary." Pu Qua, Canton,
published in London, May 4,
1799.

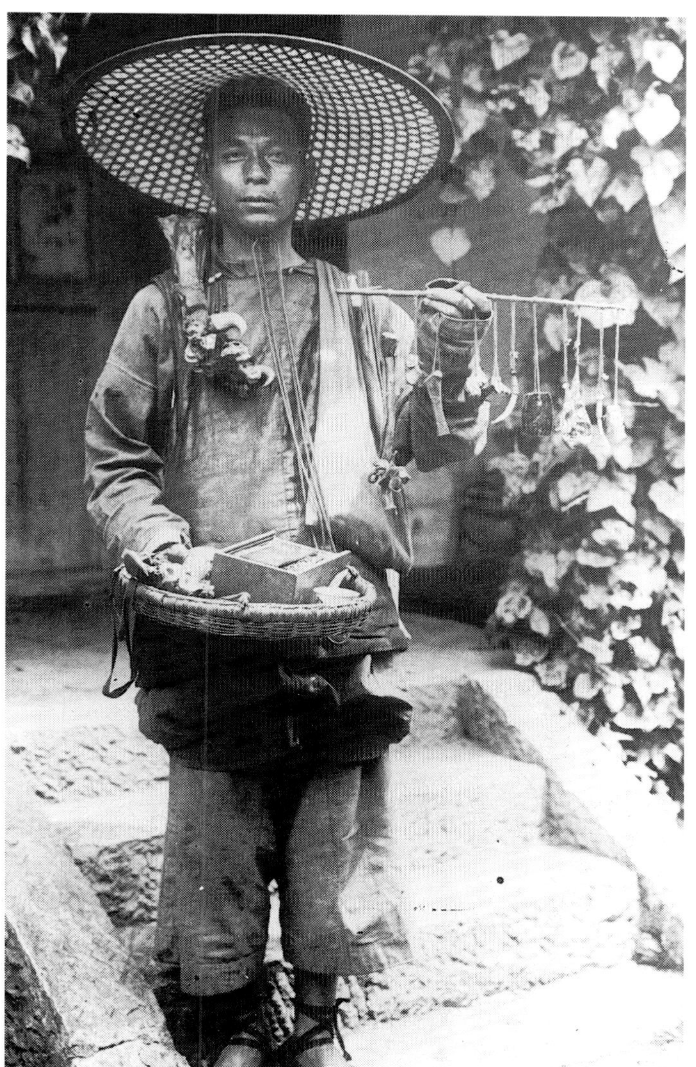

124. Itinerant doctor and medicine peddler with tiger claws,
amulets, and medicine made of
tiger parts. Yunnan, ca. 1920.

1. To be sure, reports about the peculiarities of Chinese medicine reached Europe much earlier. Initially, however, they did not suffice for conclusions about its theoretical specifics. The first known report of this kind stems from Wilhelm von Rubruk, who traveled throughout the Mongol empire from 1253 to 1255. See Wilhelm von Rubruk, *Voyage dans l'Empire Mongol*, translated from Latin by Rene Kappler (Paris: Payot, 1985) 150ff. Marco Polo's observations are also limited to merely general statements such as: "In Sugiu, one encounters many significant philosophers and famous scientists who are acquainted with the mysteries of nature." [A. C. Moule and Paul Pelliot, *Marco Polo: The Description of the World* (George Routledge and Sons, 1938)]. See also Leonardo Olschiki, *Marco Polo's Asia* (Berkeley: University of California Press, 1960), 414–432 (chapter on "Asiatic medicine in Marco Polo's book*")

2. Andreas Cleyer, *Specimen Medicinae Sinicae, Sive Opulscula Medica ad Mentem Sinensium* (Frankfurt: J.P. Zubrodt, 1682).

3. Nigel Wiseman's *Glossary of Chinese Medicine: Chinese-English, English-Chinese* (Changsha: Hunan Science and Technology Press, 1995) constitutes an important step towards a uniform way of reading and translating terms, at least for modern Chinese literature about traditional Chinese medicine.

4. For further details on the material discussed in the following sections, see Paul U. Unschuld, *Medicine in China: A History of Ideas* (Berkeley: University of California Press, 1985).

5. See also D. C. Epler, "Bloodletting in Early Chinese Medicine and Its Relation to the Origin of Acupunture," *Bulletin of the History of Medicine* 54 (1980): 337–367.

6. *Zhuangzi jicheng* 莊子集成 (Shanghai: Zhonghua shuju 上海中華書局, 1954) chapter 6, 116–119. For details, see Wolfgang Bauer, *China und die Hoffnung auf Glück* (Munich: Hanser Verlag, 1971), 70–71.

7. Xu Dachun, *Yixue yuanliulun* 徐大椿醫學源流論, 1771. Translated and commented on by Paul U. Unschuld in *Forgotten Traditions of Ancient Chinese Medicine* (Brookline, Massachusetts: Paradigm Publishing Company, 1989).

8. Volker Scheid, "Beobachtungen zur Verbindung von Chinesischer Medizin und Biomedizin in der Volksrepublik China," *ChinaMed* 4 (1994): 16–22. Thomas Ots, *Medizin und Heilung in China* (Berlin & Hamburg: Dietrich Reimer Verlag, 1987), 101 ff.

9. Donald Harper, *Early Chinese Medical Literature. The Mawangdui Medical Manuscripts* (London: Kegan Paul International, 1999)

10. Ibid. See also Paul U. Unschuld, "Die Bedeutung der Ma-wang-tui-Funde für die chinesische Medizin- und Pharmaziegeschichte (The Significance of the Mawangdui Discoveries for the History of Chinese Medicine and Pharmaceutics)" in Peter Dilg et al., ed, *Perspektiven der Pharmaziegeschichte* (*Perspectives in the History of Pharmaceutics*), Festschrift für Rudolf Schmitz zum 65. Geburtstag, (Graz: Akademische Druck- und Verlagsanstalt, 1983) 389–409.

11. Sun Simiao, *Qianjin yifang*, (Xindian: Guolizhongguo yiyao yanjiusuo 新店國立中國醫藥研究所, 1965), chapter 12,3. Paragraph "Yanglao Dali" 養老大例, 148.

12. Unschuld 1983, 409–412.

13. See Paul U. Unschuld, *Medicine in China: A History of Pharmaceutics* (Berkeley/Los Angeles/London: University of California Press, 1986).

14. Also see Okanishi Tameto, *Chongji xinxiu bencao* 岡西為人重輯新修本草 (Xindian: Guolizhongguo yiyao yanjiusuo 新店國立中國醫藥研究所, 1964).

15. The title was subsequently changed several times. The book has finally been reprinted as *Taiping huimin hejiju fang* 太平惠民和劑局方 (*Prescriptions of the Offices for the Composition of Medications for the Assistance of the Public in Great Peace*). Chen Xinqian, *Zhonghua yaoshi jinian* 陳新謙中華藥史紀年, (Beijing: Zhongguo yiyaokeji-chubanshe 北京中國醫藥科技出版社, 1994), 109.

16. Ibid., 109.

17. Zhu Yanxiu, "Jufang fahui" 朱彥俯局方發揮, in Chen Shiwen et al., *Taiping huimin hejiju fang* 陳師文太平惠民和劑局方 (Taibei: Xuanfeng Publishing Co. 臺北旋風出版社, 1975), appendix, 1.

18. David Joseph Keegan, *The 'Huang-Ti Nei-Ching': The Structure of the Compilation, the Significance of the Compilation*. Dissertation, 1988. UMI Dissertation Services Order Number 8916728. Nathan Sivin, "Huang ti nei ching", in Michael Loewe, ed., *Early Chinese Texts: A Bibliographical Guide* (Berkeley/Los Angeles/London: University of California Press, 1993), 196–215.

19. Yamada Keiji, "Kyu-ku hachi-fu setsu to shoshiha no tachiba 山田慶兒九宮八風説と少師派の立場 (The Nine-Palaces/Eight-Winds Theories and the Position of the Shao-shih School)" in *Tōho gakuho* 東方學報 52 (1980): 199–242. Also see Paul U. Unschuld, "Der Wind als Ursache des Krankseins. Einige Gedanken zu Yamada Keijis Analyse der Shao-shih-Texte des Huang-ti nei-ching (Wind as a Cause of Illness: Some Thoughts on Yamada Keiji's Analysis of the Shao-shih texts of the Huang-ti nei-ching)," *T'oung Pao* 68 (1982): 92–131.

20. Donald Harper, "The Conception of Illness in Early Chinese Medicine, as Documented in Newly Discovered 3rd and 2nd Century B.C. Manuscripts," *Sudhoffs Archiv* 74 (1990): part 1, 211–235.

21. The ancient Chinese physicians were like the natural philosophers of Greek antiquity, convinced that besides blood an invisible, vapor-like agent existed that was responsible for maintaining life and health in the body. The term qi that was chosen to refer to this agent was signified by a character composed of the two parts "steam" and "rice." It therefore corresponded to the expression *physai ek ton perittomaton* from ancient Greek texts, i.e. "vapors from left-over food." Manfred Kubny offers a comprehensive presentation of the early history of the multiple meanings of qi by Chinese philosophers and physicians in his *Qi. Lebenskraftkonzepte in China. Definitionen, Theorien, Grundlagen* (*Qi. Conceptions of Life Force in China. Definitions, Theories, Foundations*) (Heidelberg: Haug-Verlag, 1995).

22. *Nan-ching: The Classic of Difficult Issues*, translated and with 20 commentaries of Chinese and Japanese authors by Paul U. Unschuld (Berkeley/Los Angeles/London: University of California Press, 1986).

23. Ynez Violë O'Neill and Gerald L. Chan, "A Chinese Coroner's Manual and the Evolution of Anatomy," *Journal of the History of Medicine and Allied Sciences* 31 (1976): 3–16. Brian McKnight, *The Washing Away of Wrongs* (Ann Arbor: Center for

Chinese Studies [The University of Michigan], 1981).

24. Jürgen Kovacs and Paul U. Unschuld, *Essential Subtleties on the Silver Sea. The "Yinhai jingwei" Translated and Annotated* (Berkeley/Los Angeles/London: University of California Press, 1995).

25. The bibliography of the dynastic histories of the Han period mentions a formulary whose title refers specifically to the illnesses of women and children: *Furen Ying'er Fang* 婦人嬰兒方 (*Formulas for Women and Infants*) in 19 chapters. See also Barbara Volkmar, "Die Frauen-heilkunde der chinesischen Medizin (Gynecology in Chinese Medicine)," *Gynäkologie* 27 (1994): 396–402. On the history of Chinese pediatrics, B.Volkmar, medical dissertation, Freiburg 1985

26. Thomas Kuhn, *The Structure of Scientific Revolutions* (Chicago: University Press, 1965). Ludwik Fleck, *Genesis and Development of a Scientific Fact.* (Chicago: University Press, 1979).

27. Unschuld 1980, 159–175.

28. For an example in the Ming period see "Drugs Resemble Soldiers" in Zhuang Zhongfu, *Shuyizi neipan* 莊忠甫叔苴子內篇 quoted in Liu Daoqing and Zhou Yimou, *Zhongyimingyan dacidian* 劉道清周一謀中醫名言大辭典 (*Dictionary of Famous Quotes in Chinese Medicine*) (Zhongyuan nongmin chubanshe 中原農民出版社, 1991), 851. For the Qing period, see Xu Dachun and Paul U. Unschuld, 1989, 24 f., 183 f. For the twentieth century, see Yu Fengba, "Yong yao ru yong bing lun 用藥如用兵論" in Mao Jingyi, *Zhongxi yihua* 毛景義中西醫話 (Jiangdong: Maojishuju 江東茂記書局, 1922), chapter 3, 22b.

29. Paul U. Unschuld, "Das Ch'uan-ya und die Praxis chinesischer Landärzte im 18. Jh. (The Ch'uan-ya and the Practice of Chinese Country Physicians in the 18th Century)," *Sudhoffs Archiv* 62 (1978): 378–407.

30. Ursula Holler, "*Taixi renshen shuogai* - ein anatomischer Text aus dem China des frühen 17. Jh. (*Taixi renshen shuogai*: An Anatomical Text from the China of the Early Seventeenth Century)," *ChinaMed* 2 (1993): 61–62.

31. Benjamin Hobson, *Xiyi luelun* 西醫略論 (Survey of Western Medicine), (Shanghai: Renji yiguan 上海人濟醫館, 1857), 1b–2b.

32. H.T.Whitney, *Gray's Anatomy—Descriptive and Surgical*, preface to the second edition (Foochow: American Board Mission, 1889).

33. Li Jingwei 李經緯, et al., *Zhongyirenwucidian* 中醫人物詞典 (*Dictionary of Personages in Chinese Medicine*), (Shanghai: Shanghaicishu chubanshe 上海辭書出版社, 1988), 532–533.

34. Compare Paul U. Unschuld, "Epistemological Issues and Changing Legitimation: Traditional Chinese Medicine in the Twentieth Century" in Charles Leslie and Allen Young, eds., *Paths to Asian Medical Knowledge* (Berkeley/Los Angeles/London: The University of California Press, 1992), 44–61.

35. Margarete Stössl, "Vom glorreichen Gegengift. Ein Abriss zum venezianischen Theriak-monopol zwischen Legalität und Scharlatanerie. (The Glorious Detoxicant: An Outline of the Venecian Theriaca Monopoly between Legality and Quackery)," Helge Gerndt, et al., eds., *Dona Ethnologica Monacensia* (Munich: Münchner Beiträge zur Volks-kunde, 1983), 181–206.

36. Jonathan Spence, "Das Opiumrauchen im China der Ch'ing-Zeit (Opium Smoking in China During the Ch'ing Period)," *Saeculum* 23 (1972): 397–425.

37. Li Shizhen, *Bencao gang mu* 李時珍本草綱目 (Shanghai: Shangwuchubanshe 上海商物出版社, 1933), 87–88.

38. K. Chimin Wong and Wu Lien-teh, *History of Chinese Medicine*, 2nd edition (Shanghai: National Quarantine Service, 1936), 117 f.

39. Ibid., 115 f.

40. Dan Bensky, and Andrew Gamble, eds. and trans., with Ted Kaptchuk, *Chinese Herbal Medicine. Materia Medica*, revised edition (Seattle: Eastland Press, Inc., 1993), 322–324. The current experimental use of *Glycyrrhiza uralensis Fisch.* for the treatment of AIDS by Chinese doctors is based on the same traditional indication of detoxification. See "Arzneipflanzen der TCM gegen AIDS (Medicinal Plants of Traditional Chinese Medicine Against AIDS)," *ChinaMed* 4 (1994): 11 f.

41. Fu Weikang, *Zhongguo yixueshi* 傅維康中國醫學史 (*History of Medicine in China*) (Shanghai: Shanghai zhongyi-xueyuan chubanshe 上海中醫學院出版社, 1990), 120–122.

42. Ibid., 14–17.

43. Ibid., 17.

44. Chen Xinqian and Zhang Tianlu, *Zhongguo jindai yaoxueshi* 陳新謙張天祿中國近代藥學史 (*History of Medicine in China in the Modern Period*) (Beijing: Renminweisheng chubanshe 北京人民衛生出版社, 1992), 63.

45. Ibid.

46. Ibid.

47. Charles O. Hucker, *A Dictionary of Official Titles in Imperial China* (Stanford: Stanford University Press, 1985), 413, 594 f.

48. Chen Xinqian and Zhang Tianlu 1992, 64.

49. See also Paul U. Unschuld, "Die Trennung von Pharmazie und Medizin. Zur Geschichte der Pharmazie in China zur Zeit der Nördlichen Sung (960–1126). (The Separation of Pharmaceutics and Medicine. On the History of Pharmaceutics in China during the Northern Sung Period)," *Pharmazeutische Zeitung* 116 (1971): 1426–1432.

50. Ma Jixing 馬繼興, "Songdaide minyingyaoshang 宋代的民營藥商," *Zhongguo yaoxue zazhi* 中國藥學雜志 27 (1992): 1–7.

51. Zhao Zhongzhen 趙中振 and Tang Xiaojun 唐曉軍, "Qingdai 'Beijing minsu baitu' zhong yiyao yishi kao 清代北京民俗百圖中醫藥逸史考 (Investigation of the Medical-Pharmaceutical Anecdotes in the Qing period 'One Hundred Illustrations of Popular Customs in Beijing')," *Zhongguo yaoxue zazhi* 中國藥學雜志 27 (1992): 24.

52. Ma Jixing 1992, 2.

53. John Byron, *Portrait of a Chinese Paradise: Erotica and Sexual Customs* (London: Quartet Books Ltd., 1987), 28.

54. Ibid., 73.

55. Ibid., 69.

56. Ibid., 73.

57. "Wind" as a cause of illness is already attested to on Chinese oracle bones from the Shang period ca. 1200 B.C.E. The concept of wind also played a significant etiological role in the medicine of the Imperial period. "Being hit by wind" is today the terminological equivalent of the English term "stroke"; "wind dampness" is still a technical term for a complex of symptoms which includes primarily rheumatic problems. Compare Paul U. Unschuld, "Der Wind als Ursache des Krankseins (Wind as the Cause of Illness)" in *T'oung-Pao* 68 (1982), 91–131.

58. The Chinese term *lou jian feng* 漏肩風 means literally "wind flowing through the shoulder."

59. The translation of the names of the conduit openings from acupuncture is literal here, but their meanings are frequently not clear. They could be Chinese transliterations of originally non-Chinese terms.

60. Term for the condition in which the leg's girth is greatly reduced above and below the knee, while the knee itself is swollen.

61. Paul U. Unschuld, "Arzneimittelwebung und Theoriebezug in der tradi-tionellen chinesischen Medizin am Beispiel der Punktsalben (Drug Advertising and its Rela-

tion to Theory in Traditional Chinese Medicine, Illustrated by Tropical Ointments)," *ChinaMed* 3 (1994): 38-44.

62. Hans Vogel, *China ohne Maske. 20 000 km mit der schweizerischen Filmexpedition* (China Unmasked: 20,000 km with the Swiss Film Expedition) (Zürich/Leibzig: Albert Müller Verlag, 1937), 146.

63. See also Paul U. Unschuld, "Alte Werbetafeln japanischer Apotheken. Spiegelbilder chinesischer und westlicher Heilkunde (Old Advertising Boards of Japanese Pharmacies: Mirrors of Chinese and Western Medicine)," *Jahrbuch des Deutschen Medizinhistorischen Museums* 4 (1983): 101–107.

64. Paul U. Unschuld, *Medical Ethics in Imperial China. A Study in Historical Anthropology* (Berkeley, Los Angeles: Univ. of California Press, 1979)

65. Fu Weikang 1990, 218 ff.

66. Paul U. Unschuld, "Arzneimittelmissbrauch und heterodoxe Heiltätigkeit im kaiserlichen China (Medical Drug Misuse and Heterodox Medical Practice in Imperial China)," *Sudhoffs Archiv* 61 (1977): 353–386.

67. *Zhouli zhushu ji buzheng* 周禮注疏及補正 (Taibei: Shijieshuju 臺北世界書局, 1969), ch. 5. "Tianguan xia 天官下," Ia.

68. Joseph Needham, "China and the Origin of Qualifying Examinations in Medicine" in *Clerks and Craftsmen in China and the West*, (Cambridge: Cambridge University Press, 1970), 380 ff.

69. Hucker 1985, 478 f.

70. Sima Qian, *Shiji* 司馬遷史記, chapter 105, *Bian Que Canggong liezhuan* 扁鵲倉公列傳 (The Biographies of Bian Que and Canggong) (Hongkong: Zhonghua shuju 中華書局, 1969), 2793.

71. Ibid.

72. Wang Hongtu, "Cong fangyao jiajian kan Zhang Zhongjing dui 'Neijing' de jichen he fazhan 王洪圖從方藥加減看張仲景對內經的繼承和發展 (Zhang Zhongjing's Advancement and Development of the Neijing As Seen in the Increase or Reduction of Formula [Components])," *Zhejiang zhongyixueyuan xuebao* 浙江中醫學院學報 4 (1983): 1 ff.

73. Fu Weikang 1990, 178.

74. Needham 1970, 390.

75. Fu Weikang 1990, 220 f. and Joseph Needham 1970, 391.

76. See also Wu Yiyi, "A Medical Line of Many Masters: A Prosopographical Study of Liu Wansu and His Disciples from the Jin to the Early Ming," *Chinese Science* 11 (1993–94): 36–65.

77. Volker Scheid, "Meister, Lehrlinge, Lehrer und Studenten: Zur Wissensvermittlung in der chinesischen Medizin (Masters, Apprentices, Teachers, and Students: The Transfer of Knowledge in Chinese Medicine)," *ChinaMed* 5 (1995): 38–44.

78. Unschuld 1977, 360.

79. Sima Qian 1969.

80. Sun Simiao, *Beiji qianjin yaofang* 孫思邈備急千金藥方 (Xindian: Guolizhongguo yiyaoyanjiusuo 新店國立中國醫藥研究所, 1965), 1 f.

81. Robert P. Hymes, "Not Quite Gentlemen? Doctors in Song and Yuan," *Chinese Science* 8 (1987): 9–76.

82. Huang Di and Qibo are regarded as the ancestors of the tradition of Chinese medicine that is based on the yin-yang and Five Phases theory of systematic correspondence. Substantial parts of the *Huang Di neijing* are structured as dialogues between the mythological ruler Huang Di and a medical advisor of unclear origin called Qibo.

83. Xu Yanzuo, *Yicuijingyan* 徐延祚醫粹精言 (Guangzhou: Tieruyixuan 廣州鐵如意軒, 1896), 56b, 58b–60a, 61a, 63b–64a.

84. Mercedes-Andrea Riegel, "Theorie und Praxis der TCM im heutigen Taiwan (Theory and Practice of TCM in modern Taiwan)," *ChinaMed* 2 (1993): 25–30.

85. The concept of the *sha* disease has no equivalent in Western medicine and cannot be translated with a single term into English; the term *sha* 痧 refers to alternating cold and hot spells, pain and pressure in the head, breast, or stomach regions, as well as dizziness, vomiting, diarrhea, and other problems.

86. This refers to pulse diagnosis.

87. Xu Dachun and Paul U. Unschuld 1989, 242 ff. For information on the declining interest in acupuncture in China since at least the Ming dynasty, see also Christopher Cullen, "Patients and Healers in Late Imperial China: Evidence from the *Jinpingmei*," *History of Science* 31 (1993): 120, 137.

88. *Tongzhi tiaoge* 通制條格 (Regulations Throughout [the Centuries] in Individual Paragraphs) (Beijing: n.p. 1930), chap. 21, 7a–7b. See also Unschuld 1977, 360.

89. For a complete translation of this document, see Paul U. Unschuld, "Der chinesische Wanderarzt und seine Klientel im 19. Jh. Rekonstruktion eines Dialogs (The Chinese Itinerant Doctor and His Clientele in the Nineteenth Century: Reconstruction of a Dialogue)" in Helwig Schmidt-Glintzer, ed., *Das andere China* (The Other China). Festschrift für Wolfgang Bauer zum 65. Geburtstag, Wolfenbütteler Forschungen, Vol. 62. (Wiesbaden: Harrassowitz Verlag, 1995), 129–157.

90. For an alternative interpretation, see caption to figure 85.

91. Unschuld 1977, passim.

92. Xue Mo, *Jianghu neimu heihuakao* 雪漠江湖內幕黑話考 (Study of the Internal Secret Language of the Wandering Professions), (Shanghai: Wenyi chubanshe 上海文藝出版社, 1991), 31 ff. To compare the methods of the related professions of barkers and medicine swindlers in Europe, see Tomaso Garzoni di Bagnacauallo, *Piazza Universale, das ist: Allgemeiner Schauwplatz / oder Marckt / und Zusammenkunfft aller Professionen … (Universal Scene / or Market / or Congregation of All Profession…)*, (Frankfurt/Main, 1619).

93. Xue Mo 1991, 34 f.

94. Ots 1987, 155 ff., 189.

95. Ma Jixing, *Zhenjiutongren yu tongrenxuefa* 馬繼興針灸銅人與銅人穴法 (The Bronze Acupuncture Figure and the Arrangement of the Insertion Points on the Bronze Figure) (Beijing: Zhongguo zhongyiyao chubanshe 北京中國中醫藥出版社, 1993), 5 ff.

96. A different source mentions "mercury."

97. In order to find the insertion points that were situated proportionally closer or further apart in thinner or larger persons, the "individually standardized inch measure" served as the standard. Chinese acupuncture teaches that the length of the middle joint of the bent middle finger is longer or shorter in proportion to the body girth. It is therefore suited as the individual standardized body measurement in order to find the relative distances between the insertion points on the surface of the body.

98. Fu Weikang 1990, 259. Compare also Lu Gwei-djen and Joseph Needham, *A History and Rationale of Acupuncture and Moxibustion*, (Cambridge: Cambridge University Press, 1980), 131 f.

99. Nathan Sivin, *Chinese Alchemy. Preliminary Studies*, (Cambridge, Mass.: Harvard University Press, 1968).

100. Ibid., 144.

101. Unschuld 1980, 40 f.

102. Sivin 1968.

103. Jürgen Kovacs and Paul U. Unschuld, 1995.

104. Ma Kanwen et al., "Tangdai mingyi Sun Simiao guli diaochaji 馬堪溫唐代名醫孫思邈故里調查記 (Records of an Inspection of the Home of the Famous Tang Dynasty Physician Sun Simiao)," *Zhonghua yishizazhi* 中華醫史雜志 (1954), 253–257.

105. An Yumin, "Yaoxian yaowangshan jianjie 安玉民 耀縣藥王山簡解 (Brief Comments to the Medicine King Mountain in Yaoxian)," *Zhonghua yishizazhi* 中華醫史雜志 (1989), 109–111.

106. Anon., *Shaanxi zhongyi shihua* 陝西中醫史話 (*About the History of Chinese Medicine in Shaanxi Province*), (Xi'an: 1987), 103.

107. Anon., "Sun Simiao guli jinian jianzhu xianzhuang ji yange 孫思邈故里紀念建 築現狀及沿革 (The Current Condition and Historical Development of Memorials in the Home of Sun Simiao)," *Zhonghua yishizazhi* 中華醫史 雜志 (1981): 205–207. See also anon., *Yaowang Sun Simiao* 藥王 孫思邈 (*The Medicine King Sun Simiao*), (Xi'an: 1990).

108. Paul U. Unschuld, "Arzneigott und Zement (Medicine God and Concrete)," *ChinaMed* 4 (1994): 41–44.

109. This is not comprehensible as a place name (Shang xian yi du 上賢一都). It might be a formulaic expression since similar formulations are used in many of the investigated petition and donation slips.

110. Allusion to an occurence, supposedly from the Han dynasty, which is recorded in the *Biographies of Mountain Recluses* (*Liexianzhuan* 列仙傳, second chapter). In it, a hermit called Su 蘇 predicted an epidemic for the coming year (to his mother before leaving her house). He claimed that she could protect herself with a simple recipe prepared from the water from the well in her courtyard and from the leaves of the orange tree.

111. Allusion to the apricot forest that was, according to tradition, created by an immortal healer called Dong Feng 董奉 from the state of Wu in the third century C.E. Dong Feng refrained from billing his patients and, instead, asked those with serious illnesses to place five apricot stones in the ground after being cured and those with less serious illnesses to plant one. After several years, a forest with hundreds of thousands of apricot trees had grown. Compare Ge Hong, *Shenxianzhuan* 葛洪神 仙轉 (*Biographies of Spirits and Recluses*), tenth chapter. Also, Gertrud Güntsch, *Das Shen-hsien chuan und das Erscheinungsbild eines Hsien* (*The Shen-hsien chuan and the Appearance of a Hsien*). Würzburger Sino-Japonica 16. (Frankfurt/Main/Bern/New York/Paris: Lang, 1988), 198.

112. The reference to the southeastern province of Jiangxi is incomprehensible, since there are no indications that the historical Sun Simiao, who came from Northern China, ever spent time in this region. Maybe the leaflets that were reproduced with this block were sold in Jiangxi, in which case the reference to Jiangxi suggested a particular affinity of the "Medicine King" to the residents of this province.

113. See anon., 1990, 58.

114. Li Guangdi, ed., *Zhuzi quanshu* 李光地朱子全書 (*Master Zhu [Xi's] Collected Works*), (Hongdaotang 宏道堂, 1714), chapter 19, 23a. See also Unschuld 1975, 27 ff.

115. Liu Dunyuan, "Han huaxiangshishangde zhenjiutu 劉 敦願 漢畫像石上的針灸圖 (Depictions of Acupuncture in Han Reliefs)," *Wenwu* 文物 (1972): 47–51.

116. Kano Yoshimitsu, "Isho ni mieru kiron" 加納喜光醫書 に見える氣論 in: Onozawa Seiichi et al., eds., *Ki no shiso* 小 野澤精氣の思想 (*The Concept of Qi*), (Tokyo: Tokyo University Press, 1980), 284 ff.

117. Petra Klose, *Der Shuilu-Ritus und seine Bilder* (*The Shuilu Ritual and its Depictions*). Dissertation, (Heidelberg: 1992).

118. Kongzi, *Lunyu* 孔子論 語, book X, chapter 11.

119. See Robert Herrlinger, *Geschichte der medizinischen Abbildung* (*History of Medical Illustrations*): "The medical illustration is also part of art history. All doubts that this, on the other hand, is part of intellectual history have been dispelled long ago." (Munich: Heinz Moos Verlag, 1967), 7.

120. Ibid., 9–28.

121. *Huang Di hamajing* 黃帝 蝦蟆經, (Beijing: Zhongyiguji chubanshe 北京中醫古籍出 版社, 1984). See Ma Jixing, *Zhongyiwenxianxue jichu* 馬繼興 中醫文獻學基礎 (*Foundations of the Literary Studies of Chinese Medicine*), (Shanghai: Shanghai kexue jishu chubanshe 上海科 學技術出版社, 1990), 300. Also see Lu Gwei-djen and Joseph Needham 1980, 120. Detailed quotations from the "Frog Classic" in *Ishinpo* 醫心 方, chapter 2.

122. Karl Sudhoff, *Kurzes Handbuch der Geschichte der Medizin* (*Short Handbook of the History of Medicine*) (Vienna: Karger-Verlag, 1922), 129.

123. Herrlinger 1967, 10 ff.

124. Guo Shiyu, *Zhongguo zhenjiushi* 郭世余中國針灸史 (*History of Acupuncture in China*), (Tianjin: Tianjin kexuejishu chubanshe 天津科學技術出 版社, 1989), 62 ff. Also see Lu Gwei-djen and Joseph Needham 1980, 120, annotation g: "A text with the abbreviated title, almost impossible to date, is still allegedly extant in Japan."

125. E.T. C. Werner, *Myths & Legends of China*, (London: George G. Harrap & Co. Ltd., 1958), 184–188. Also see Werner, *A Dictionary of Chinese Mythology* (New York: The Julian Press, Inc., 1969), 43, 320.

126. Herrlinger 1967, 30.

127. Ibid., 118 ff. Lu Gwei-djen and Joseph Needham 1980, 128.

128. Unschuld 1986, 48.

129. Zheng Jinsheng, "The Collation and Annotation of the Rare Book *Lü Chanyan Bencao*: A Medical Literature Research Project" in Paul U. Unschuld, ed., *Approaches to Traditional Chinese Medical Literature*, (Dordrecht: Kluwer Academic Publishers, 1989), 29–40.

130. Unschuld 1986, 128 ff.

131. Ralph Croizier, *Traditional Medicine in Modern China: Science, Nationalism, and the Tensions of Cultural Change*, (Cambridge, Mass.: Harvard University Press, 1968), 72.

132. Ibid., 73.

133. Ibid.

134. Ibid.

135. Ibid., 74.

136. Stephen H. West and Wilt L. Idema, eds., *The Moon and the Zither: The Story of the Western Wing* (by Wang Shifu), (Berkeley/ Los Angeles/Oxford: University of California Press, 1991), 417–428.

137. Chinese 醫不三世不服 其藥.

138. Yoshimoto Akiharu (Shoji), "Jinpingmei ni miru chugokuyigaku 金瓶梅にみる 中國醫學 (References to Chinese Medicine in the Jinpingmei)," in *Nihon yishigakuzasshi* 日本醫史學雜志 (1992), 133–163. Ibid., *Jinpingmei to dokyoyigaku* 金瓶梅と道教醫 學 (*The Jinpingmei and Daoist Medicine*), 36–52. Christopher Cullen 1993, 99–150.

139. Daria Berg, *The Xingshi yinyuan zhuan: A Study of Utopia and the Perception of the World in Seventeenth Century Chinese Discourse*. Dissertation, (University of Oxford, 1994).

140. Cullen 1993, 121.

141. Ibid., 110.

142. Berg 1994, 107–112.

143. Wilt L.Idema, "Diseases and Doctors, Drugs and Cures: A Very Preliminary List of Passages of Medical Interest in a Number of Traditional Chinese Novels And Related Plays," *Chinese Science* II (1977), 37–63.

# Plates

The approximately thirteen thousand texts about traditional Chinese medicine, that are still preserved and date from the second century B.C.E. through the end of the Imperial period, are impressive because of their diverse contents and the wide spectrum of information. Only a small number of these texts has so far been evaluated for content or translated into Western languages in a philologically exacting fashion. Therefore, a thorough comparison to Western medical literature, in terms of size or content, from the past two millennia is not yet possible.

Extensive bibliographical catalogues from the earliest time permit what appears to be an almost complete overview of the titles and locations of the antique texts that are available in printed form. Medical literature in manuscript form, however, has yet to receive sufficient attention either inside or outside of China. The printing technology in China has such a long tradition that it seems as if, for centuries, every significant work has found a publisher. Many manuscripts are, in fact, copies of already published texts by readers who could not afford to purchase them. In addition, uncounted manuscripts exist that were not printed for a variety of reasons. Secret knowledge has been highly relevant in China until the present and contributes to the status of a doctor of traditional medicine.

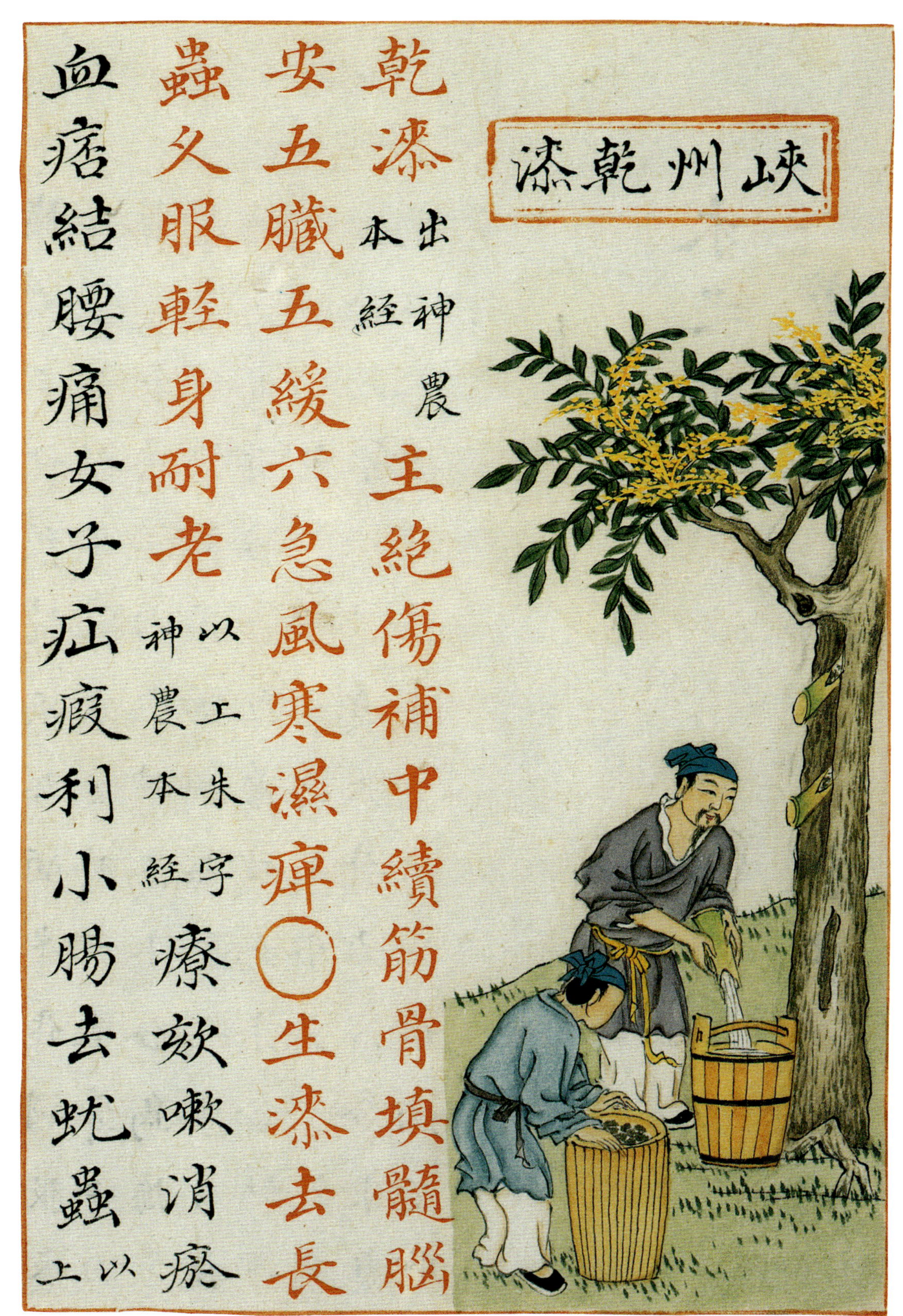



1. The production of lacquer from the juice of certain trees and the beginning of the description of the drug *xiazhou ganzi* (dried lacquer from Xiazhou). From *Yuzhi bencao pinhui jingyao* 御製本草品彙經要 (*Materia Medica Written on Imperial Orders, Containing the Essential and Important in Classified Order*), 1505. Identical copy of the original, created in the nineteenth century or earlier. Staatsbibliothek, Berlin.

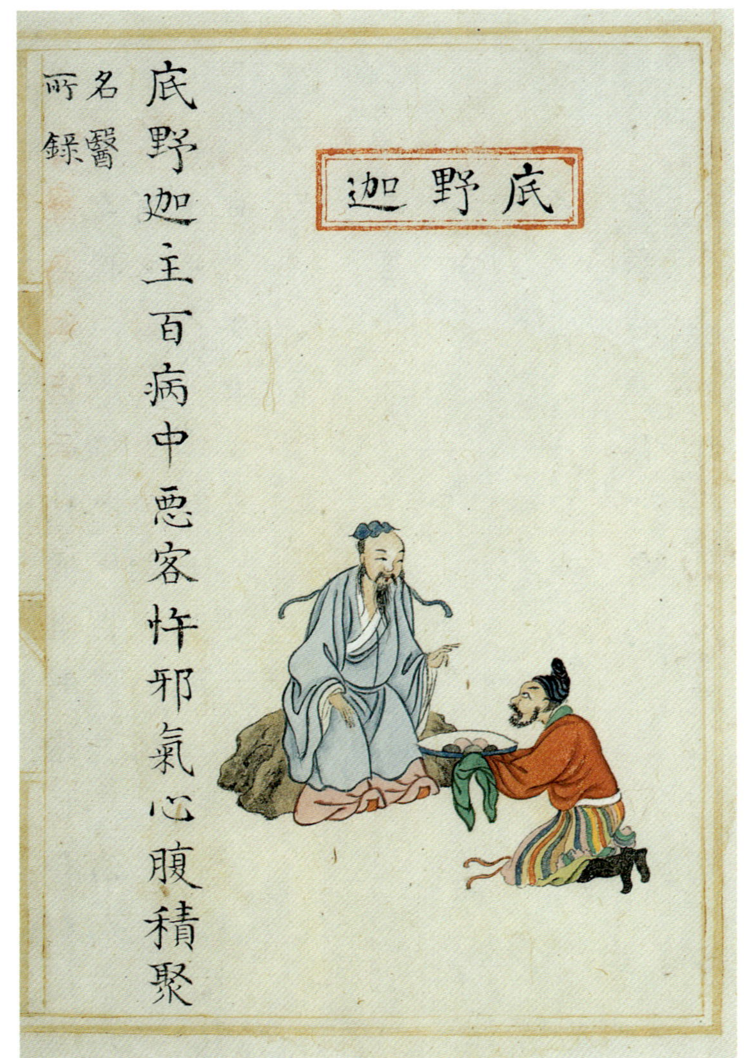



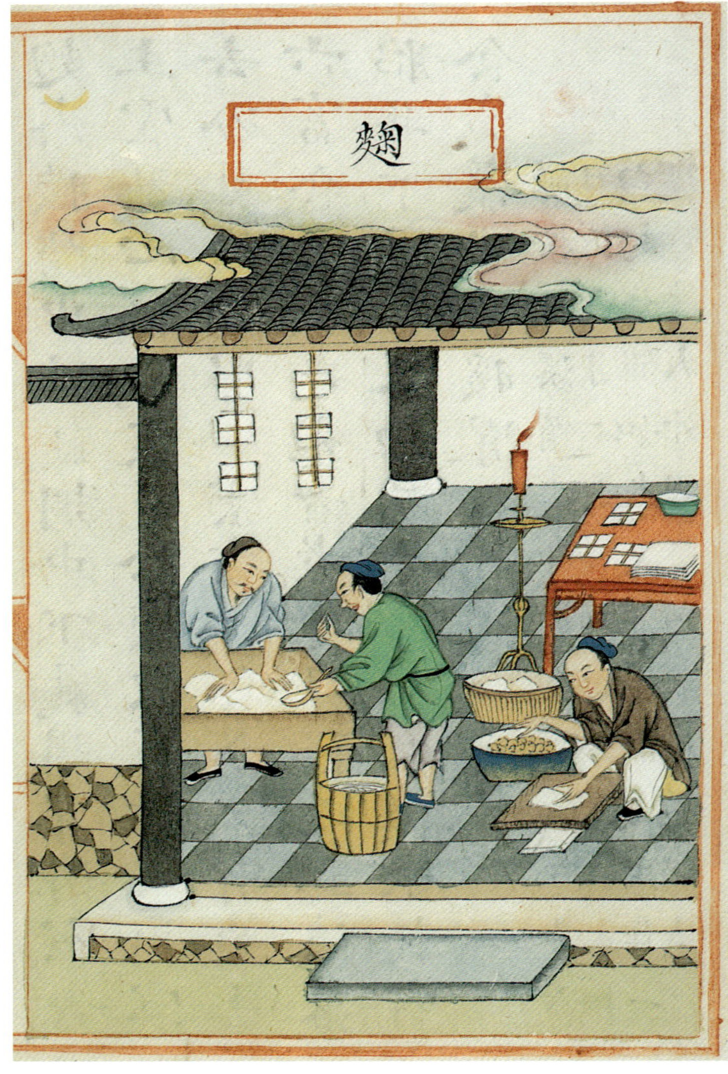



2. A foreigner presents a bowl of *diyejia* (theriaca) to a Chinese. From *Yuzhi bencao pinhui jingyao* 御製本草品彙經要 (*Materia Medica Written on Imperial Orders, Containing the Essential and Important in Classified Order*), 1505. Identical copy of the original, nineteenth century or earlier. Staatsbibliothek, Berlin.

3. The production of yeast. From *Yuzhi bencao pinhui jingyao* 御製本草品彙經要 (*Materia Medica Written on Imperial Orders, Containing the Essential and Important in Classified Order*), 1505. Identical copy of the original, nineteenth century or earlier. Staatsbibliothek, Berlin.

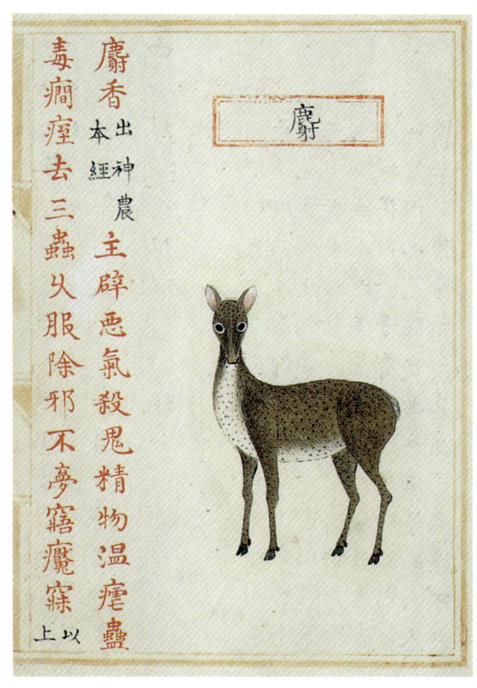


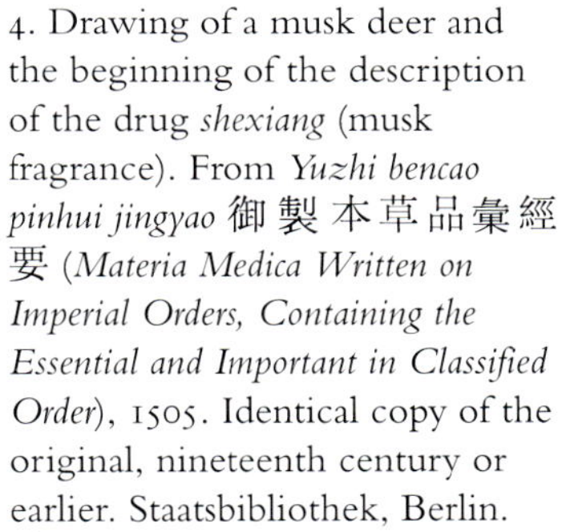

4. Drawing of a musk deer and the beginning of the description of the drug *shexiang* (musk fragrance). From *Yuzhi bencao pinhui jingyao* 御製本草品彙經要 (*Materia Medica Written on Imperial Orders, Containing the Essential and Important in Classified Order*), 1505. Identical copy of the original, nineteenth century or earlier. Staatsbibliothek, Berlin.

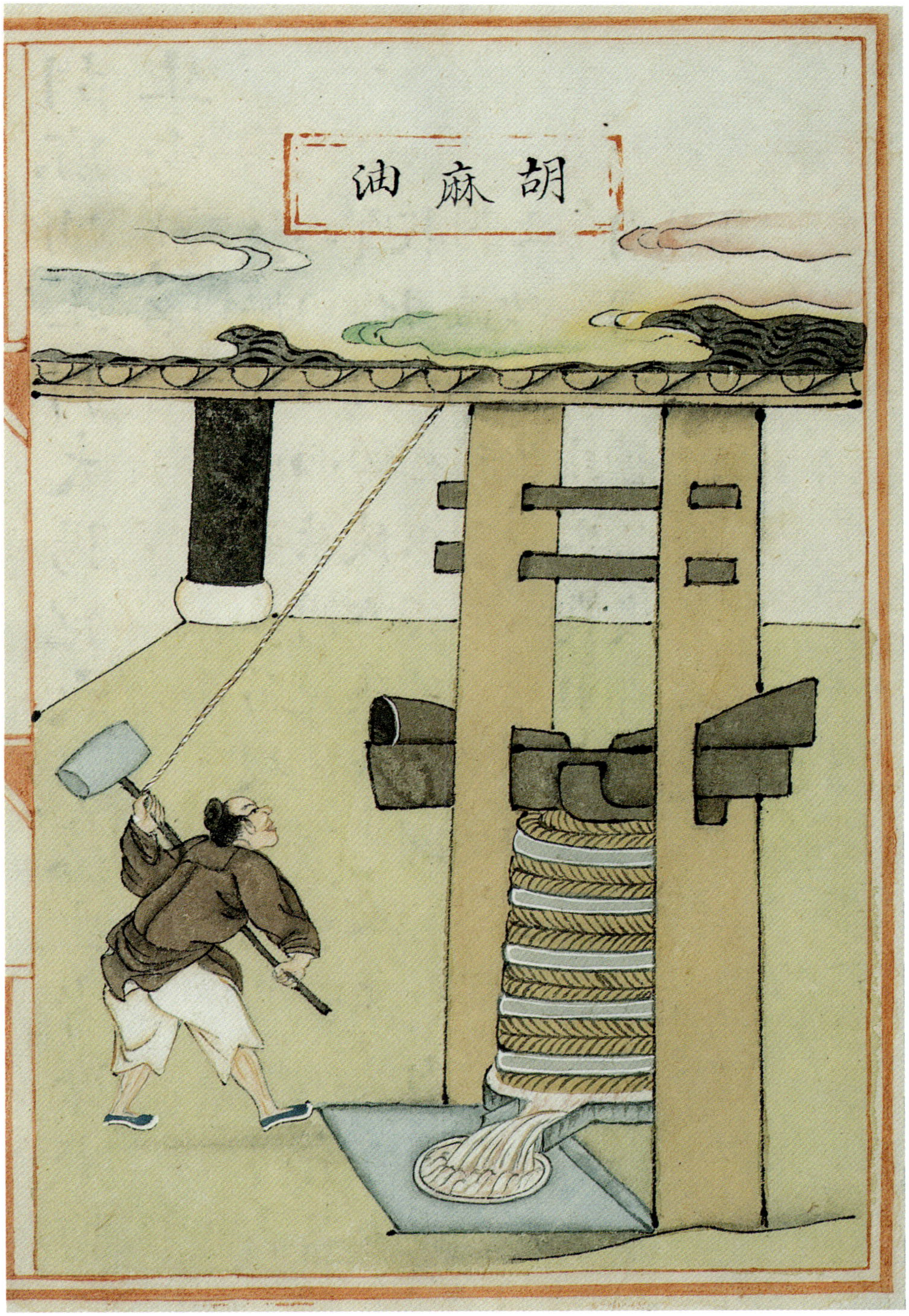

5. The production of sesame oil in a press. From *Yuzhi bencao pinhui jingyao* 御製本草品彙經要 (*Materia Medica Written on Imperial Orders, Containing the Essential and Important in Classified Order*), 1505. Identical copy of the original, nineteenth century or earlier. Staatsbibliothek, Berlin.

6. "Illustration of how to apply the technique of splinting a fracture with a bamboo mat or fir lattice." From *Yucuan yizongjinjian* 御纂醫宗金鑑 (*Imperially Decreed Golden Mirror of Medical Ancestors*), 1742. Edition n.p., publisher Jiangxi shuju 江西書局, 1876.

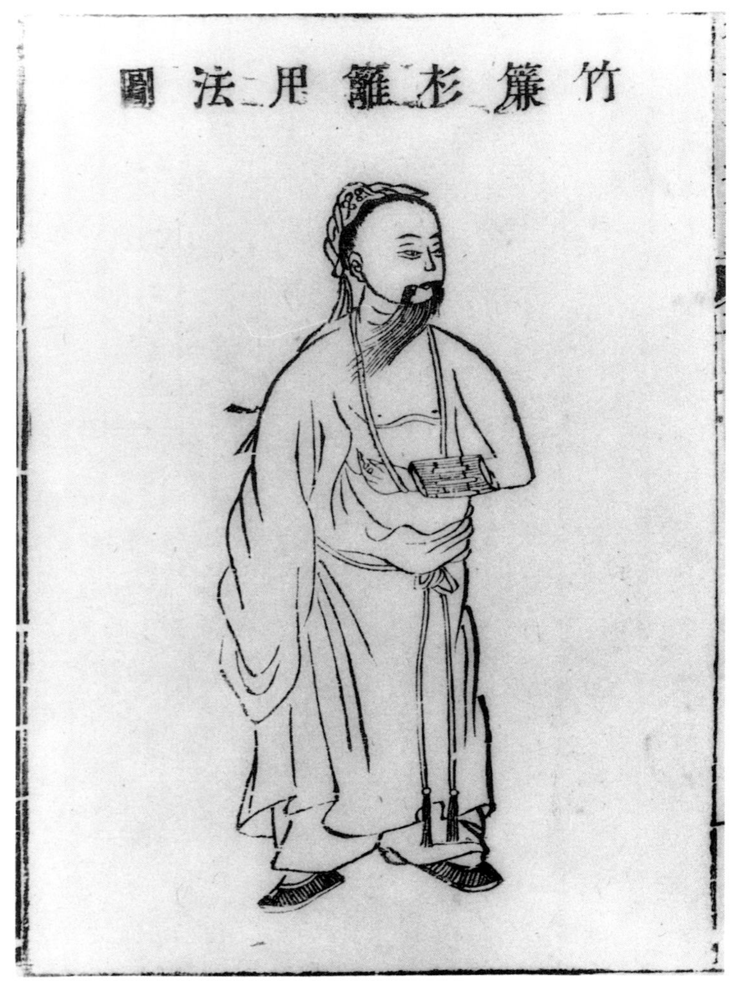

7. From right to left: "Illustration of the use of the rope-pull and brick-stack techniques," "illustration of the stretching block," "illustration of the use of the stretching block on the back." From *Yizongjinjian* 醫宗金鑑 (*Golden Mirror of Medical Ancestors*), 1742. Publisher Jinzhang 錦章, Shanghai, early twentieth century.

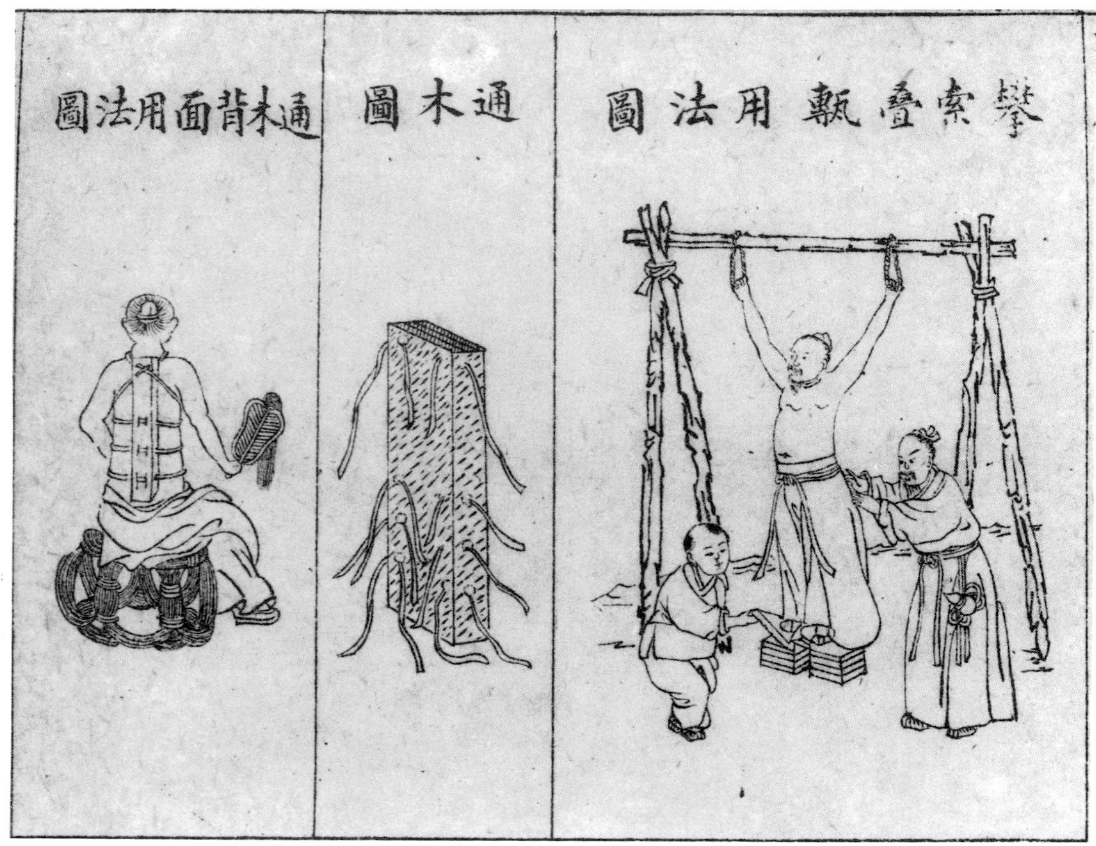

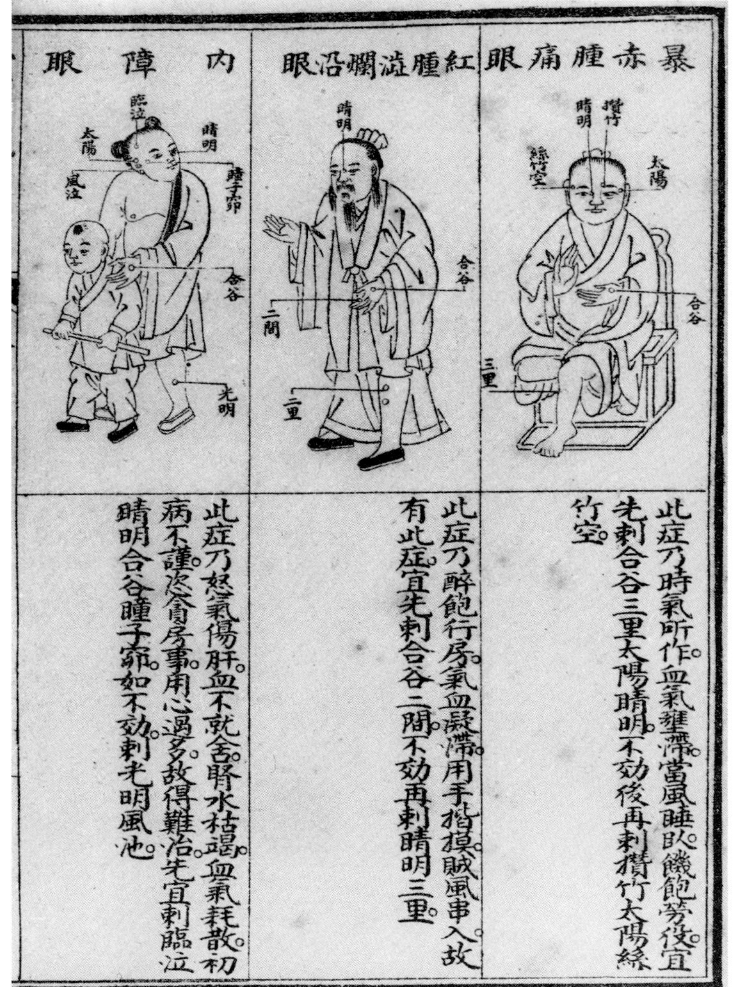

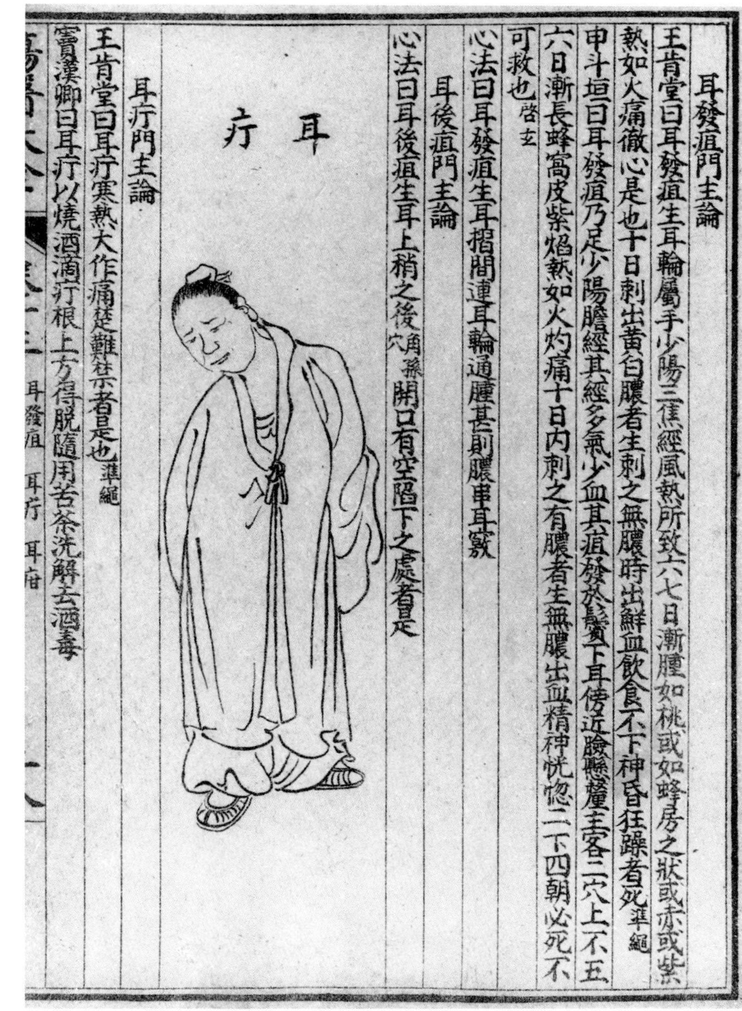

8. Drawing and description of the causes of three eye disorders as well as the skin openings to be needled in regards to them. From right to left: "Sudden reddening, swelling, and pain in the eye. This condition is caused by seasonal qi. The flow of blood and qi is blocked. [The afflicted person] laid down to sleep in the wind. Hunger and satiating, exhaustion and leisure [follow each other without order. For the treatment] it is appropriate to pierce first [the openings] *hegu*, *sanli*, *taiyang*, and *qingming*. If this is without effect, also pierce the openings *zanzhu*, *taiyang* and *sizhu*." "Reddening, swelling, roughness, and suppuration at the eye. This condition is caused by sexual intercourse when drunk or on a full stomach. The flow of blood and qi is blocked. One rubs [the eyes] with the hands. Robber Wind has invaded. Therefore this condition is caused. [For the treatment] it is appropriate to pierce first [the openings] *hegu* and *erjian*. If there is no effect, also pierce [the openings] *qingming* and *sanli*." "Internal cataract. This condition is caused by anger qi that has damaged the liver. The blood is unable to return to its resting point. The water of the kidneys has dried out. Blood and qi are dispersed. In the beginning, people do not pay attention to this illness. They indulge in their pleasures and engage in sexual intercourse. This results in over-exertion of the mind. Therefore [the disorder] becomes difficult to cure. [For the treatment] it is appropriate to pierce first the openings *linqi*, *qingming*, *hegu*, and *tongzi*. If there is no effect, also pierce [the openings] *guangming* and *fengchi*." From *Shenshi yaohan yanke daquan* 審視瑤函眼科大全 (*Careful Observation of the Jade Vessel—Complete Ophthalmology*), 1642. Undated, unmarked edition, early twentieth century.

9. Drawing and explanations of "ear abscesses." From *Yangyi daquan* 瘍醫大全 (*Complete Abscess Medicine*), 1760. Edition from 1920, unknown publisher.

診婦人有妊歌
肝為血兮肺為氣。血為榮兮氣為衛。陰陽配偶不參差。兩臟通和皆類例。
氣升血亦升氣降血亦降陰陽配偶無一毫之參差三陽三陰舉皆二臟通和而類其例焉
肝藏血肺主氣血屬陰為榮而行脈中氣屬陽為衛而行脈外
血衰氣旺定無娠。血旺氣衰應有體。
素問曰金木者殺之木始木多而生金多則殺
寸微關滑尺帶數。流利往來并雀啄。小兒之脈已見形。數月懷妊猶不覺。
女人此脈一見乃血旺氣衰經閉不行懷孕之脈已見形也
左疾為男右為女。流利相通速來去。兩手關脈大相應。已形亦在通前語。左手帶縱兩個男。右手帶橫一
診婦人有妊之圖
婦人血旺氣衰
應有體
左脈
太陽浮大男
帶縱兩個男
疾爲男
逆主三男
右脈
太陰沉細女
帶橫一變女
病爲女
順主三女
寸微關滑尺帶數
流利往來并雀啄
小兒之脈已見形
數月懷胎猶未覺
滑疾不散胎三月
汗出不食吐逆時
小兒月足胎成聚
精神聚結其中住
身熱脈亂無所苦
但病不散五月母
弦緊牢強滑者安
沉細而微歸泉路

10

氣痔
血攻痔
蓮子痔
翻花痔
子母痔
搭腸痔
脫肛痔
蜆肉痔
雌雄痔
內痔
泊腸痔
懸珠痔
雞冠痔
櫻桃痔
雞心痔
盤腸痔
蜂窠痔
珊瑚痔
牛奶痔
栗子痔
蓮花痔
菱角痔
鼠尾痔
核桃痔

11

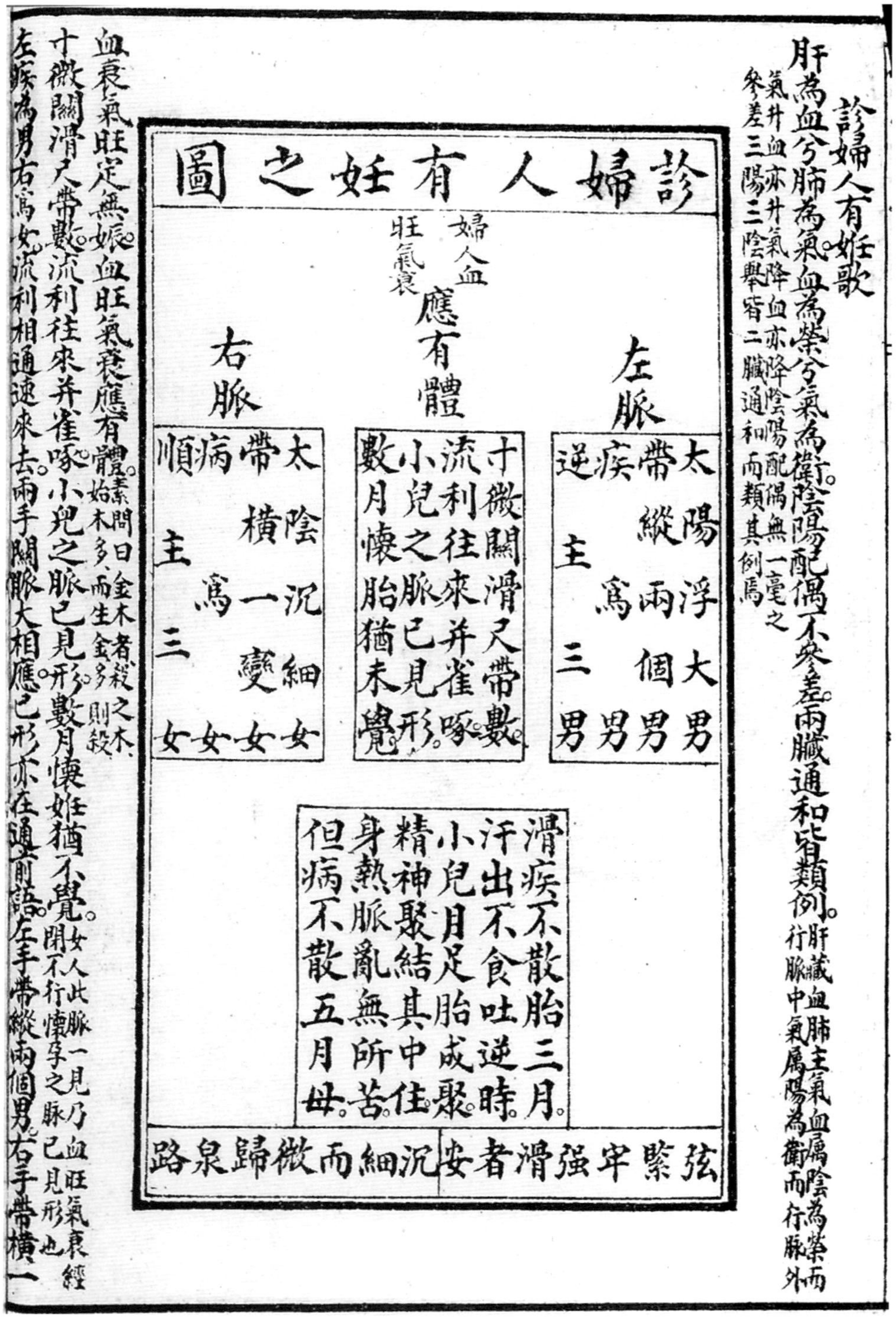

10. "[Memorization] song for diagnosing a woman's pregnancy," with text and schematic representations of the pulse qualities on the left and right wrist from which a pregnancy—as well as the gender and number of fetuses—can be recognized. From *Tuzhu nanjing maijue* 圖注難經脈決 (*Commented and Illustrated [Edition of the Classic] of Difficult Issues and Pulse Doctrine*), 1683. Undated edition, publisher *Guangyi shuju* 上海廣益書局, Shanghai, early twentieth century.

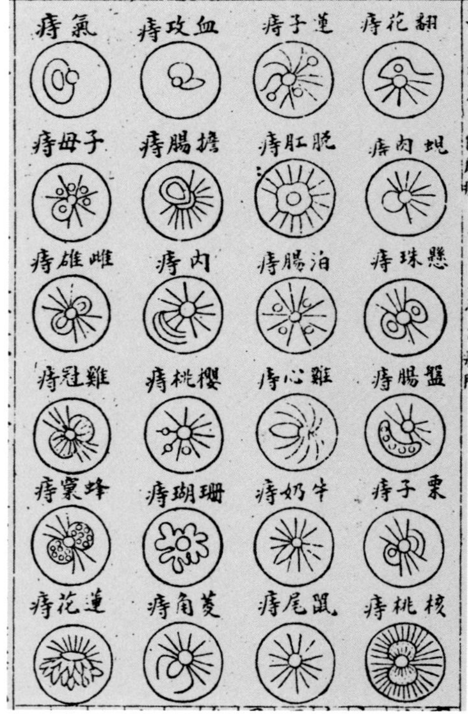

11. "Illustration and explanation of the twenty-four types of hemorrhoides." From *Yucuan yizongjinjian* 御纂醫宗金鑑 (*Imperially Decreed Golden Mirror of Medical Ancestors*), 1742.

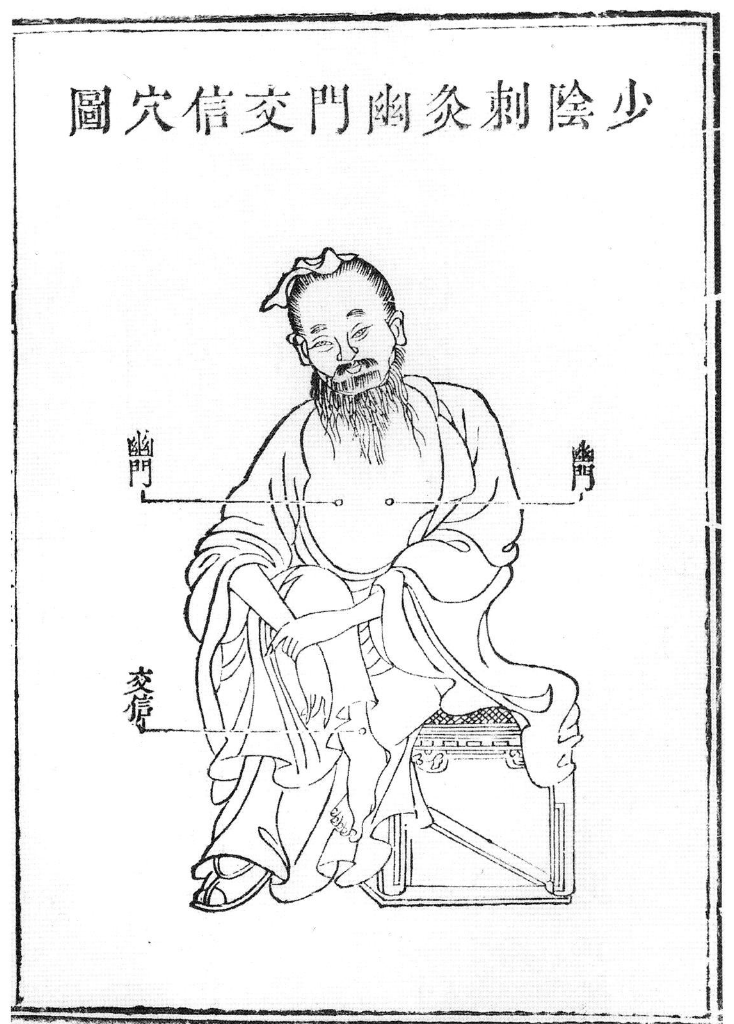


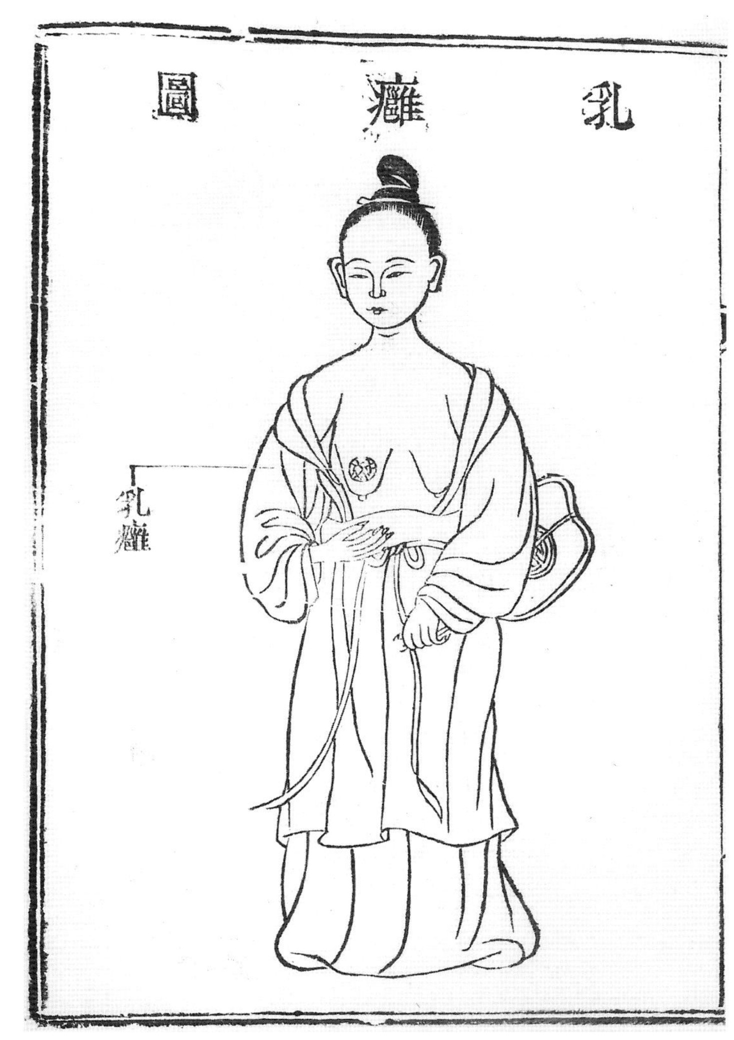


12. "Siteplan of the openings *youmen* and *jiaoxin* for piercing and cauterizing on the Small Yin [Conduit]." From *Yucuan yizongjinjian* 御纂醫宗金鑑 (*Imperially Decreed Golden Mirror of Medical Ancestors*), 1742. Edition n.p., publisher Jiangxi shuju 江西書局, 1876.

13. "Depiction of an abscess on the female breast." From *Yucuan yizongjinjian* 御纂醫宗金鑑 (*Imperially Decreed Golden Mirror of Medical Ancestors*), 1742. Edition n.p., publisher Jiangxi shuju 江西書局, 1876.

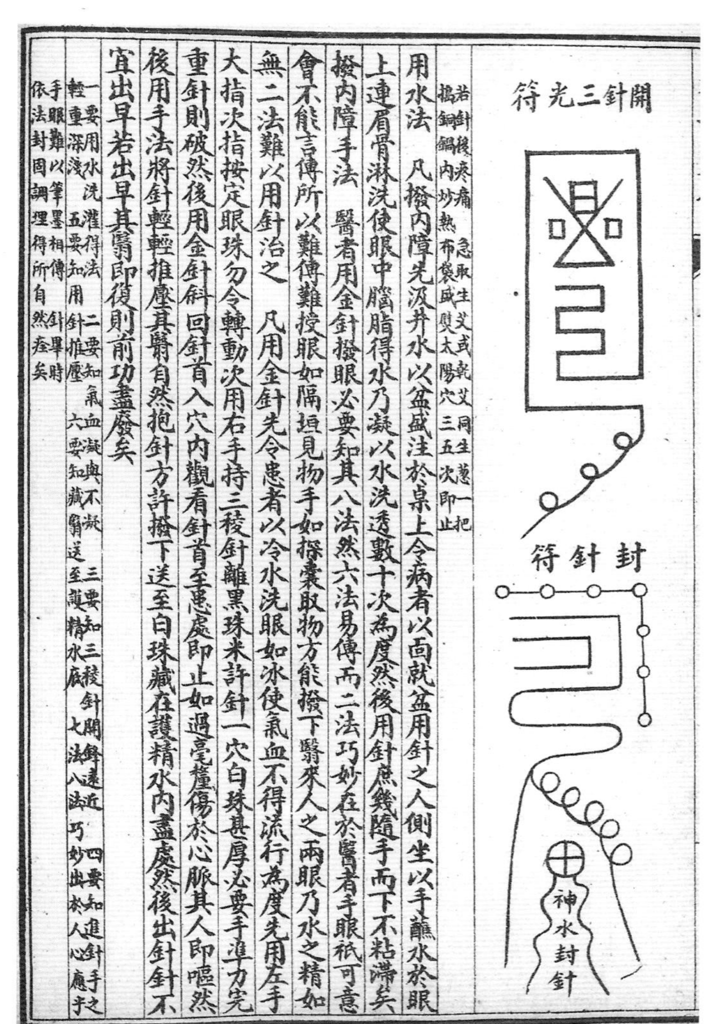


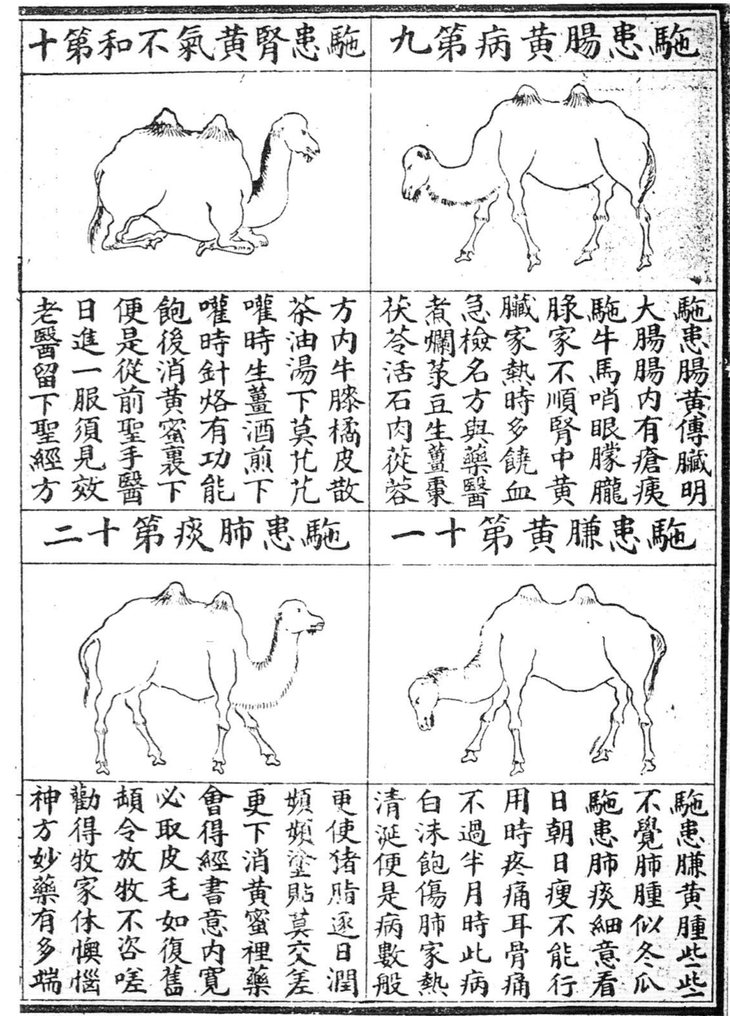


14. Right: Buddhist charm diagrams for increasing the effect of needles during cataract operations. Top: "Charm for exposing the needle and [bringing in] the three lights (i.e. light of the sun, light of the mind, light of the eyes)." Bottom: "Charm in which to wrap the needle [prior to surgery]." Left: text explaining the use of water in preparation of the eyes for cataract surgery. From *Yangyi daquan* 瘍醫大全 (*Complete Abscess Medicine*), 1760. Edition from 1920, unknown publisher.

15. Text and illustration of the illnesses of camels. From right to left: "No. 9: Camel suffering from yellowness [originating in the] intestines." "No. 10: Camel suffering from yellowness [originating in the] kidneys and a disharmony of qi." "No. 11: Camel suffering from yellowness in the lower flank." "No. 12: Camel suffering from lung phlegm." From *Yuan Heng liaomaji* 元亨療馬集 (*Collection of Horse Diseases by [Yu Ben]yuan and [Yu Ben]heng*), 1608. Undated edition, publisher Saoyeshanfang 掃業山房, Shanghai.

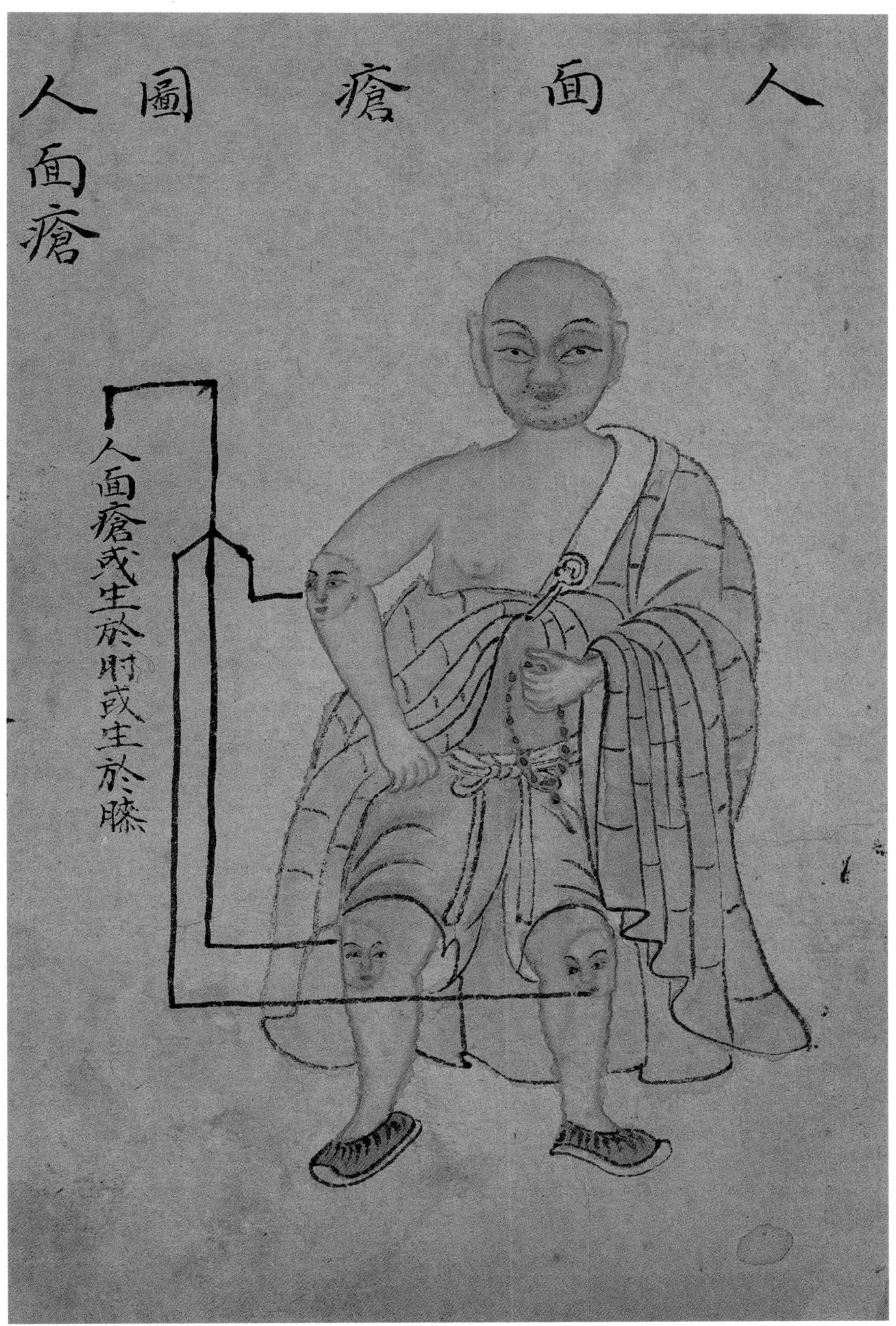



16. "Depiction of abscesses with human faces. Abscesses with human faces appear on the elbows or knees." *Yucuan yizongjinjian* 御纂醫宗金鑑 (*Imperially Decreed Golden Mirror of Medical Ancestors*), 1742. Undated manuscript version.

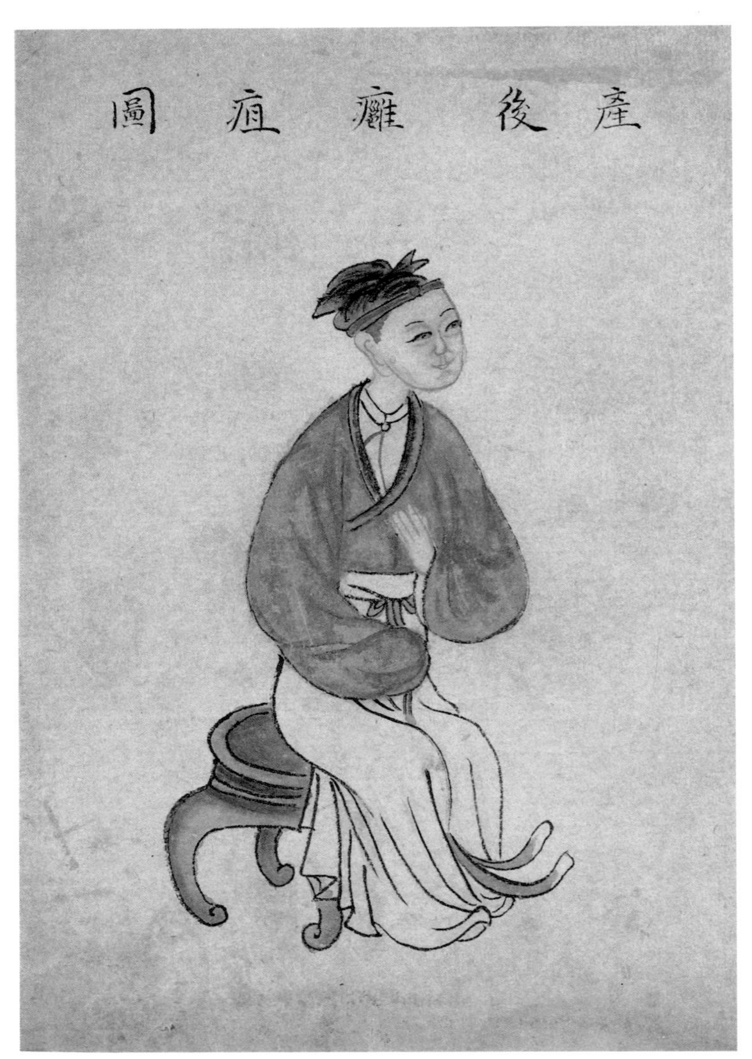



17. "Depiction of the *yong* and *ju* abscesses which appear after childbirth." From *Yucuan yizongjinjian* 御纂醫宗金鑑 (*Imperially Decreed Golden Mirror of Medical Ancestors*), 1742. Undated manuscript version.

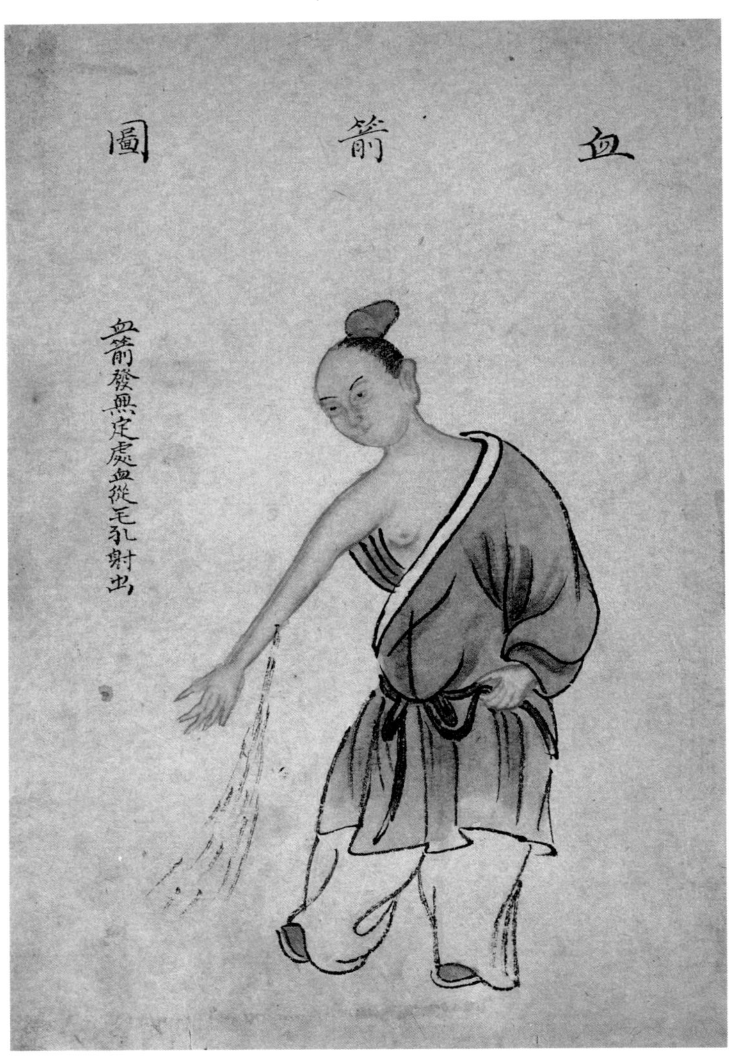



18. "Depiction of the blood arrow. The blood arrow is not discharged at a specific place. The blood shoots out from the hair openings." From *Yucuan yizongjinjian* 御纂醫宗金鑑 (*Imperially Decreed Golden Mirror of Medical Ancestors*), 1742. Undated manuscript version.

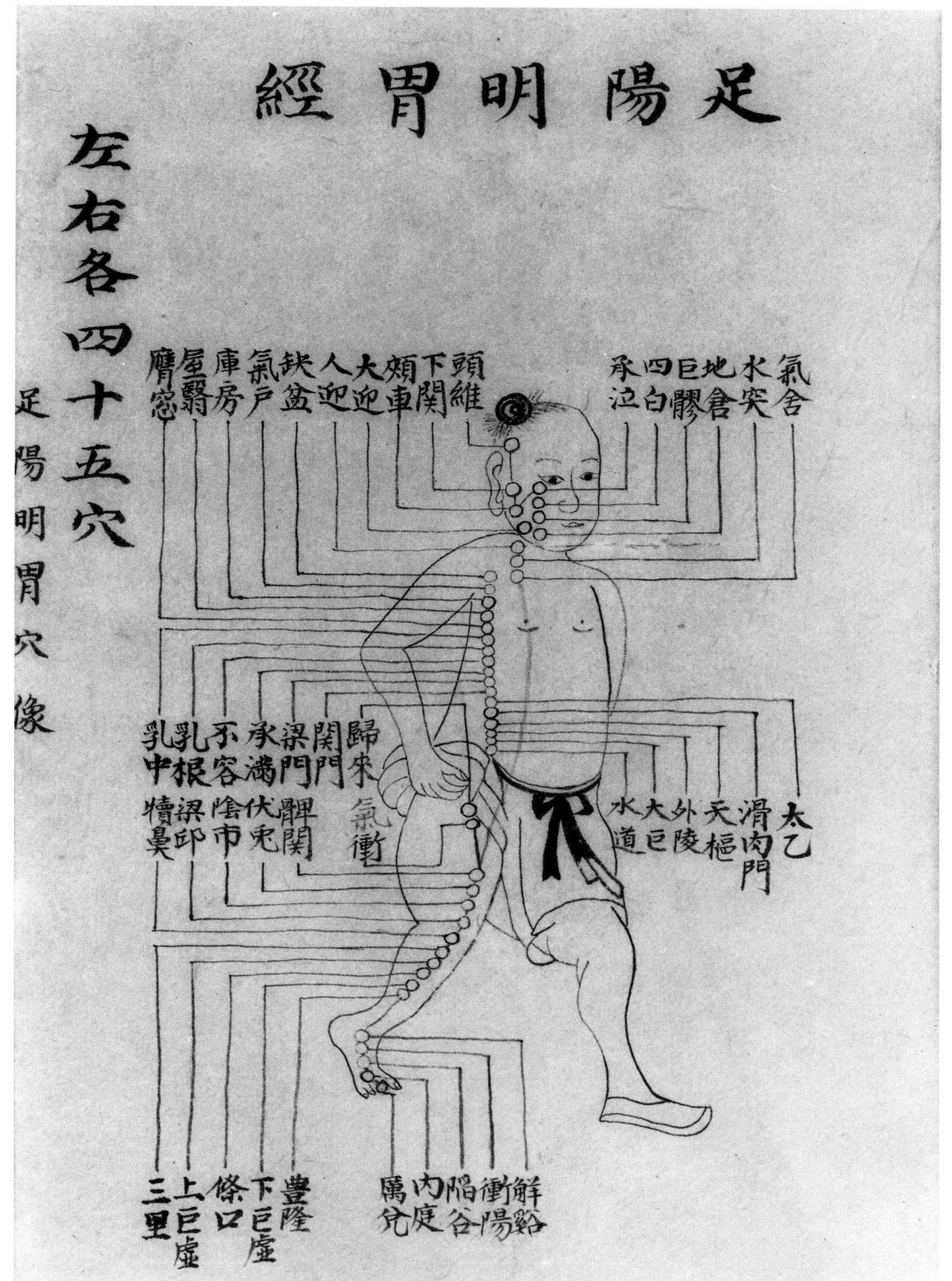


19. "The Foot Bright Yang Conduit of the Stomach" with information regarding the position and names of the forty-five insertion points on the right side of the body. Private medical handbook, undated manuscript.

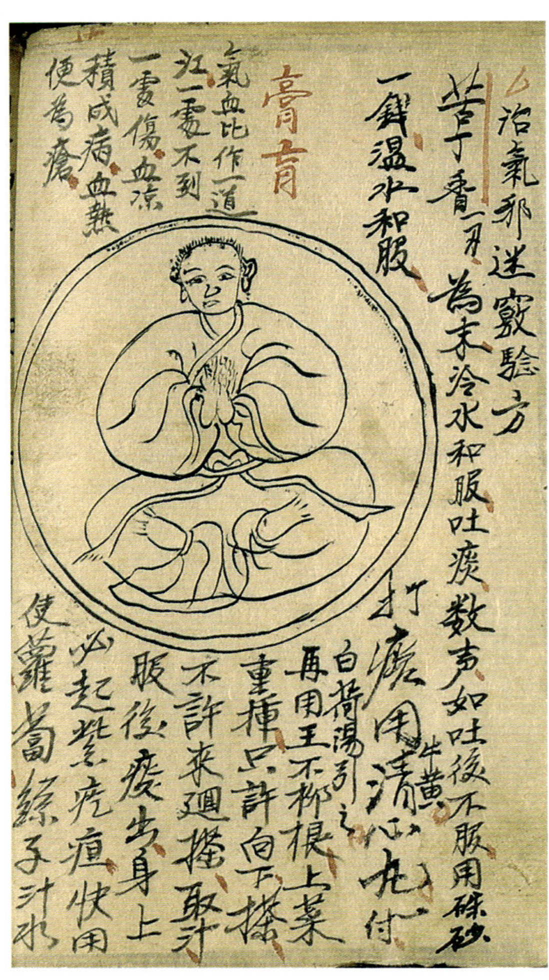

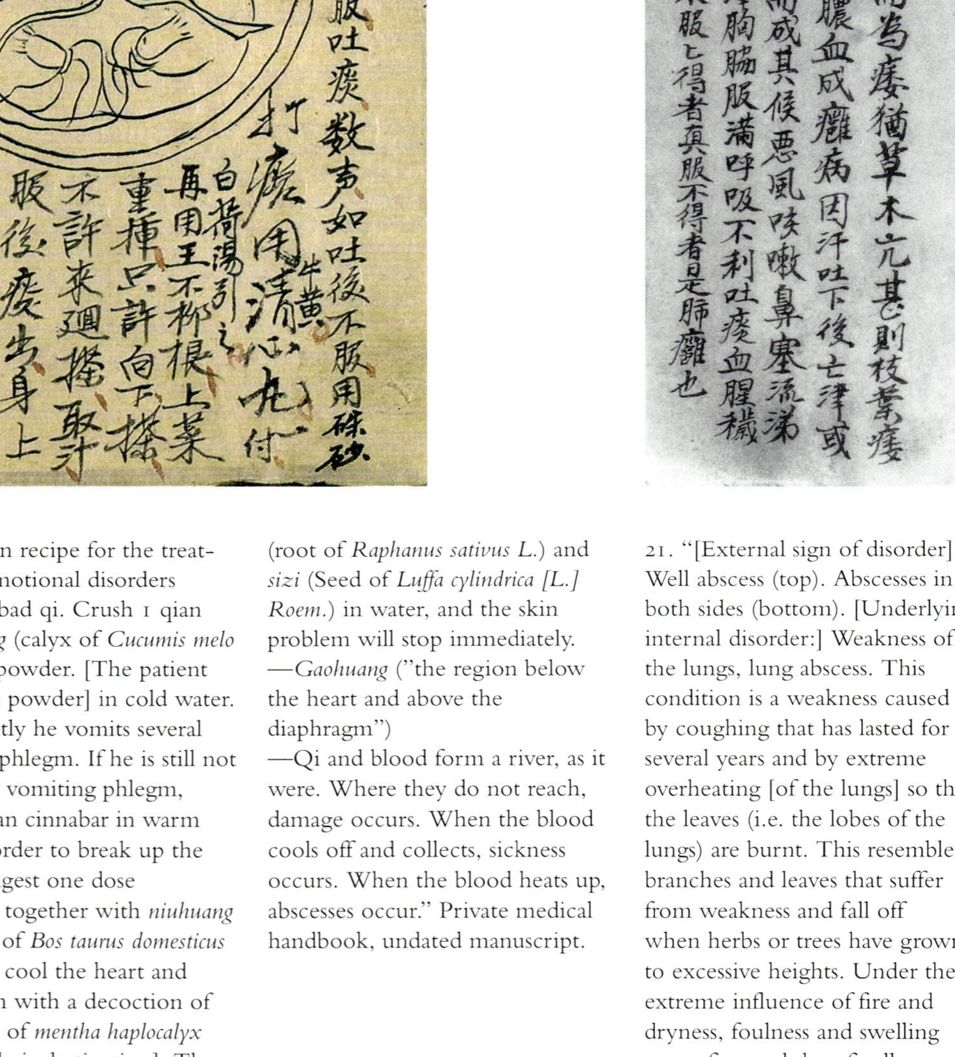

20. "Proven recipe for the treatment of emotional disorders caused by bad qi. Crush 1 qian *kudingxiang* (calyx of *Cucumis melo L.*) into a powder. [The patient ingests this powder] in cold water. Subsequently he vomits several bushels of phlegm. If he is still not cured after vomiting phlegm, ingest 1 qian cinnabar in warm water. In order to break up the phlegm, ingest one dose of the pills together with *niuhuang* (gallstones of *Bos taurus domesticus Gmelin*) to cool the heart and guide them with a decoction of *baihe* (herb of *mentha haplocalyx Briq.*) [to their destination]. Then take the herb of *wangbuliu* (*Vaccaria segetalis [Neck.] Garcke*) above the root and crush it vigorously. Only pound downwards; it does not work to pound sideways back and forth. Take the juice. After ingestion, the phlegm will come out. Red pustules have to form on the body. Then quickly ingest the juice of *luobo* (root of *Raphanus sativus L.*) and *sizi* (Seed of *Luffa cylindrica [L.] Roem.*) in water, and the skin problem will stop immediately.
—*Gaohuang* ("the region below the heart and above the diaphragm")
—Qi and blood form a river, as it were. Where they do not reach, damage occurs. When the blood cools off and collects, sickness occurs. When the blood heats up, abscesses occur." Private medical handbook, undated manuscript.

21. "[External sign of disorder] Well abscess (top). Abscesses in both sides (bottom). [Underlying internal disorder:] Weakness of the lungs, lung abscess. This condition is a weakness caused by coughing that has lasted for several years and by extreme overheating [of the lungs] so that the leaves (i.e. the lobes of the lungs) are burnt. This resembles branches and leaves that suffer from weakness and fall off when herbs or trees have grown to excessive heights. Under the extreme influence of fire and dryness, foulness and swelling occur first and then finally suppuration of the blood. This causes a [lung] abscess. This illness is caused by the loss of fluids after sweating, vomiting, or purgation. Another cause is a flaming up of fire due to emptiness of the kidneys. Or [this condition is caused by foods with] a strong aroma, leading to the development of hot vapors. The [illness] is expressed in an aversion to wind and in coughing. The nose is stuffed up and runny. The neck is stiff and [the head] cannot be moved to the side. The skin loses its moisture; a sensation of fullness arises in the chest and in the sides. The flow of breathing is interrupted. Vomiting of phlegm and blood with foul odor occurs. To differentiate whether this is in fact [a weakness of the lungs] or not, have [the patient] ingest ground roots of the Yellow Bean in water. If he can take it, it is in fact [a weakness of the lungs]; if not, it is a lung abscess." Private medical handbook, undated manuscript.

22. Drawing with formulae. From right to left: "When the corners of the eyes are reddened and swollen, it is a case of heart fire. [For therapy,] a decoction of *jing*[*jie*] (herb of *Schizonepeta tenuifolia Briq.*) and *fang*[*feng*] (root of *Saposhnikovia divaricata [Turcz.] Schischk.*) is recommended, with the addition of 8 qian *huangqin* (root of *Scutellaria baicalensis Georgi*), 8 qian *mutong* (stem of *Akebia trifoliata [Thunb.] Koidz.* and other types of akebia) and 9 leaves of bamboo. When the white eyeball is completely red, swollen, and sore to the extent of blurred vision, tear flow, and dread of light, this is a case of an excess of fire. [For therapy,] the decoction that cools the blood and disperses the fire is recommended. For [the treatment of] adults, give a double dose. If [the patients] pass hardened stools, further add 1 qian *shengjun* (raw root of *Rheum palmatum L.*). Decoction that cools the blood and disperses the fire: *shengdi* (rhizome of *Rehmannia glutinosa [Gaertn.] Libosch.*), 1 qian; *huangqin* (root of *Scutellaria baicalensis Georgi*), 8 fen; *jingjie* (herb of *Schizonepeta tenuifolia Briq.*), 8 fen; *cheqian* (entire plant of *Plantago asiatica L.*), 1 qian; *chantui* (*Cryptotympana atrata Fabricius*), 6 fen; *danpi* (root bark of *Paeonia suffruticosa Andr.*), 8 fen; *fangfeng* (root of *Saposhnikovia divaricata [Turcz.] Schischk.*), 8 fen; *guiwei* (secondary roots of *Angelica sinensis [Oliv.] Diels.*), 8 fen." Private medical handbook, undated manuscript.

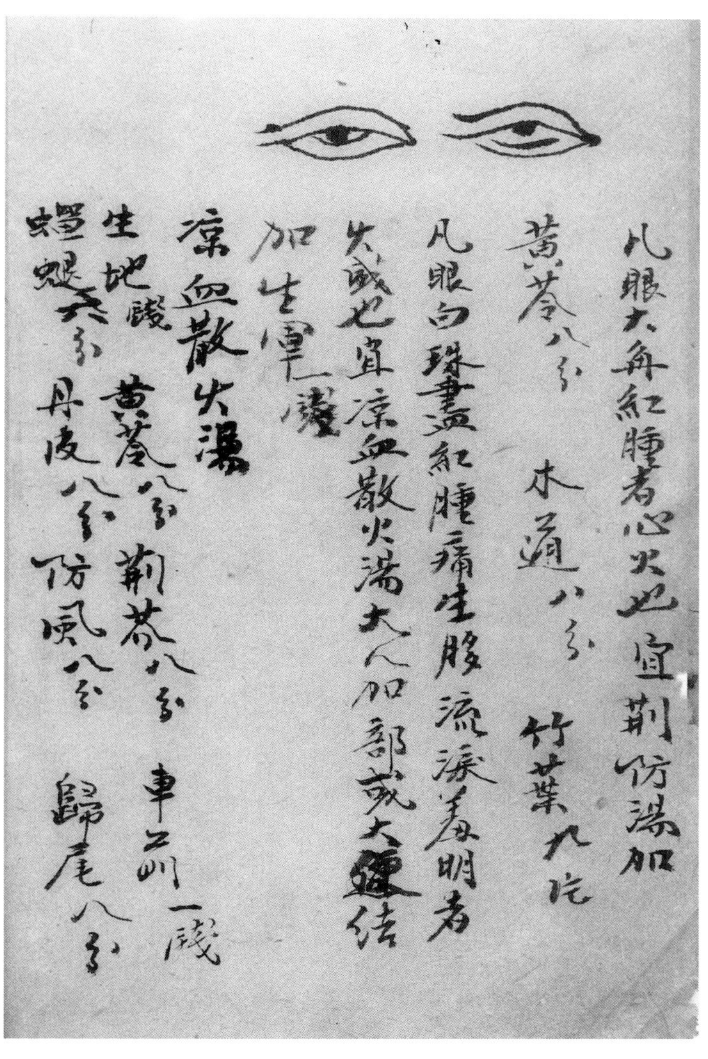

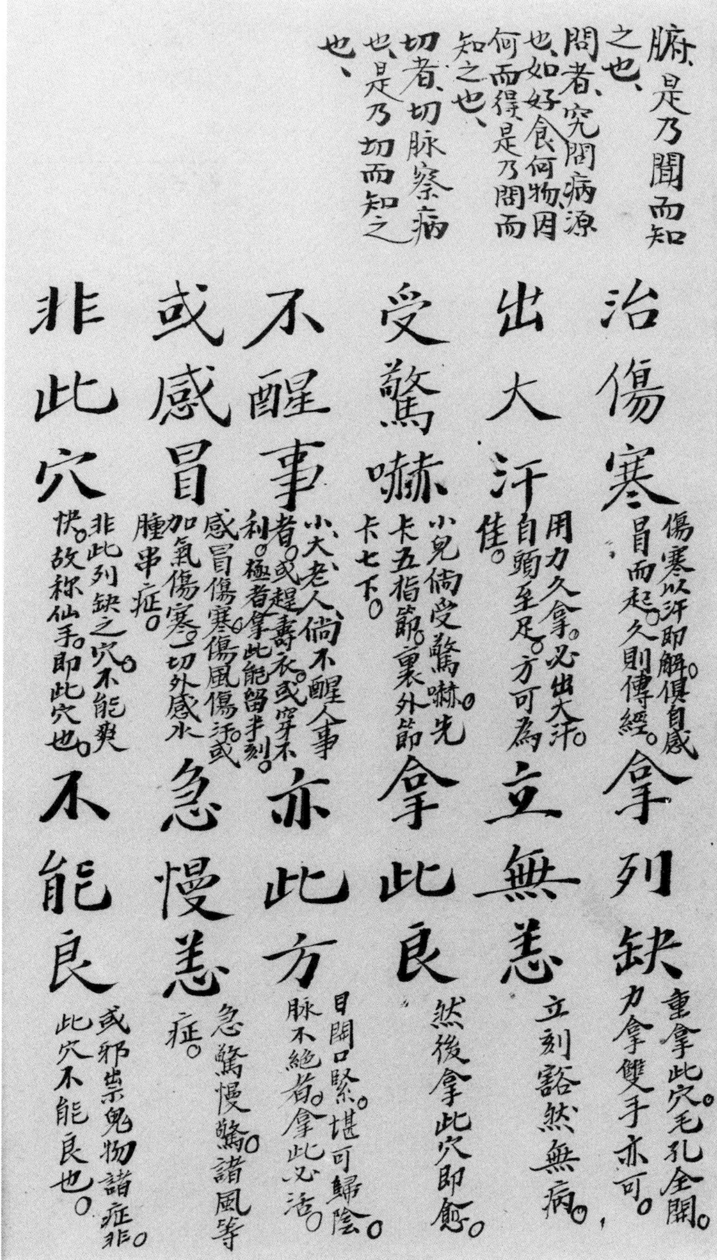

23. Page from a teaching and memorization book on the push and pull massage of children, following the structure of the classical antique textbook *Sanzijing* 三字經. Arranged in rhymes of three characters each, with additional commentaries: *Zhishanghan / nalieque // chudahan / liuwuyang // shoujinghe / naciliang // buxingshi / yicifang // huoganmao / jimanyang // feicixue / bunengliang.*
"For the treatment of cold-related damages, massage at the *lieque* [opening] (a skin opening which in acupuncture is related to the function of the lungs). Profuse sweating will occur, and the illness is over immediately. If [the child] has suffered a fright, it is [also] beneficial to massage this [point]. In case of unconsciousness, also [apply] this formula. If one fails [to massage] this opening in a case of flu, whether acute or chronic, then it cannot improve." *Tuina sanzijing* 推拿三字經 (*Three Character Classic of the Push and Pull Massage*), origin unknown, undated manuscript.

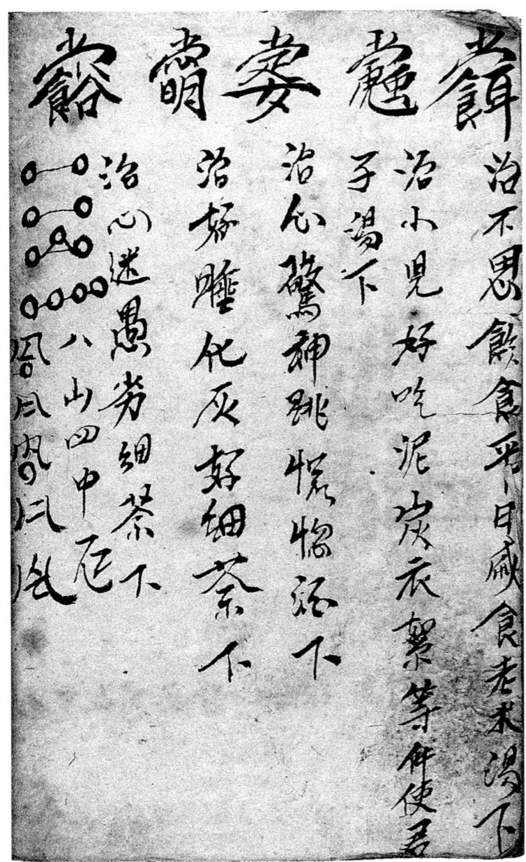

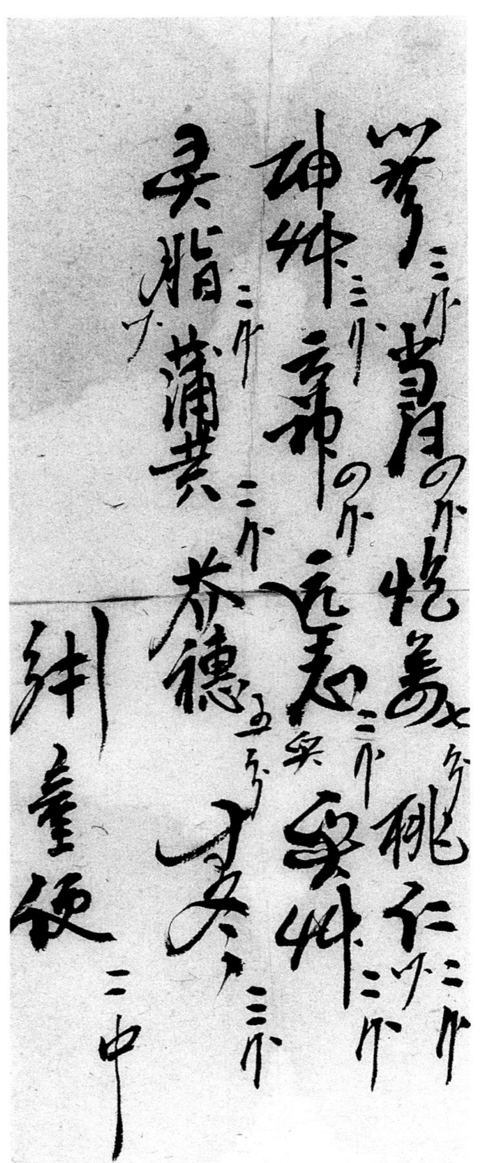

25. Handwritten formula for an individual case of illness. Twelve drug names and their prescribed amounts. Undated.

24. Exorcistic characters that are assumed to remove the indicated problems when ingested as ash. From right to left: "For treatment if someone does not think of food or drink and fasts on very ordinary days: ingest in a decoction of old rice. For treatment if small children like to eat such things as mud, coal, or fabric scraps: ingest in a decoction of *shijunzi* (fruits of *Quisqualis indica L.*). For treatment of frightened emotions, unsteady mind, and absentmindedness: ingest in wine. For treatment if someone likes to sleep: Burn to ashes and ingest in fine tea of good quality. For the treatment of disturbances of consciousness: ingest in fine tea of lesser quality." Private medical handbook, undated manuscript.

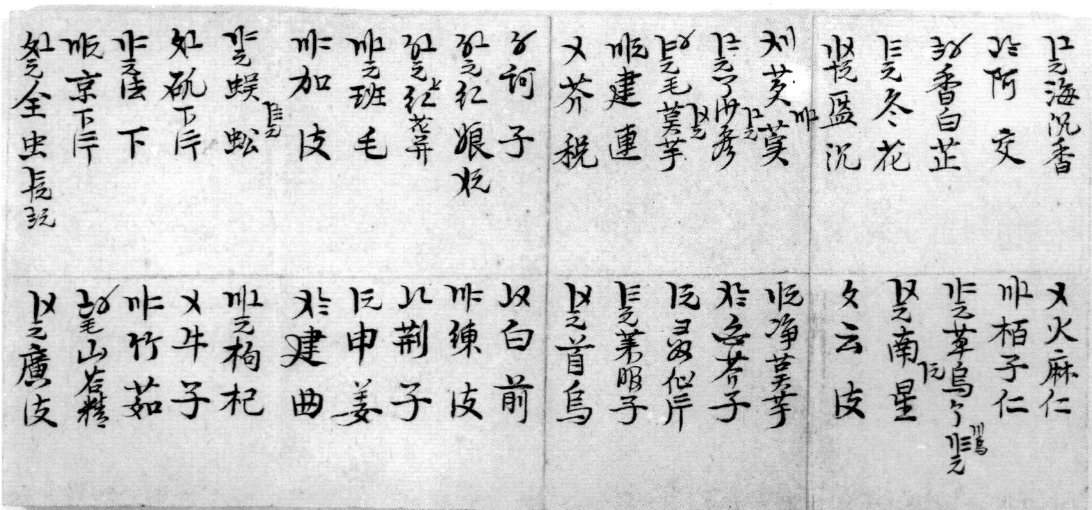

26. Leporello manuscript belonging to a pharmacist or medicine merchant listing drug names and information regarding price or amount often added above in secret notation. Undated.

Acupuncture is a technique for therapeutically influencing physical conditions in humans or animals by inserting needles of various sharpnesses and lengths. The historical origins and further development of this procedure have been researched only superficially. The current state of knowledge permits, however, the following statements. Until the second century B.C.E., bleeding was widespread in China; no archaeological or literary references exist that prove acupuncture existed prior to this point in time. At the beginning of the Han dynasty, attempts to externally influence the vessels of the body—through the skin—were abstracted and refined. The visible blood, previously manipulated by bleeding, was complemented by notions about the physiological significance of invisible vapors, qi. Thus, the knowledge of the blood vessels on the surface of the body was expanded by the assumption that deeper canals existed in which qi circulated continuously. The crude lancing stone used for bleeding was complemented, and later completely replaced, by the narrow needle.

This needle therapy was intended to direct the flow of qi through its conduits with various insertion techniques—in order to treat slight changes in a patient's condition at a point before the onset of illness. Initially, it seemed that acupuncture might affect the entire conduit, similar to the bleeding of a blood vessel. Only in a second stage were very specific body parts defined at which needles could be inserted for specific therapeutic purposes.

The development of acupunctural teaching charts, with information regarding the position of the conduits inside the body and the insertion points on the body, is probably the result of the construction of the first model of the entire body—with replicas of the internal organs—for the instruction of acupuncture in 1027. The conduits and insertion points marked on this model helped standardize the application and transmission of the practice.

As a rule, acupunctural teaching charts consist of four drawings: front, back, and side views of the body as well as a view of the body's organs. Since the morphology of the interior of the body was not considered significant in China between the Song period and the nineteenth century, no systematic change in the representation of the bodily organs is visible on the teaching charts during this period of seven centuries.

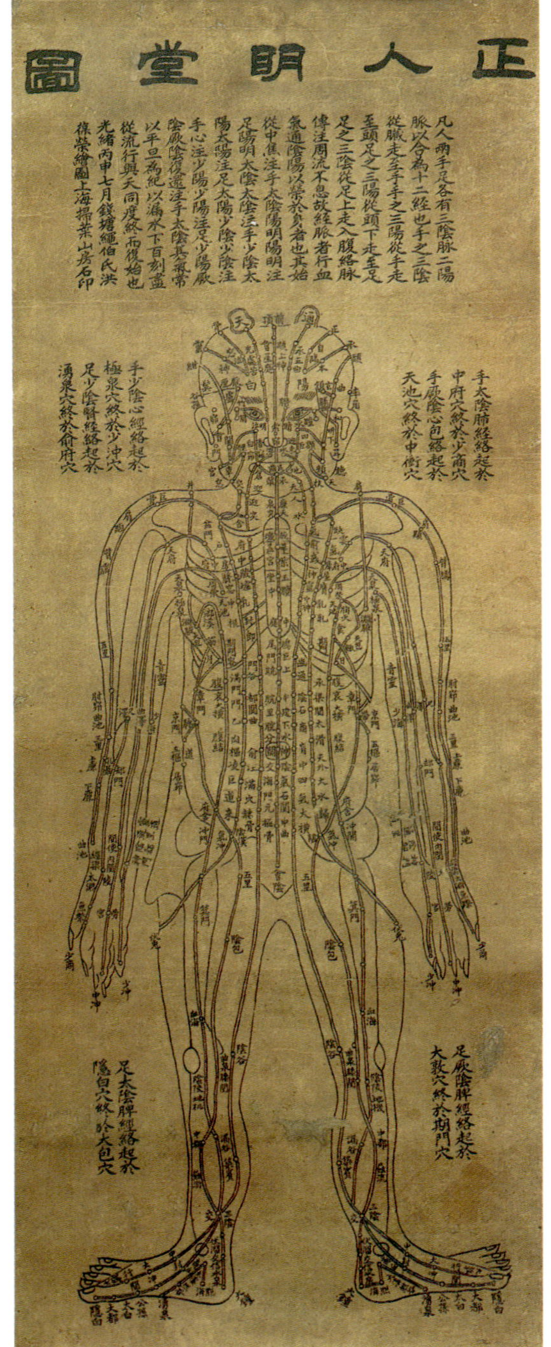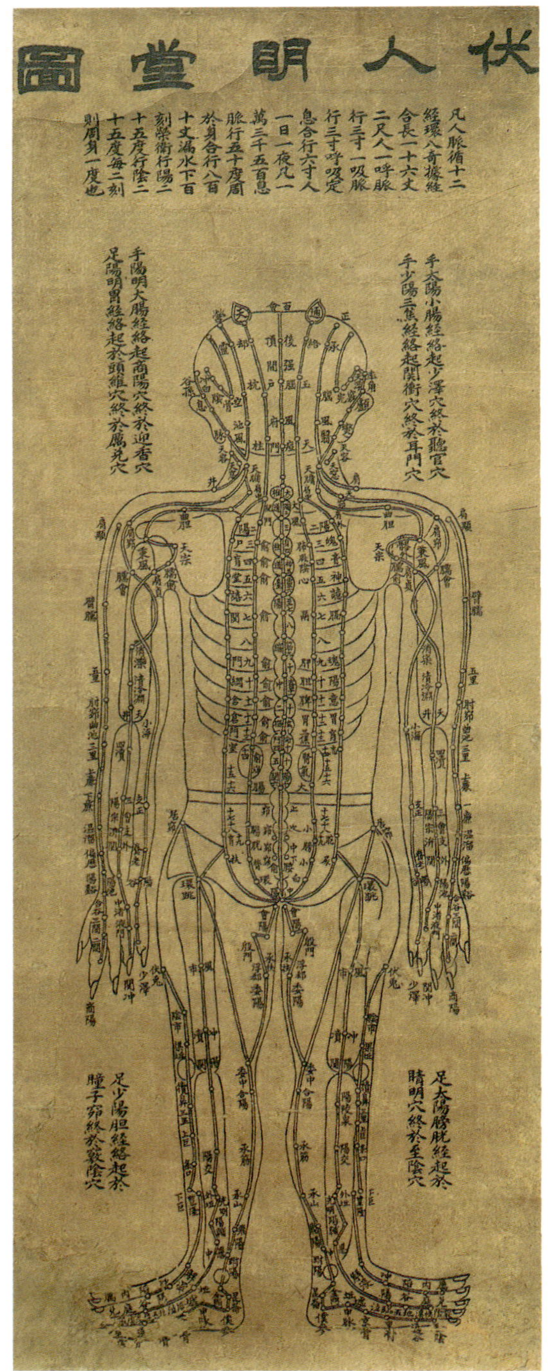

27a-b

27a-d. Four teaching charts for acupuncture. Front, back, and side views of the body. Transparent representation of the conduits and insertion points in relation to the skeletal structure. Text from *Huang Di neijing* 皇帝內經 (*Huang Di's Inner Classic*) regarding the position of the conduits and the movements in the vessels. The fourth chart illustrates a morphology of the bodily organs, with text on the position and function of the bodily organs. Print with hand-written texts, Qing period. 60.3 x 22.4 cm.

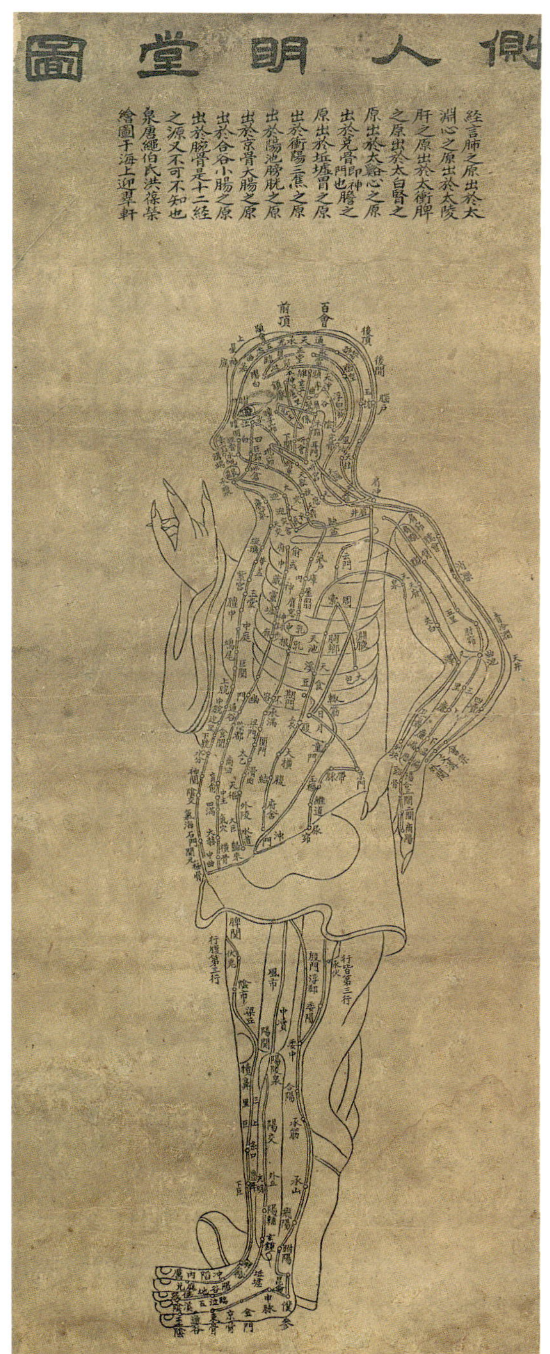

側人明堂圖

經言肺之原出於太
淵心之原出於太陵
肝之原出於太衝脾
之原出於太白腎之
原出於太谿心之原
出於兌骨即神門也膽之
原出於坵墟胃之原
出於衝陽三焦之原
出於陽池膀胱之原
出於京骨大腸之原
出於合谷小腸之原
出於腕骨是十二經
之源又不可不知也
泉唐繩伯氏洪祿榮
繪圖于海上迎翠軒

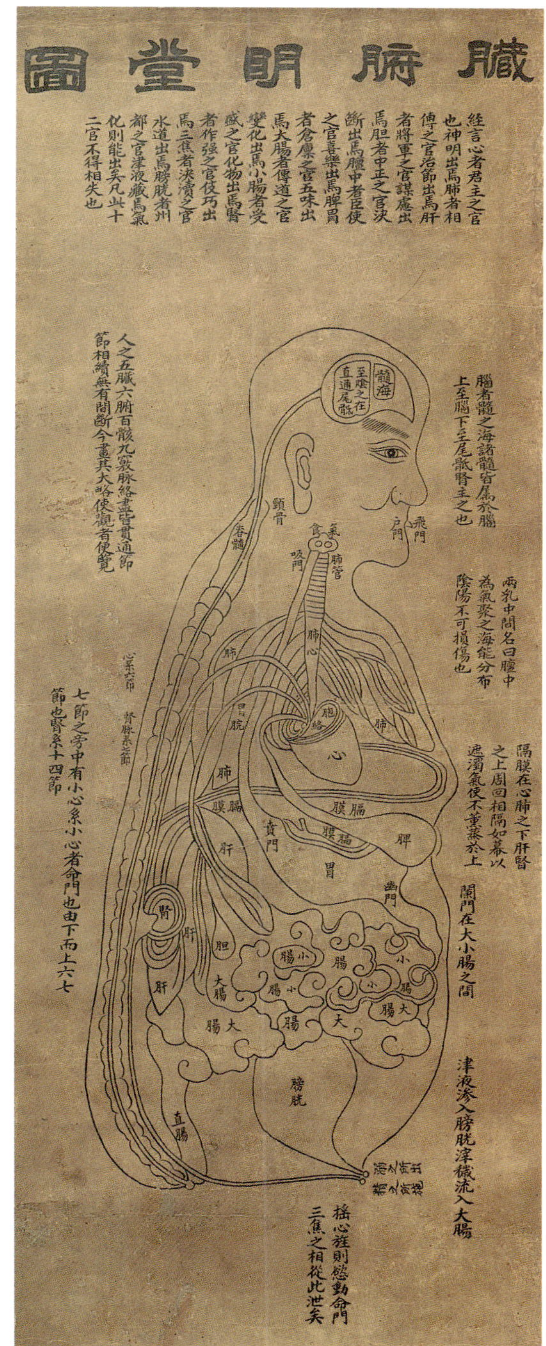

臟腑明堂圖

經言心者君主之官
也神明出焉肺者相
傅之官治節出焉肝
者將軍之官謀慮出
焉膽者中正之官決
斷出焉膻中者臣使
之官喜樂出焉脾胃
者倉廩之官五味出
焉大腸者傳道之官
變化出焉小腸者受
盛之官化物出焉腎
者作強之官伎巧出
焉三焦者決瀆之官
水道出焉膀胱者州
都之官津液藏焉氣
化則能出矣凡此十
二官不得相失也

27c-d

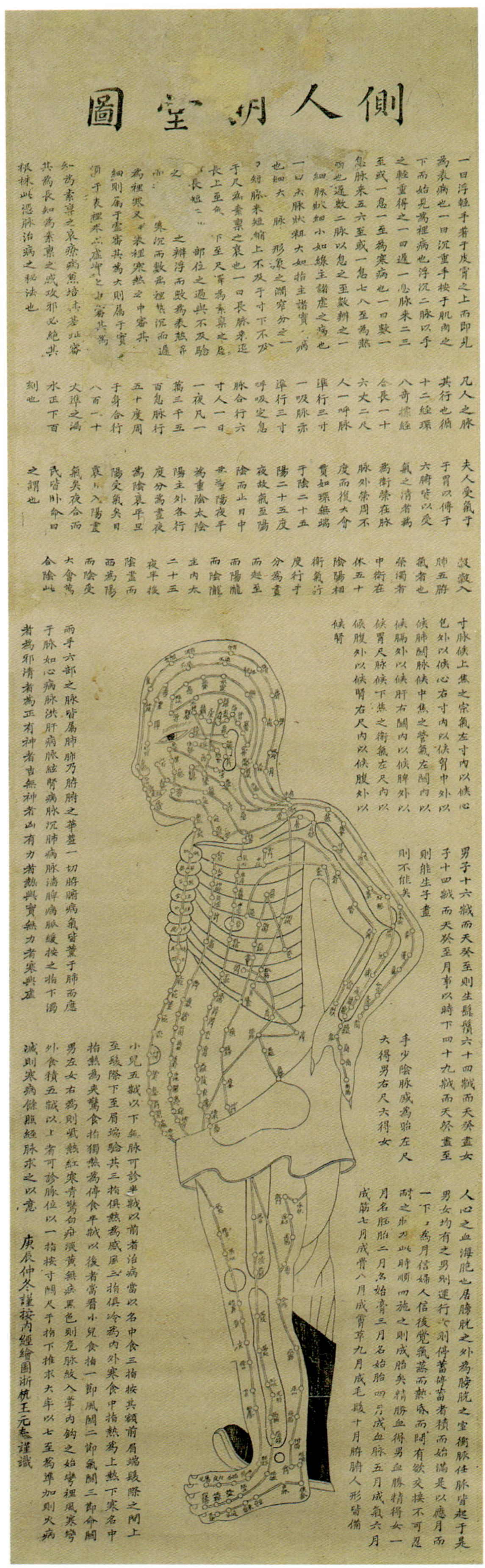

28. Teaching chart for acupuncture. Side view of the body. Transparent representation of the conduits and insertion points in relation to the skeletal structure. Text on the movements in the vessels and the physiological peculiarities of adults and children. Handwritten dedication at bottom left: 庚辰仲冬謹按內經繪圖浙杭王元泰謹識, "In the year gongchen, middle winter month, drawn under careful consideration of [Huang Di's] Inner Classic. In [the province of] Zhe[jiang], in Hang[zhou] by Wang Yuantai." Print, Qing period. 107.5 x 30.6 cm.

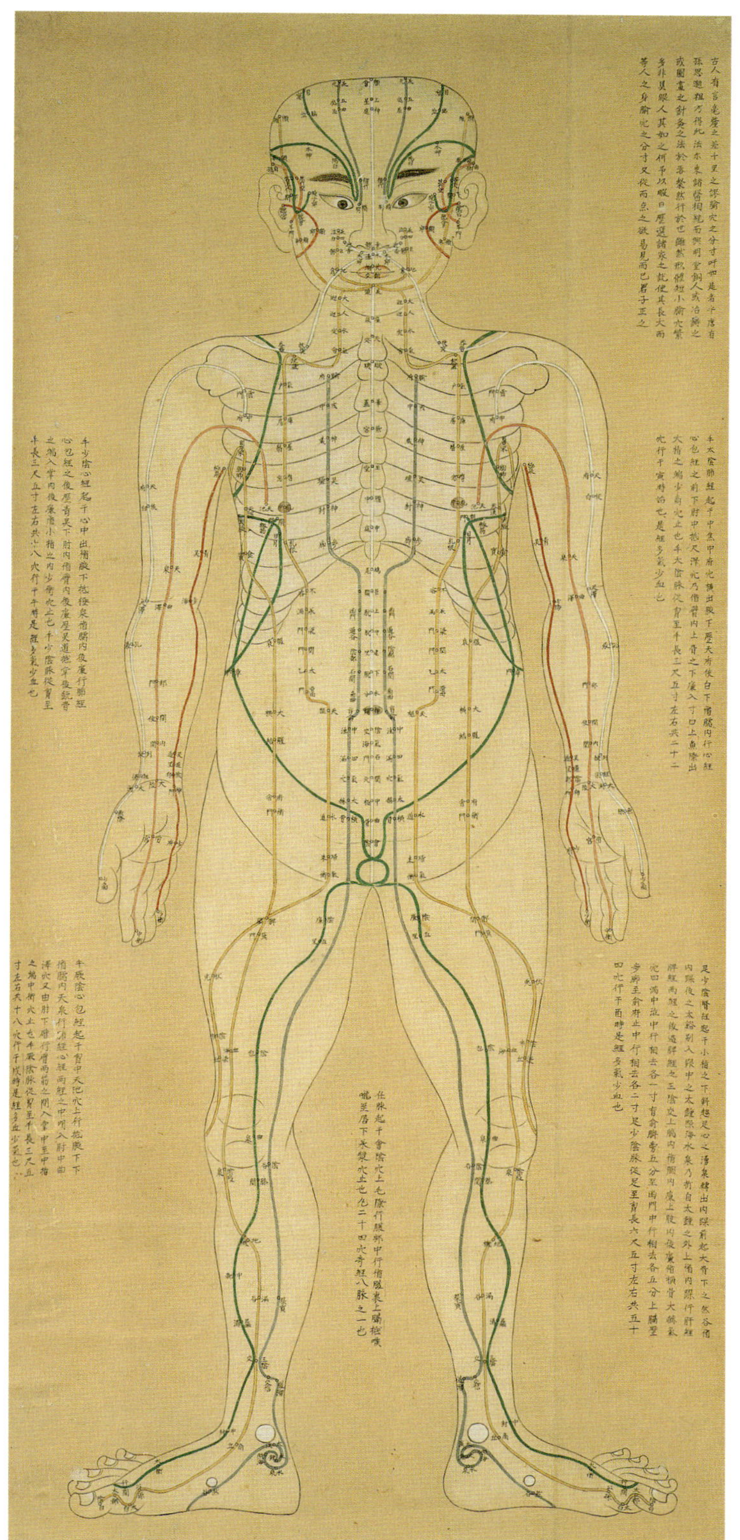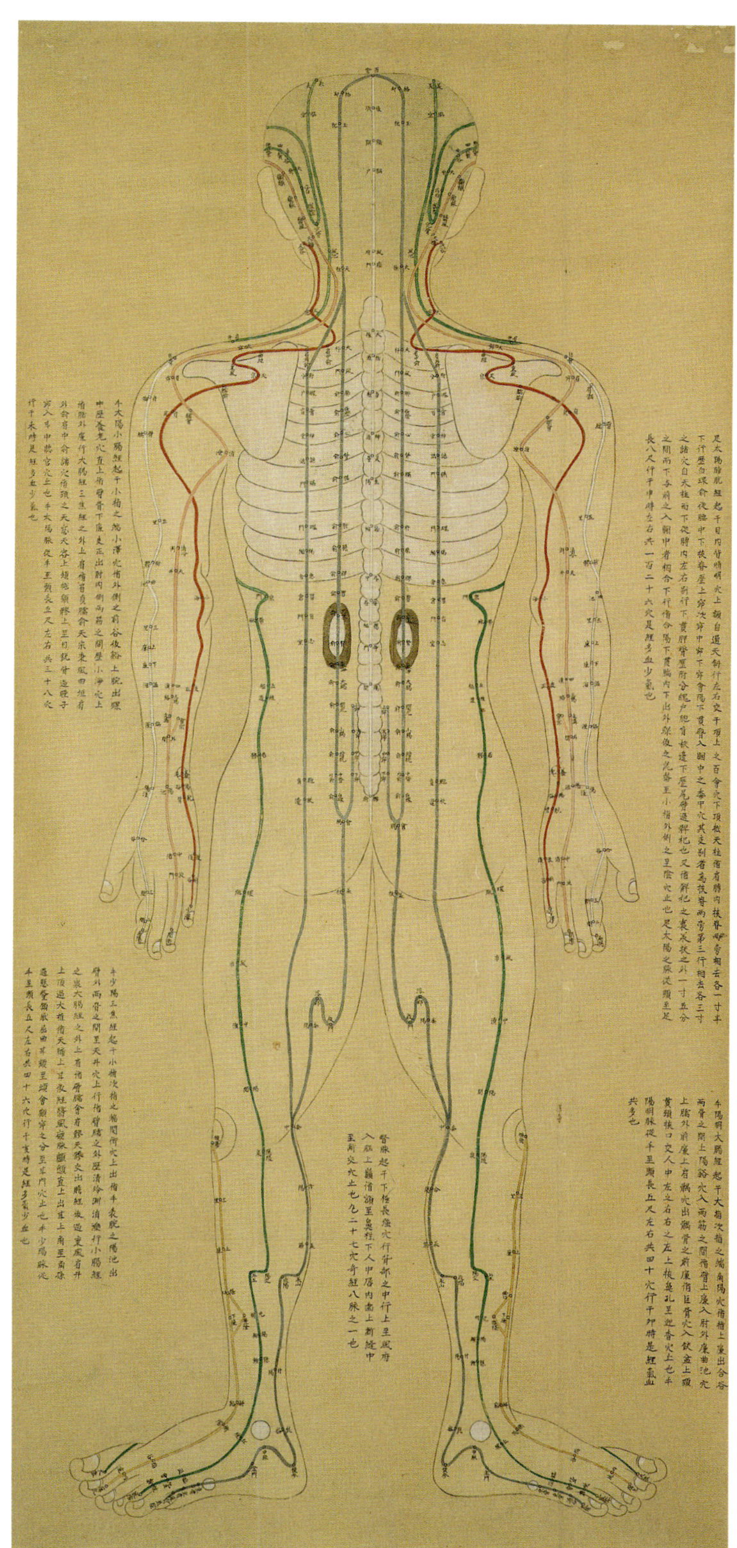

29a–d. Four teaching charts for acupuncture. Front, back, and side views of the body. Semi-transparent representation of the conduits and insertion points in relation to the skeletal structure. Texts on the course of the conduits and on the position and number of insertion points. Chinese text with Japanese reading marks. The third chart illustrates a morphology of the bodily organs. Hand-colored drawings, 175 x 78 cm; third illustration 140 x 50 cm, nineteenth century or earlier.

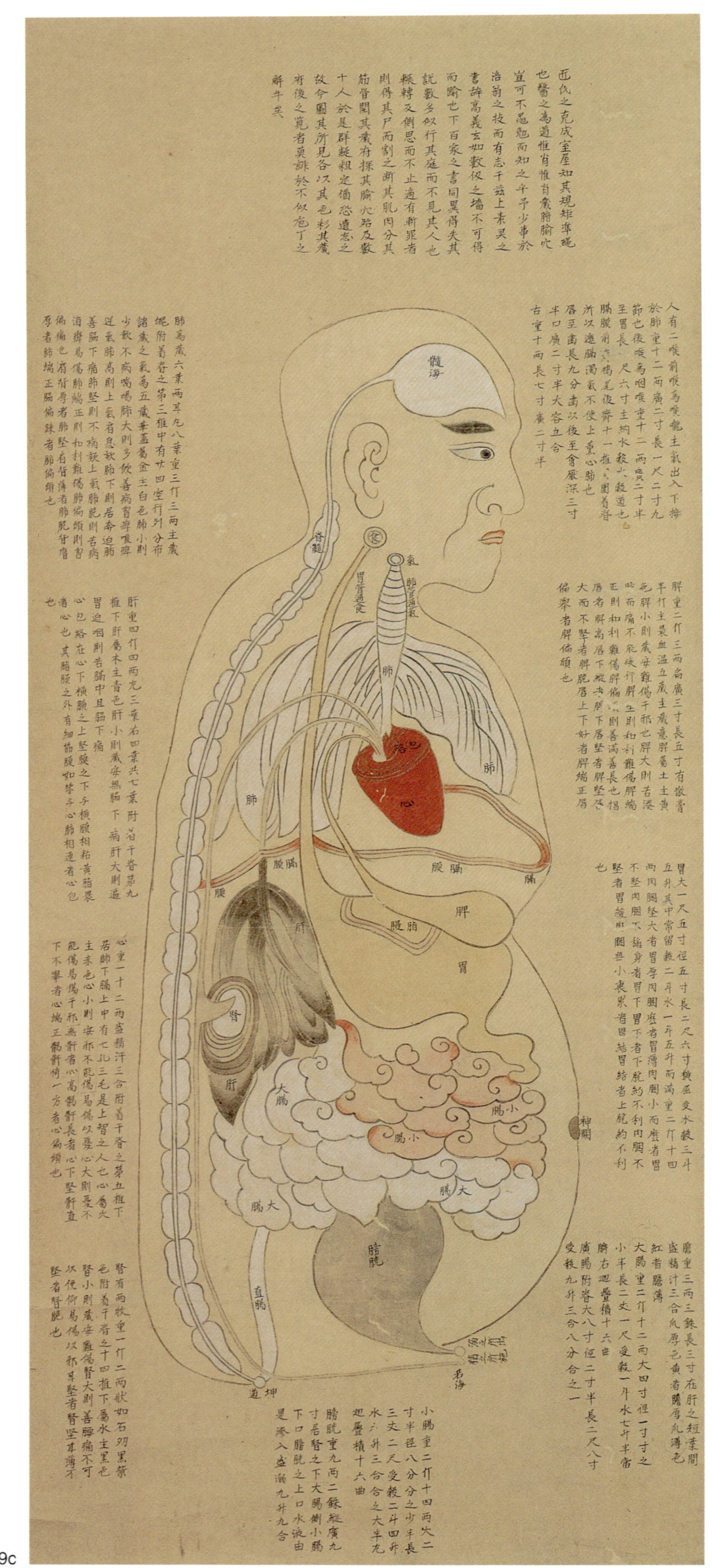


29c

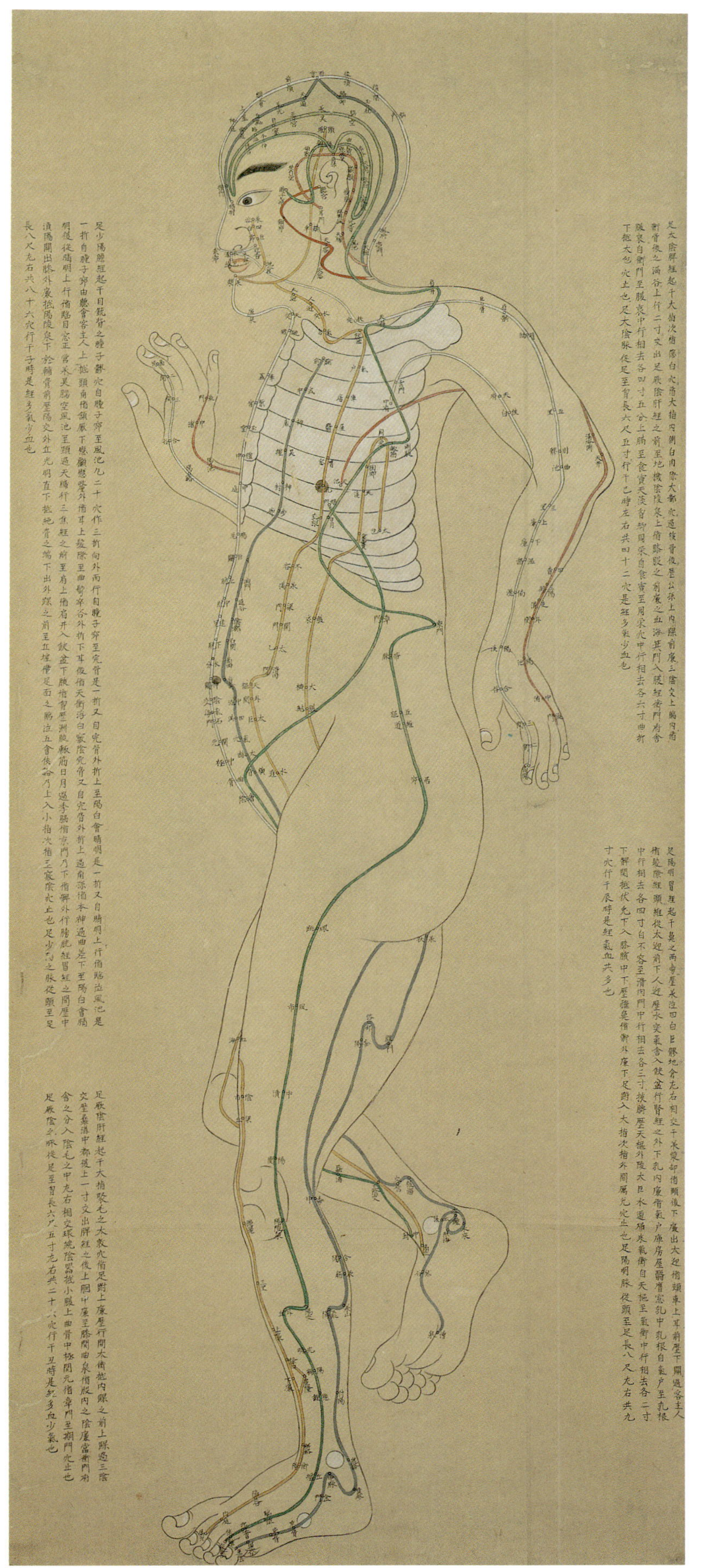

Since the late-Song period, traditional Chinese pharmacists have been familiar with the practice of adjusting a medical treatment to the needs of individual patients. For the most part, however, they have used numerous individual drugs and formulas from antiquity that have proven again and again, over the course of time, their efficacy in treating well-defined illnesses, regardless of patients' individual histories. Against this background, famous drug combinations were developed for patients to purchase and even apply without a doctor's diagnosis.

By giving a formula a new name or labeling a prescription with their own name, pharmacies introduced specialties that customers could only purchase from them. Advertising for these products was done by way of handbills, printed from wooden blocks and distributed in the area around the pharmacy. Before the introduction of mass media, this was apparently the most efficient way to reach literate clientele.

These handbills offer information that occasionally cannot be found in the medical literature. This includes the advertising bills for point ointments (see p. 58f.), a type of application that has not been described before.

Pharmacy advertising boards from China and Japan are also remarkable. The latter advertise for traditional Chinese recipes and, at the same time, for modern ready-made preparations of Western medicines that have been for sale in Japanese pharmacies since the end of the nineteenth century. Thus, these advertising boards serve as expressive and simultaneously aesthetically appealing examples of the early coexistence of Western and Chinese medicine.

Not only the producers of medicines, but also the physicians in China engaged (and engage) in advertising. Some doctors used hand-printed bills to praise the medicines they sold, while others used them to announce their own medical skills.

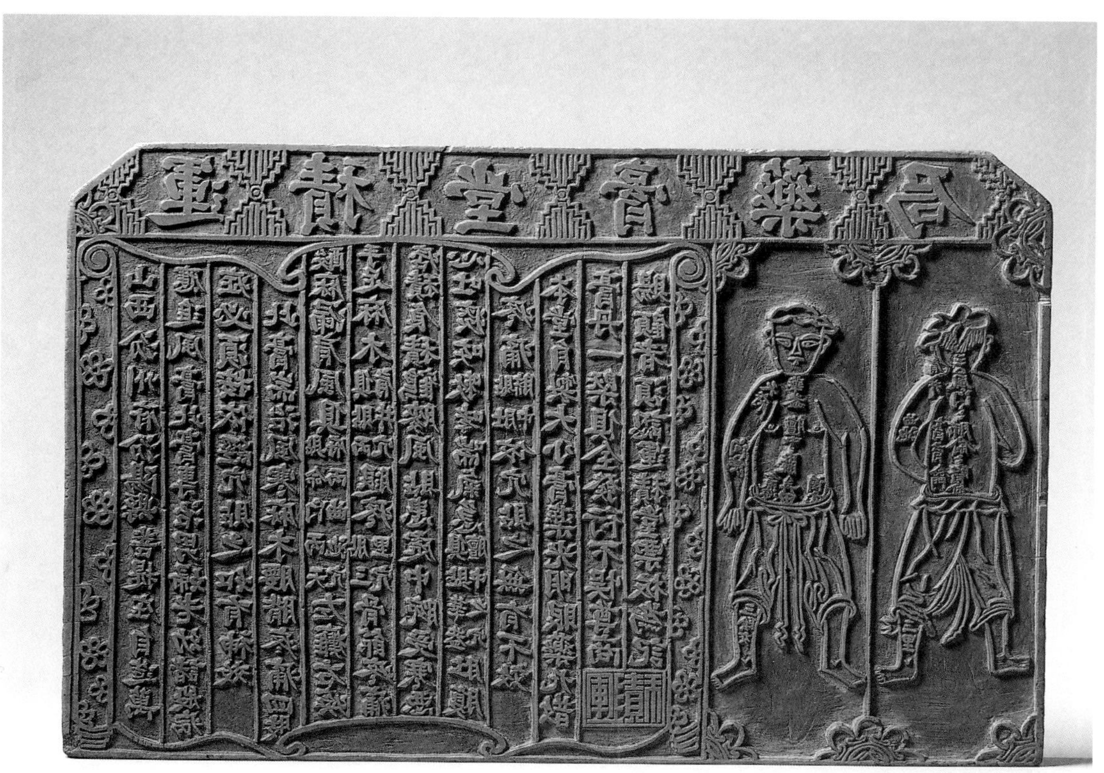

30. Printing plate for advertising bills for point ointments. 運積堂膏藥局 (Yunjitang Ointment Pharmacy). Wood, 19.5 x 30 cm (see ill., p. 58).

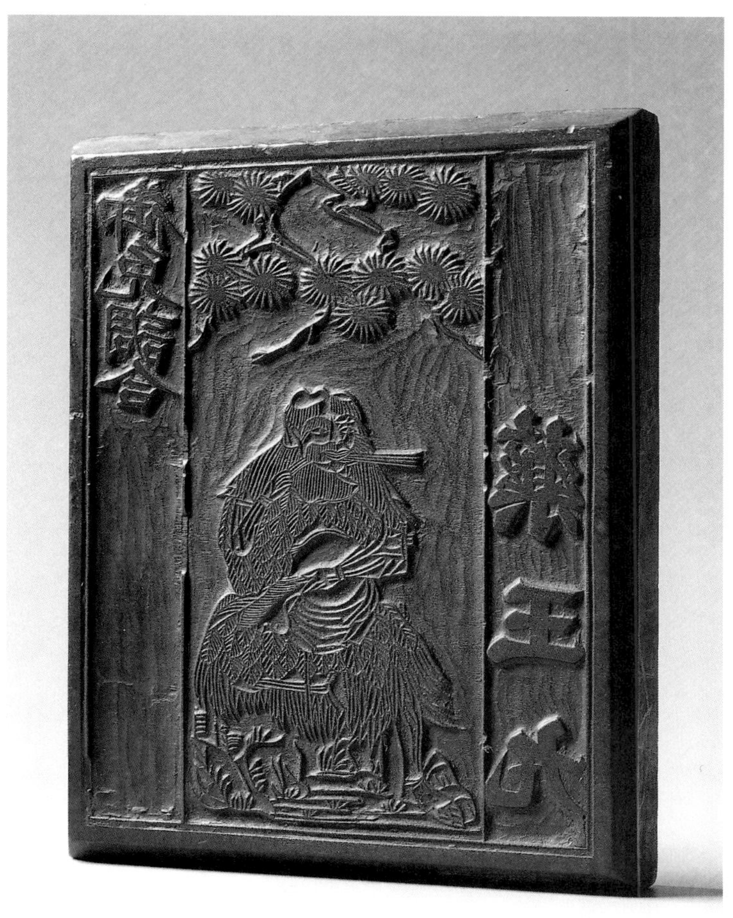

31. Printing plate for advertising bills for Medicine King Pills, Japan. Wood, 18.2 x 12.6 cm (see ill., p. 23).

撥雲散

專治男婦連年近日一切風
眼火眼氣眼或痛或瘼或目
起紅絲翳障昏盲由心肝瘫
熱目赤腫痛或白膜遮睛攀
睛努肉忽然兩目失明或風
毒上攻暴作目腫痛澀難開
眵淚不絕視物昏睛欲成内
障並皆熙之

32

京都
直隸蔚縣

針藥堂

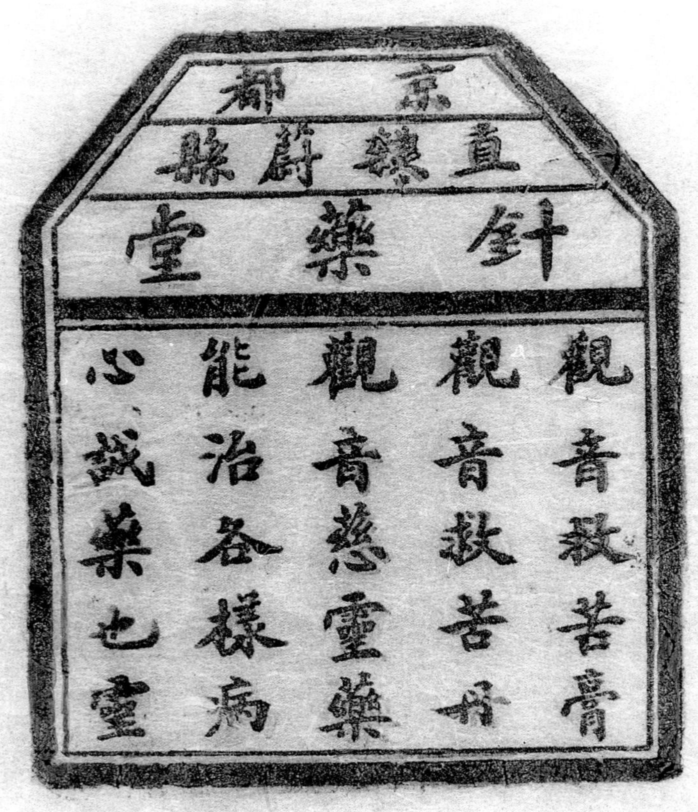

觀音救苦膏
觀音救苦丹
觀音慈靈藥
能治各樣病
心誠藥也靈

33

湧順堂

本堂自造海馬追風膏
風寒腫毒膏及打虫子
藥小兒驚瘋丸咳嗽補
肚丸散膏丹一概俱全
貨真價實不悮主顧
開設西合營西莊本堂
此膏世代祖傳　謹啟

34

天成德記　　内

本號向在東阿監製黑
驢皮九天貢膠加料精
製不惜工本并親身採
取阿井之水慶製良藥
誠心濟世凡福商賜
顧者認明本號同印為
記庶不致悮
謹識

35

32. Advertising bill for a "powder which disperses the clouds": "Especially [suited] for the treatment [of the following problems]: chronic or acute wind eyes, fire eyes, and qi eyes, if they hurt or itch or if red threads protrude. Cataracts and clouded vision. Reddening, pain, or swelling of the eyes caused by cataracts or heat in the heart or liver. A white membrane covering the eyeball. Fleshy growths creeping over the eyeball. Sudden loss of vision in both eyes. Wind poison rises up [in the body], attacks [the eyes there], and causes sudden swelling of the eyes with itching and [the sensation of] rawness, so that they can only be opened with difficulty, cloudy vision, and continuous tearing. Objects are perceived only blurred. It is possible that an internal cataract will form. In all these cases, sprinkle this [powder into the eyes]." Wood-block print, nineteenth or early twentieth century.

33. Advertising bill of the Zhenyaotang Pharmacy in Beijing: "Capital (= Beijing). (Main establishment in) Zhili (Hebei), district of Wei. Pharmacy for needles and medicines. The paste by which Guanyin saves from suffering, the elixir by which Guanyin saves from suffering, and the miraculous remedy which procures Guanyin's compassion are trust-worthy and, at the same time, miraculous medicines which are able to cure any kind of illness." Text in verse form a-b-a-c-c. Wood-block print, nineteenth or early twentieth century.

34. Advertising bill of the Yongshuntang Pharmacy: "This pharmacy manufactures: the ointment out of sea horses which expels wind, the ointment against swellings and poison due to wind cold, the medicine that strikes down insects, the pills against fright and wind disorders in small children, as well as pills, powders, ointments, and elixirs against coughing and for strengthening the abdomen. Anything will be cured. The merchandise is genuine, the price is real. The customer suffers no disadvantages. This ointment has been transmitted by descendants for generations. To be noted with care." Wood-block print, early twentieth century.

35. "This company is located in East A and manufactures gelatin of the highest quality from black donkey skin in a nine-day procedure under supervision. The processing is done with the greatest care. We save neither in expenditures of labor nor money. Moreover, we haul our own water from the A well and do not spare any effort to produce good medicines in order to provide assistance to humanity with a sincere mind. All well-off customers should memorize our company seal as trade-mark in order to avoid being misled." Seal: "To be noted with care." Early twentieth century.

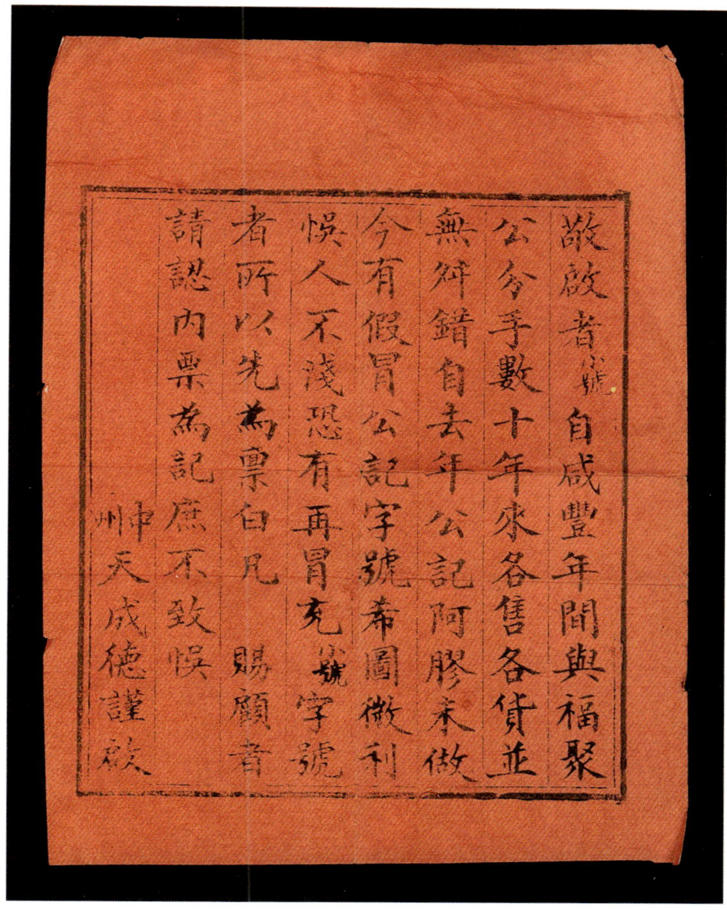

36. "Announcement by the [Pharmacy] Virtue Created by Heaven in Zhongzhou. To be announced herewith: Our company separated from the Fuju Partnership in the reign period Xianfeng (1851–1861). For several decades, each sold their merchandise separately, and no overlapping ever occurred. Because we failed to register the public trademark A gelatin in the past year, our company name has now appeared [on the market] with a counterfeit public trade-mark. The profit to be expected [by the competition] is slight, but the misleading of the population is not slight. Since we fear that the company name will again be abused for criminal purposes, we notified the authorities as a precaution. All clients should memorize the package insert as trade-mark in order to prevent being misled—Zhongzhou. By the [Pharmacy] Virtue Created by Heaven, to be noted with care." Package insert, early twentieth century.

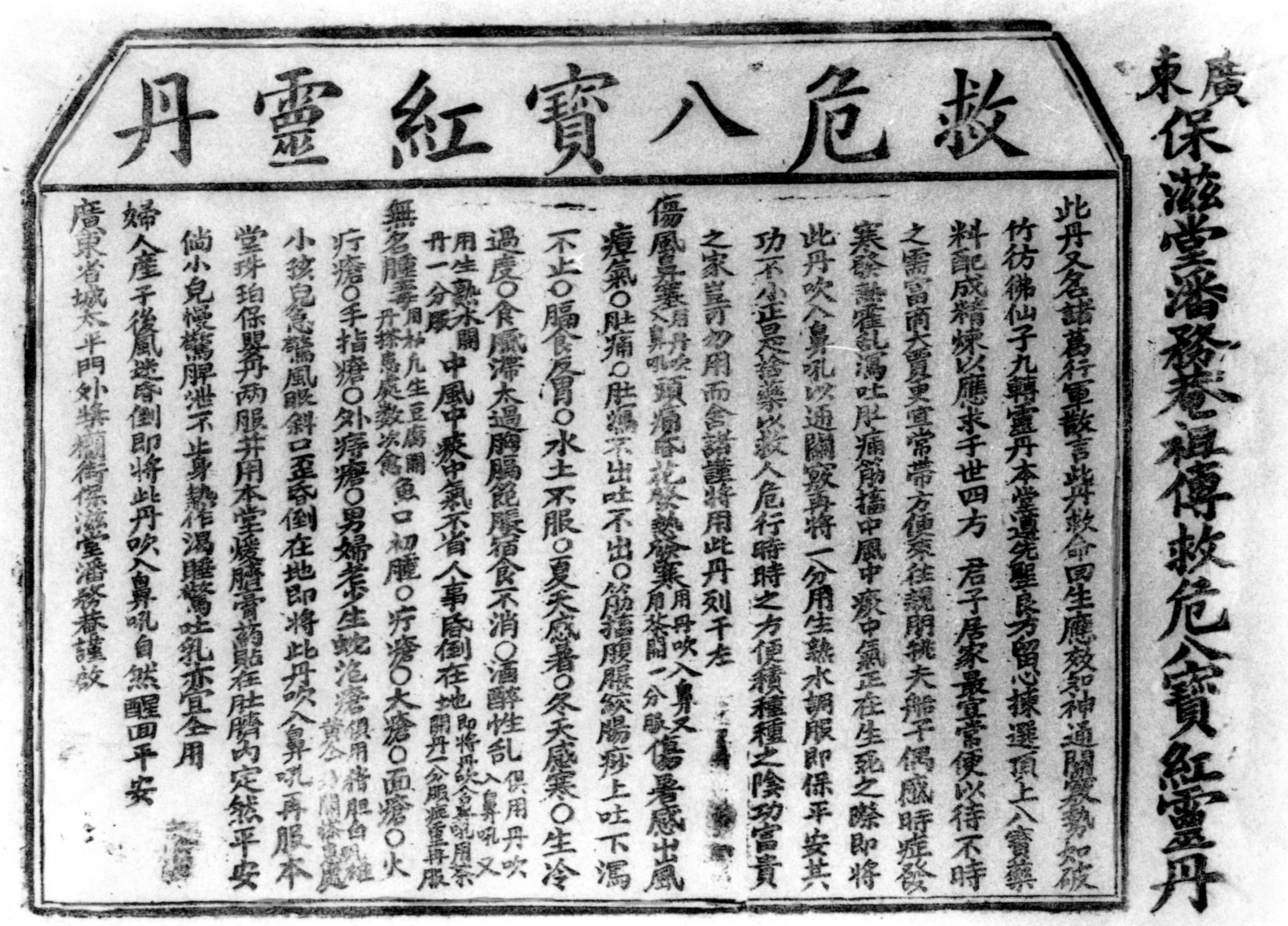



37. Advertising bill for "Pan Wuan's Red Miracle Elixir with Eight Precious [Ingredients] for Saving from Danger," transmitted by the ancestors, from the Pharmacy for Protection and Strength in Canton. This elixir is also called Zhuge [Liang]'s Powder Which Causes the Soldiers to Run. This means, this elixir saves one's existence and brings back life. Its effects are divine. It penetrates gates and openings with strength as if it was [merely] breaking through bamboo. ... Our pharmacy honors the fine formulas of the ancient sages and takes care to only choose the best. The combination and processing of the Eight Precious Ingredients satisfied the needs of a thousand generations in all four directions.

For the gentleman residing in his house, it is of the greatest importance to always have [this remedy] on hand in order to be prepared for any unforeseeable events. For the well-off merchant, it is even more important to always carry [this remedy] on him in order to be able to receive his relatives and friends without worries or travel to them.

Mr. Yao Fuchuan was unexpectedly affected by a seasonally caused illness. By turns, he felt cold and feverish. [He suffered from] cholera [with] diarrhea and vomiting, abdominal pain and spasms of the tendons, wind stroke, phlegm stroke, and qi stroke. He had in fact reached the border between life and death. Then, someone blew this elixir into his nose opening in order to penetrate the gates and openings and made him ingest another dose in hot water. With this, his health was protected. The effect of this [elixir] was not slight. ...

[It is suited] for bringing well-being at any time and collecting secret merits of all kinds. How could wealthy families renounce its application. All of its uses are noted below. ..."

Zhuge Liang 諸葛亮 (181–234) was the political and military advisor of Liu Bei 劉備 (162–223), the founder and first emperor of the Shu dynasty. Contemporaries attributed superhuman abilities to Zhuge Liang; he was regarded as a mathematical genius and seemed to be able to not only forecast, but even control natural events. He invented, for example, a bow which could shoot several arrows simultaneously, and made decisive improvements to the "eight military strategies". The powder which causes the soldiers to run (*xingjunsan* 行軍散), and its eight ingredients, alluding to the eight military strategies of Zhuge Liang, was published for the first time in the revised edition of the cholera book *Huoluan lun* 霍亂論 (On Cholera)(1862) by Wang Shixiong 王士雄 (1808–1866), first edition 1838. Ever since, it has been mass-produced and marketed by numerous pharmacies. It is also known under the name *Wuhou xingjunsan* 武侯行軍散 (The Military Lord's Powder to Make the Soldiers Run); *wuhou* (military lord) is a posthumous honorary title of Zhuge Liang.

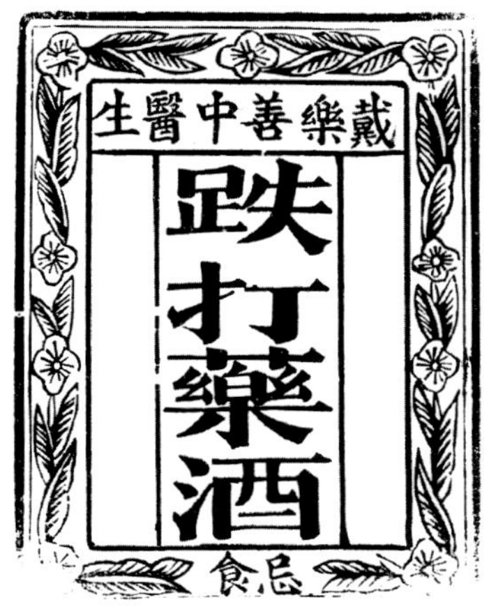

38. Advertising bill by a "doctor of Chinese medicine [called] Dai Leshan" for a "medicinal wine [for the treatment of] falling and hitting [injuries]." Wood-block print, early twentieth century.

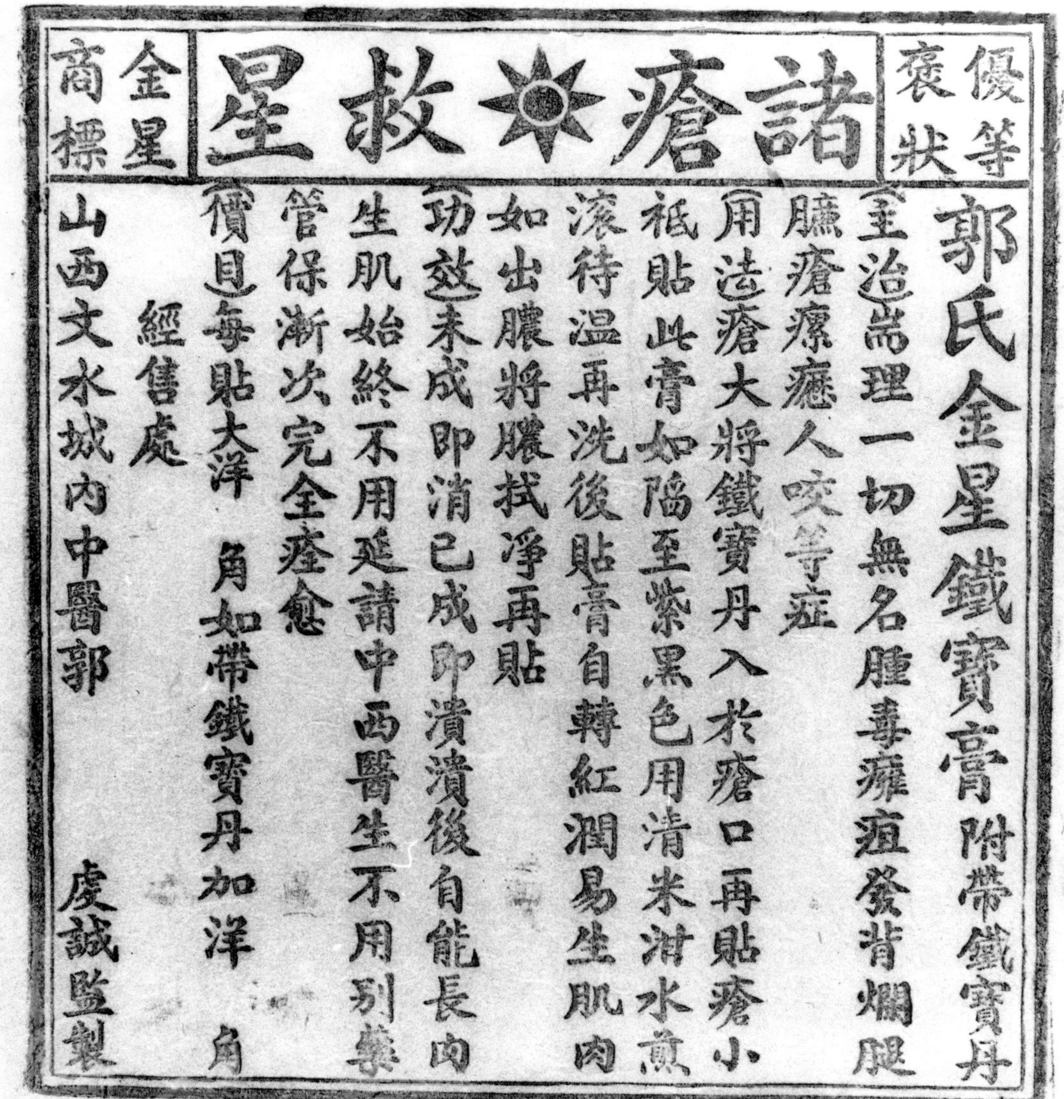

39. Advertising bill of a "doctor of traditional Chinese medicine" for medicines sold by him: "First class and commendable. The savior from all ulcer problems. Trade-mark Golden Star. The Golden Star Iron Treasure Ointment by Sir Kuo. In addition: the elixir for guiding the iron treasure. Main indications: Especially suited for the treatment of any unspecified swellings, toxic *yong* and *ju* ulcers, open back, scrofulous ulcers on legs and thighs, as well as bites by humans. Application: For extensive ulcers, put the Iron Treasure Elixir directly on the ulcer opening and then apply [the ointment on top of it]. For small ulcers, merely apply the ointment. When [the ulcer] has sunk in and turned a purplish black color, bring clear rice-washing water to a simmer, let it cool to a warm temperature and wash [the ulcer] repeatedly with it. Then apply the ointment. Afterwards, [the ulcer] will turn a shiny red and will easily form [new] flesh. If [the tumor] discharges pus, wipe it off and then apply [the ointment]. Effects: When [the tumor] has not yet erupted, it will reduce [the swelling]. When [the tumor] has already erupted, then it will flow out. When it has flown out, then it will form [new] flesh on its own. From beginning to end, there is no need to consult a doctor of Chinese or Western medicine or to apply any other medicines. Step by step, a complete recovery is guaranteed. Prices: Each application: [ ] silver dollar. If the elixir for guiding the iron treasure [is also used], in addition [ ] silver dollars. Locations where [the medicines] are sold: [ ]. Produced under [government] supervision by the doctor for Chinese medicine Kuo Chucheng in Shanxi [Province], Wenshui City." Wood-block print, early twentieth century.

40. Street sign-board of a pharmacy. Front: 回春堂尚治一切瘋科疑難雜症 "Pharmacy Return to Spring. Cures especially any problematic conditions from the area of wind problems"; Back: 趙振康尚治一切傷科疑難雜症 "[Owner:] Zhao Zhenkang. Cures especially any problematic conditions from the area of injuries."

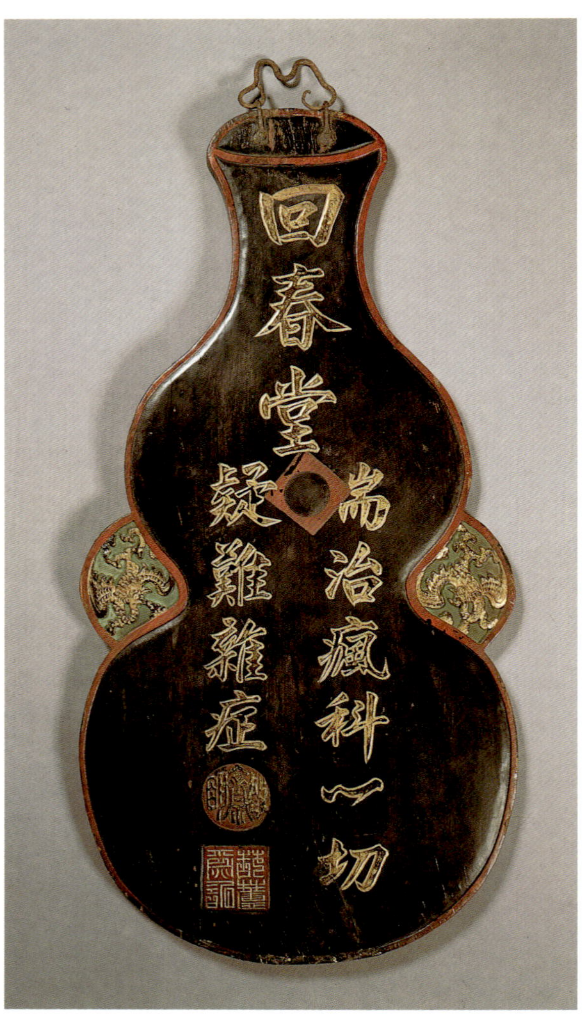

41. Advertising board (Kanban) of a Japanese pharmacy for Chinese and Western medicines. Right border: "Main establishment in Ise." Right rectangle: "Pills for the treatment of illnesses. Expel one hundred kinds of poisons." Circle in center: "To be applied externally. New drug for any inflammations of the skin." Middle of center circle: (German technical term in Katakana) "Hauto (= skin)." Small circle top center: Trade-mark with pine and crane. Left rectangle: "Miraculous drug from gynecology. Decoction of the Dragon King for harmonizing and adjusting with ginseng." Left border: "Contracted shop Yamaguchi Pharmacy." Gold and black lacquer on wood with broad frame of black lacquer and rounded edges, 50.5 x 90 cm. Types of writing: Kanji/Chinese characters, Hiragana, Katakana, Western letters. Some of the characters are filled-in with red, late-nineteenth, early twentieth century.



*Opposite page:*

42. Advertising board (Kanban) of a Japanese pharmacy for Chinese and Western medicines. Right border: "Main establishment in Tokyo, Ushiko. Product of the Shiseido [Company]." Right oval (Latin): "Shiseido. Recor. Geisteskranken (German: the mentally ill)." Chinese characters right and left: "Illnesses of the brain and the nervous system. Reliably effective sedative." Katakana center: "Recoru." Chinese characters center: "Special water. Eye medicine." Left oval (Latin): "Shiseido. Prosin. Magen-Darmkatarrh (German: gastric-enteritis)." Chinese characters right and left: "Problems of the digestive system. Brand-new high-quality preparation." Katakana center: "Puroshin." Left border: "Contracted shop Daikokuya Pharmacy". Gold, red, and black lacquer on wood with broad frame of black lacquer and rounded edges, 42 x 121 cm. Types of writing: Kanji/Chinese characters, Hiragana, Katakana, Western letters, late-nineteenth, early twentieth century.

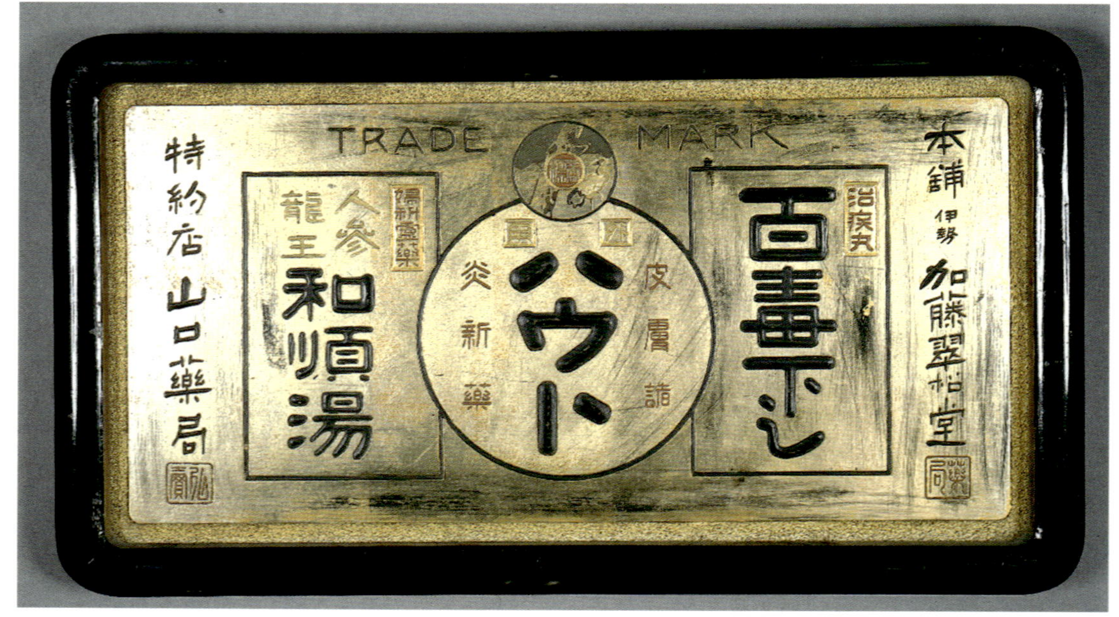

43. Advertising board (Kanban) of
a Japanese pharmacy for Chinese
and Western medicines. Right
border: "Main establishment: Red
Cross Pharmacy." Black plate on
right: "Miraculous stomach medicine guides downwards what
adversely rises to the top." Gold
plate right: "Strengthens the
stomach: Pills which penetrate
quickly." Top center: Globe with
red cross. "Registered trademark."
Center: "Suppresses the pain. Pills
that treat diarrhea. Miraculous
medicine for all types of diarrhea."
Black plate left: "Special cough
medicine." Gold plate left:
"Suppresses coughing. Powder
which removes phlegm." Left
border: "Wholesale firm Tsukada
Pharmacy." Gold, red, and black
lacquer on wood with broad frame
of black lacquer and rounded
edges, 42 x 121 cm. Types of
writing: Kanji/Chinese characters,
Hiragana late-nineteenth, early
twentieth century.

44. Advertising board (Kanban)
of a Japanese pharmacy for
Chinese and Western medicines.
Red circle right: "Special water.
Eye medicine."
Left oval: "Capsulae Gonor"
(Latin); "Treat gonorrhea"
(Chinese); "Gonoru"( Katakana);
"Innerlichen (Interior)"
(German). Right border: "Main
establishment in Tokyo,
Ushigome, Shiseido." Left border:
"Contracted shop Nagasawa
Pharmacy." Gold, red, and black
lacquer on wood with broad
frame of black lacquer and
rounded edges, 42 x 112 cm.
Types of writing: Kanji/Chinese
characters, Hiragana, Katakana,
Western letters late-nineteenth,
early twentieth century.

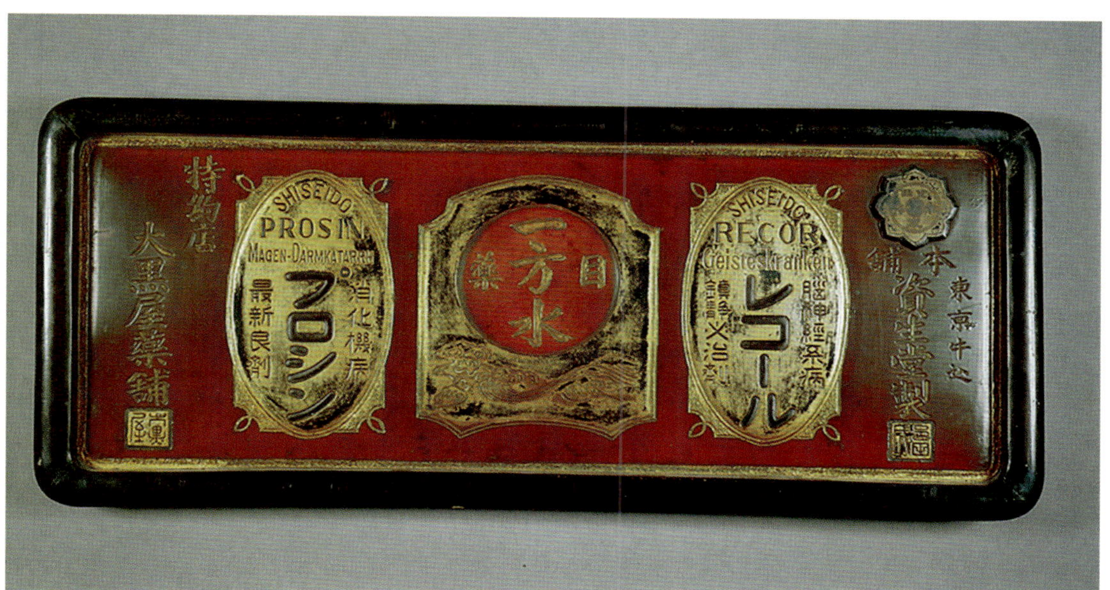

42

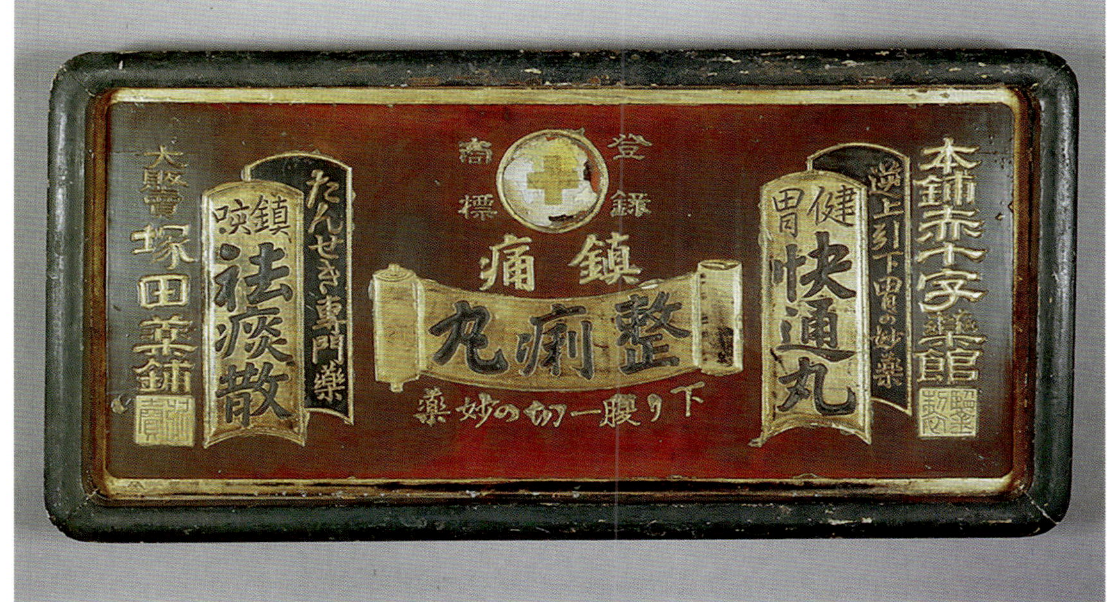

43

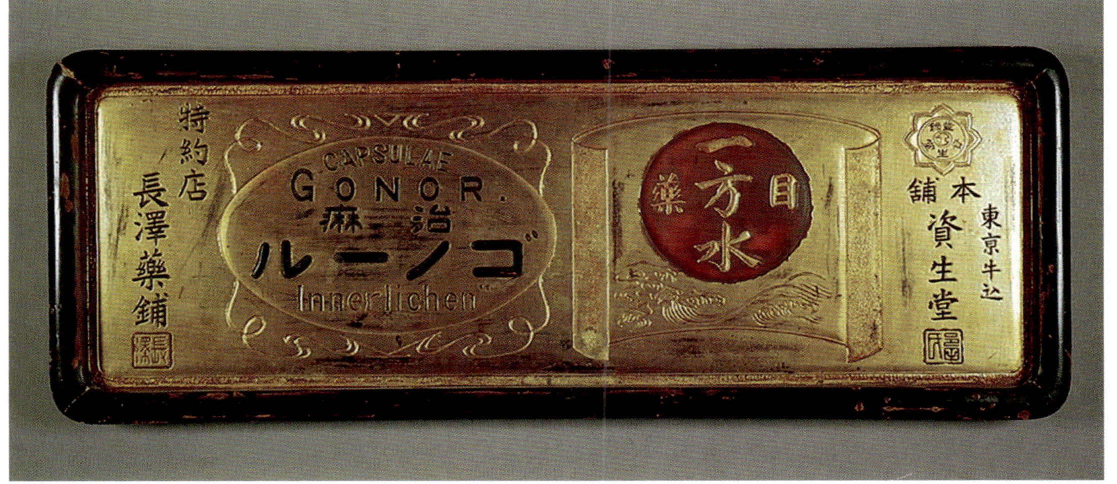

44

The oldest preserved medical texts in China date from the second century B.C.E. In these manuscripts, pharmaceutical drug lore plays an eminent role among the various methods of treatment, as seen in several hundred drugs recommended in several hundred formulas for fifty-two internal and external illnesses of the human body. Of special interest is the level of sophistication of the pharmaceutical technology, apparent from the numerous techniques for drug preparation and processing as well as the use of a differentiated terminology.

Several centuries later, detailed information was already being published in textbooks regarding the synergistic effects of various drugs when used in combination; pharmaceutical procedures served to alleviate or avoid undesired side effects altogether. During the development of materia medica, from the twelfth to the fifteenth centuries, pharmaceutical processing was responsible for the modification of active and guiding drugs in complicated recipes by treating them with different fluids or types of fire—the assumption being that medications would reach specific locations in the body and cause highly specific and theoretically determined results.

Pharmacies purchased (and purchase) the drugs, generally pre-dried and pre-treated, from gatherers and wholesale traders. They then processed them for distribution as individual drugs or extensive combinations. Specialized implements were used by the pharmacies to facilitate the drying and steaming of the raw drugs as well as their pulverization and processing into pills, powders, pastes, or medicinal fluids. With the exception of mass-produced preparations, often intended for use during travel, medications that had been composed for individual illnesses were generally taken as decoctions.

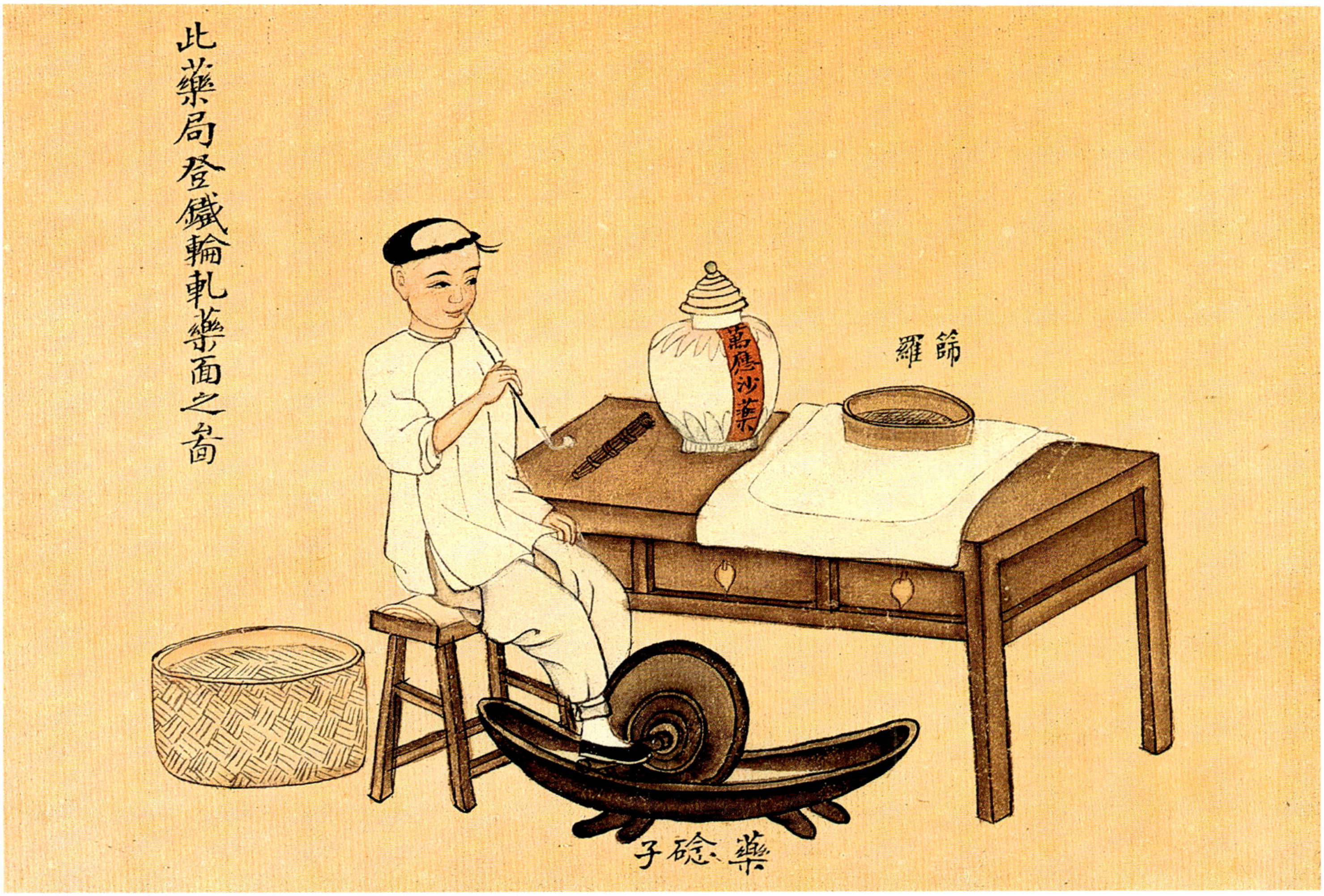

45. "This illustration shows the pulverization of medicine in a pharmacy with the iron wheel." Gouache, second half of the nineteenth century. Museum für Völkerkunde, Berlin.

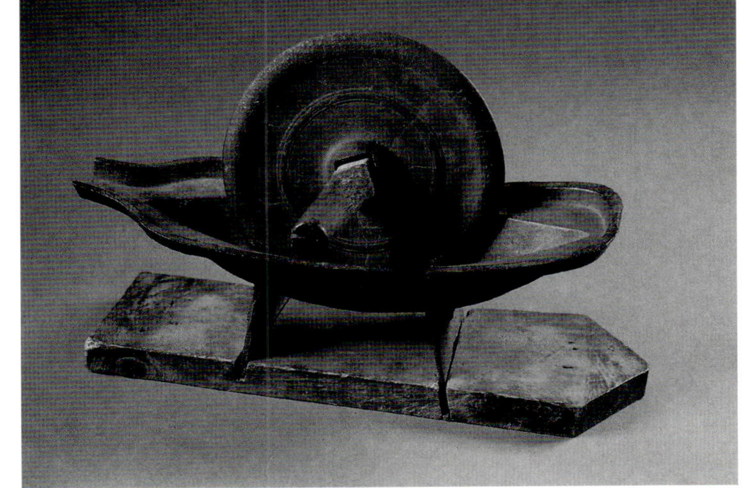

46. Pharmacy implement for the pulverization of plant-based drugs. Iron boat on wooden board with iron wheel and wooden handle, height 14.3 cm, South China.

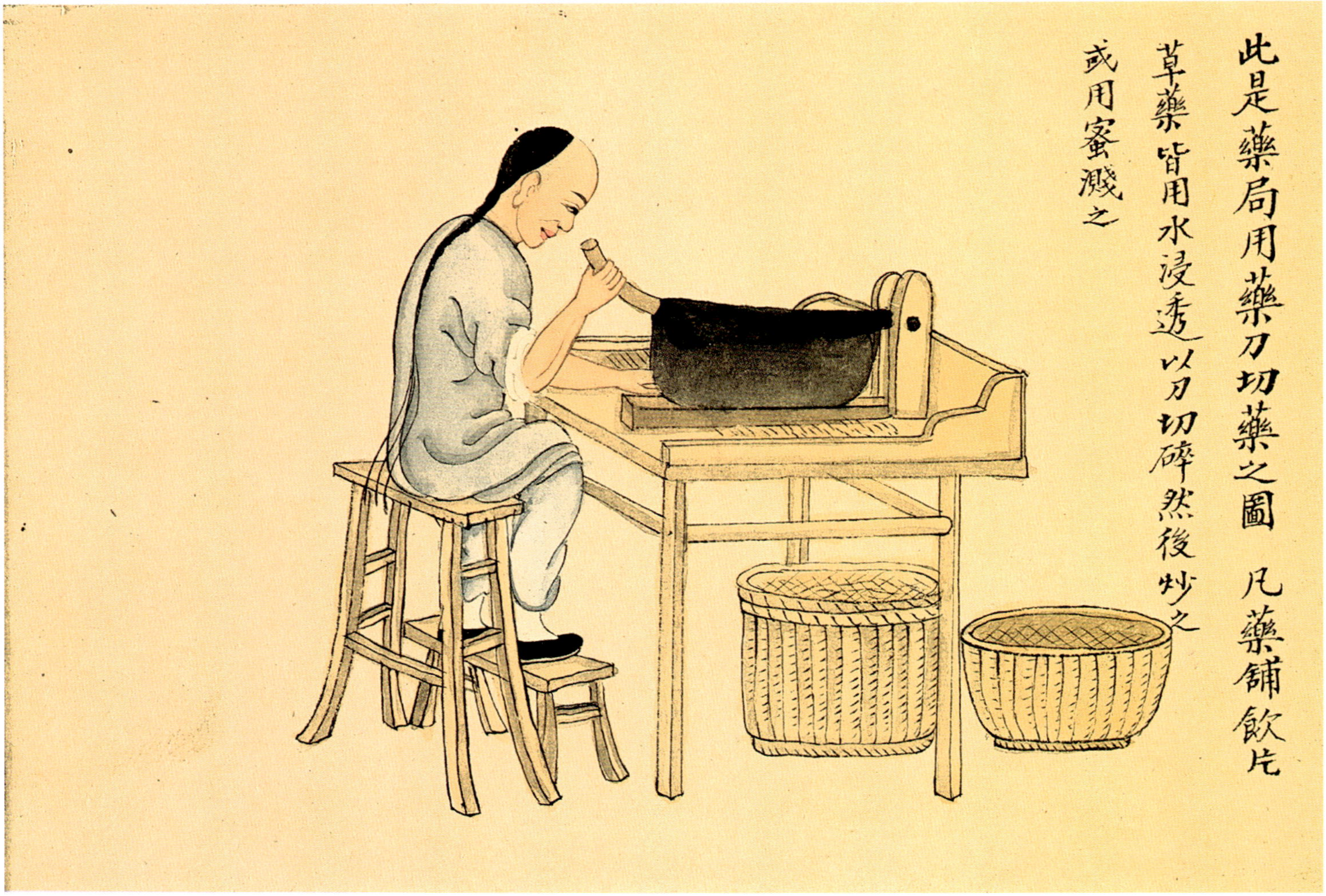

47. "This illustration shows how drugs are cut up in a pharmacy with the drug knife. All herbal tablets and herbal medicines are softened in water in the pharmacy and cut up with the knife. Then they are roasted. Some are coated in honey." Gouache, second half of the nineteenth century. Museum für Völkerkunde, Berlin.

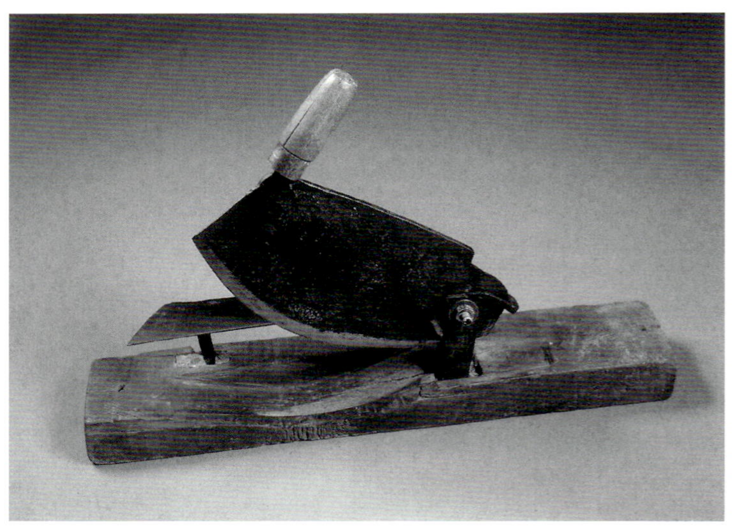

48. Pharmacy implement for cutting plant-based drugs, height 26.5 cm, Shanghai.

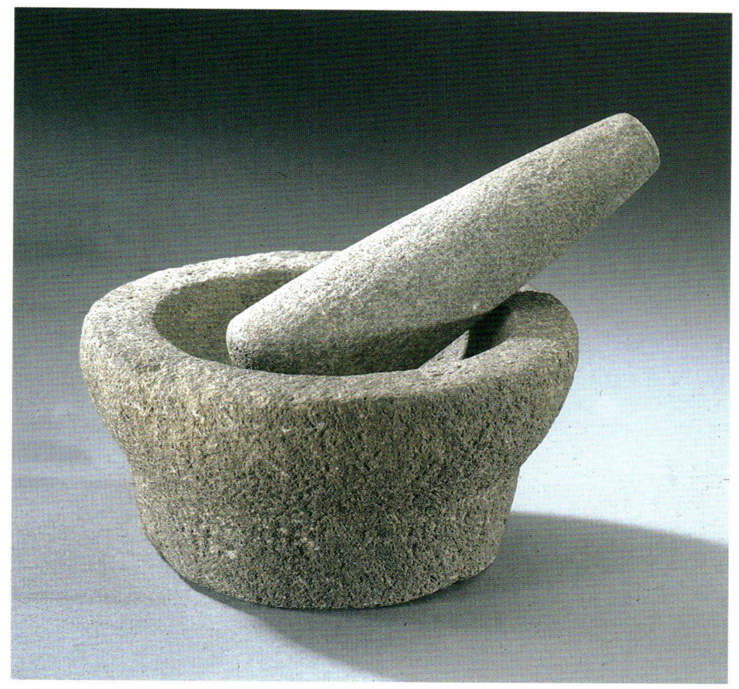

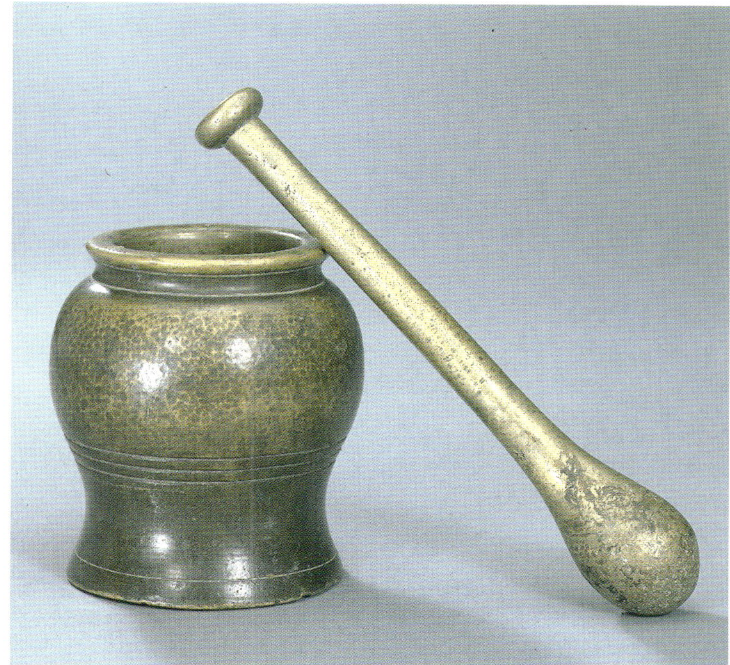

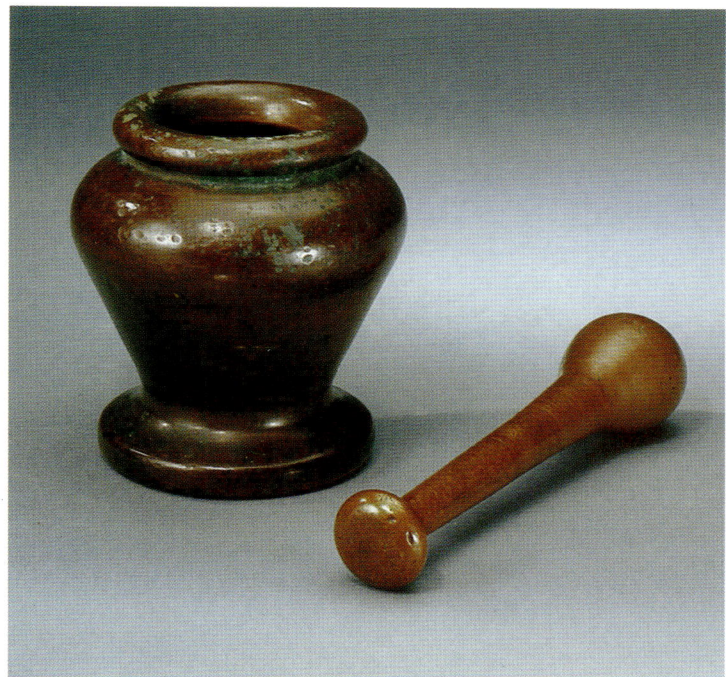

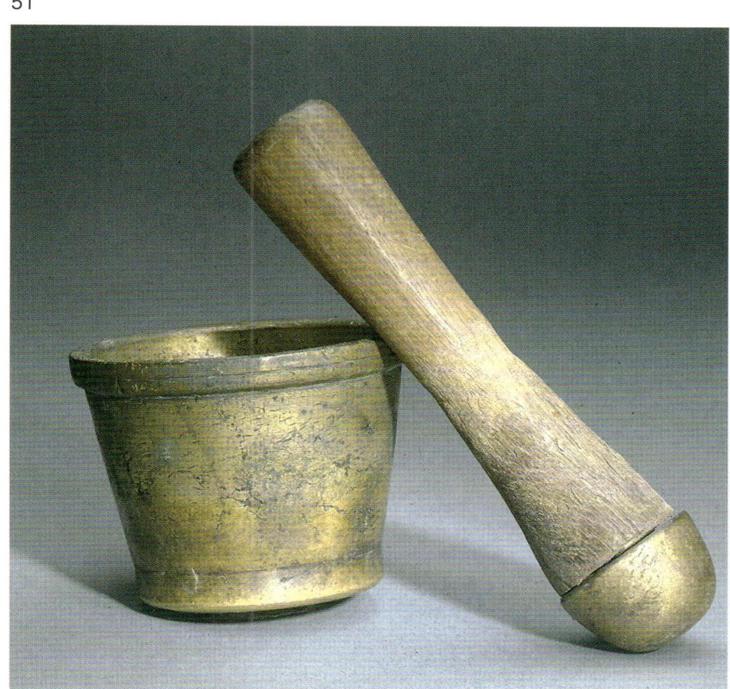

49. Pharmacy mortar and pestle. Stone, height 7.7 cm, South China.

50. Pharmacy mortar and pestle. Brass, height 13 cm, North China, nineteenth century or earlier.

51. Pharmacy mortar and pestle. Brass, height 12 cm, North China, nineteenth century or earlier.

52. Pharmacy mortar and pestle. Brass, wooden pestle handle with brass tip, height 9 cm, South China.

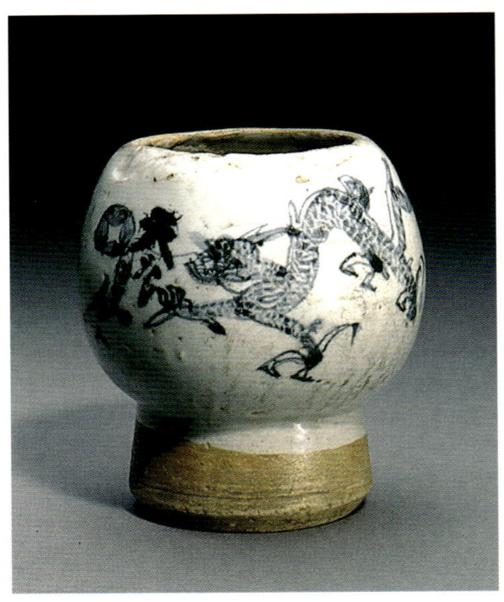 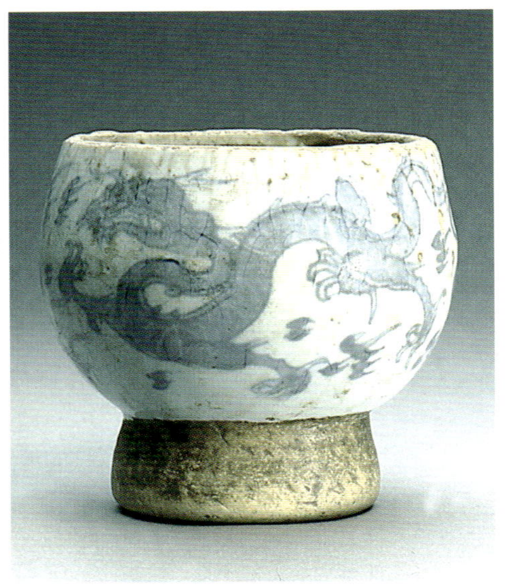

53. Pharmacy mortar decorated with dragon and plant. Porcelain, Fujian ware, blue underglaze on a white background, height 12 cm, seventeenth–eighteenth centuries.

54. Pharmacy mortar decorated with dragon and clouds. Fujian ware, blue underglaze on a white background, height 10.6 cm, seventeenth–eighteenth centuries.

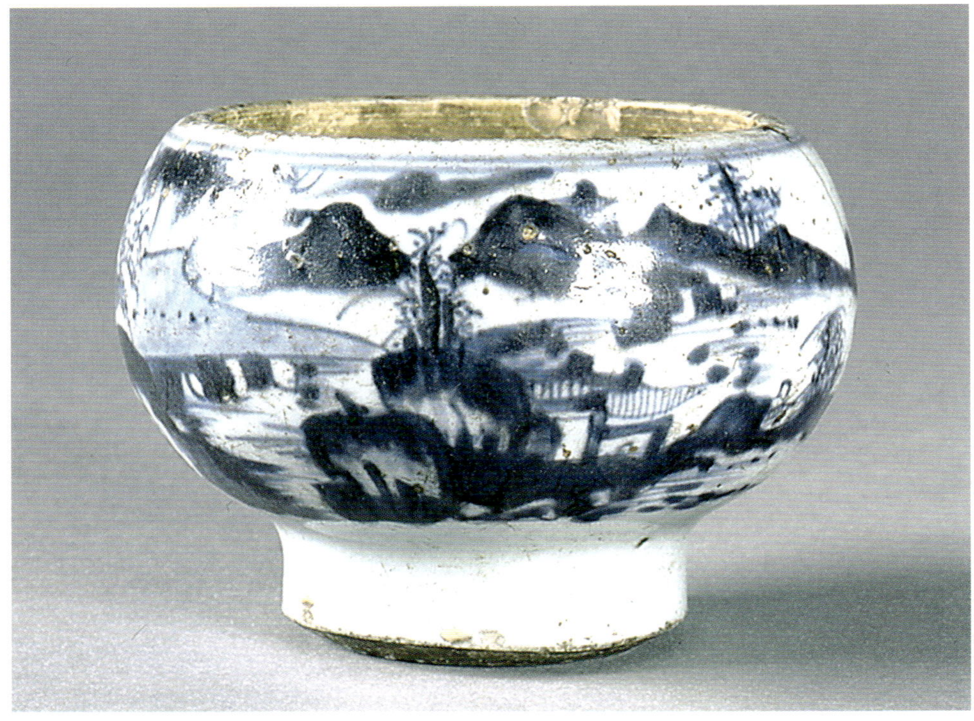

55. Pharmacy mortar decorated with landscape, human figures, boats, and houses. Porcelain, Fujian ware, blue underglaze on a white background, height 9 cm, eighteenth century.

56. Pharmacy mortar decorated with a child among plants. Porcelain, Fujian ware, blue underglaze on a white background, height 7.6 cm, eighteenth–nineteenth centuries.

57. Pharmacy mortar with plant decor. Porcelain, Fujian ware, blue underglaze on white background, height 8 cm, nineteenth century.

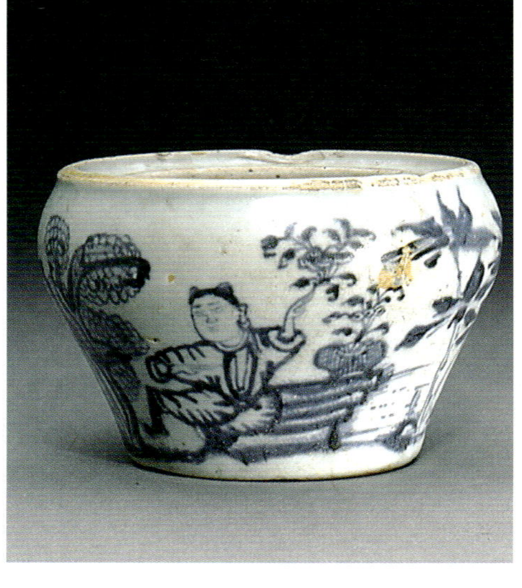 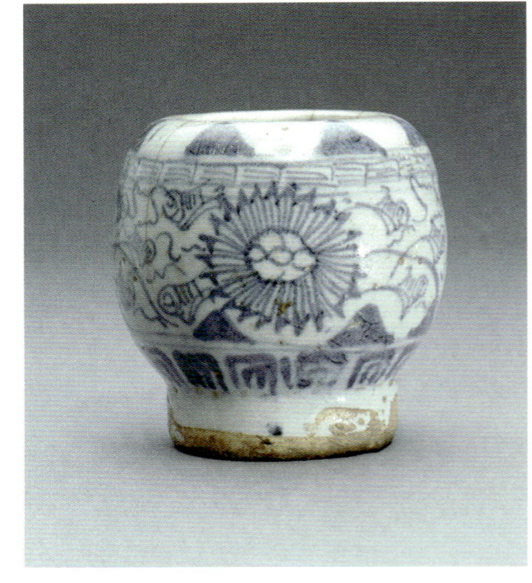

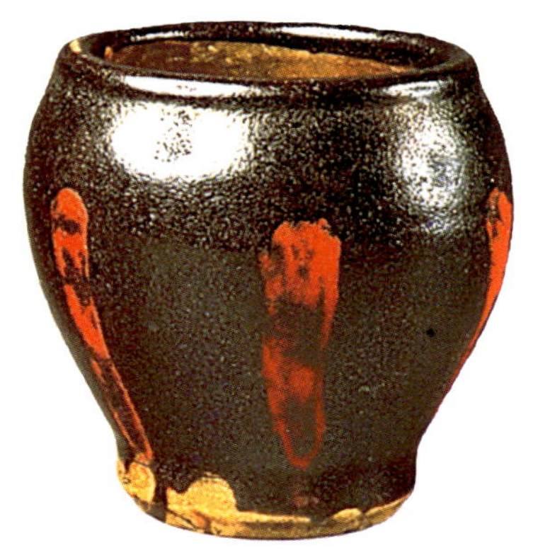

58. Pharmacy mortar with red stripes on a blackish-brown ground. Porcelain, Fujian ware, height 9 cm, nineteenth century.

59. Pharmacy mortar decorated with *Fo* dog and plants. Porcelain, blue underglaze on a white background, height 8 cm, South China

60. Three pharmacy grinding bowls decorated with landscapes. Porcelain, early eighteenth through early twentieth centuries.

61. Pharmacy grinding bowl decorated with a landscape. Porcelain. Wooden pestle handle with porcelain tip, height 7.6 cm.

62. View of the base of a pharmacy grinding bowl decorated with peonies. Signed: Eighth year of the Republic (1919), "Pharmacy which lets everybody partake in spring." Porcelain, height 7.1 cm.

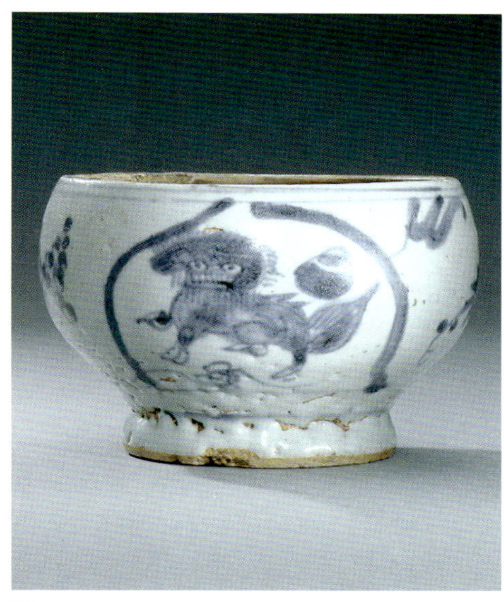

59

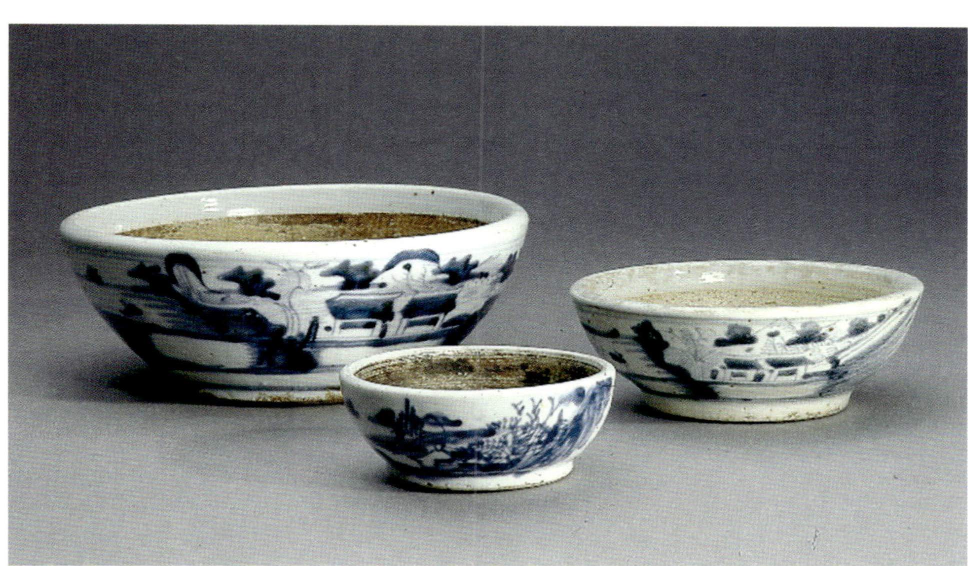

60

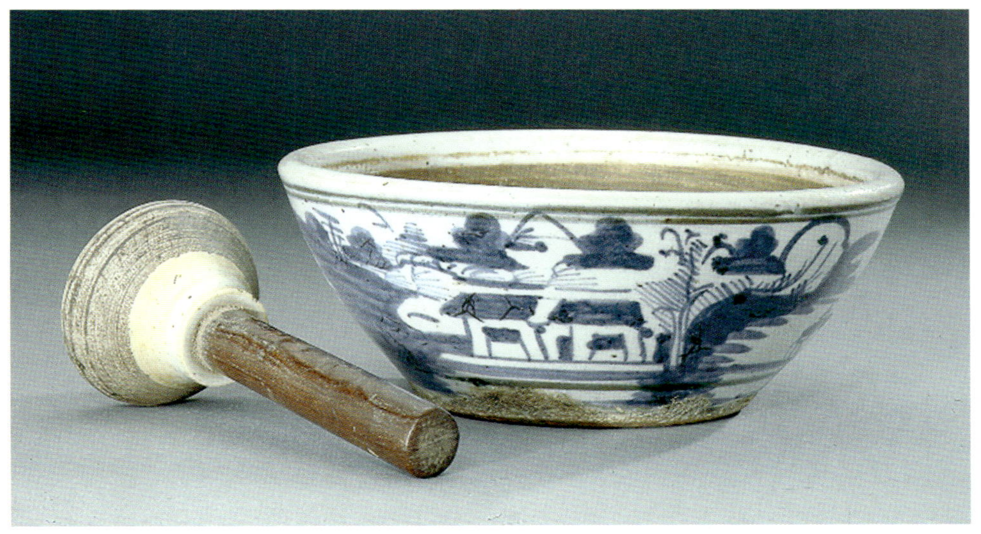

61

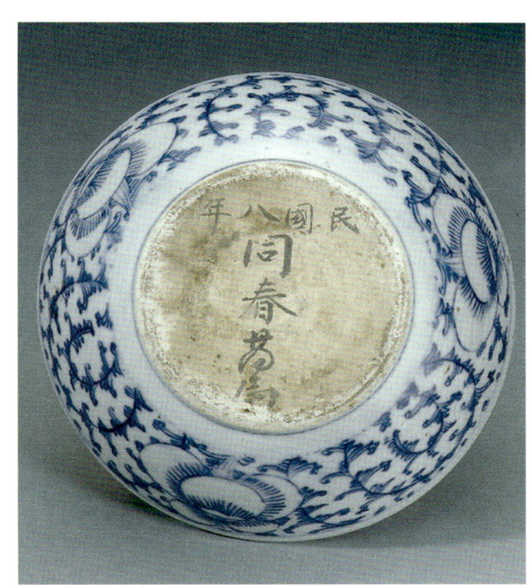

62

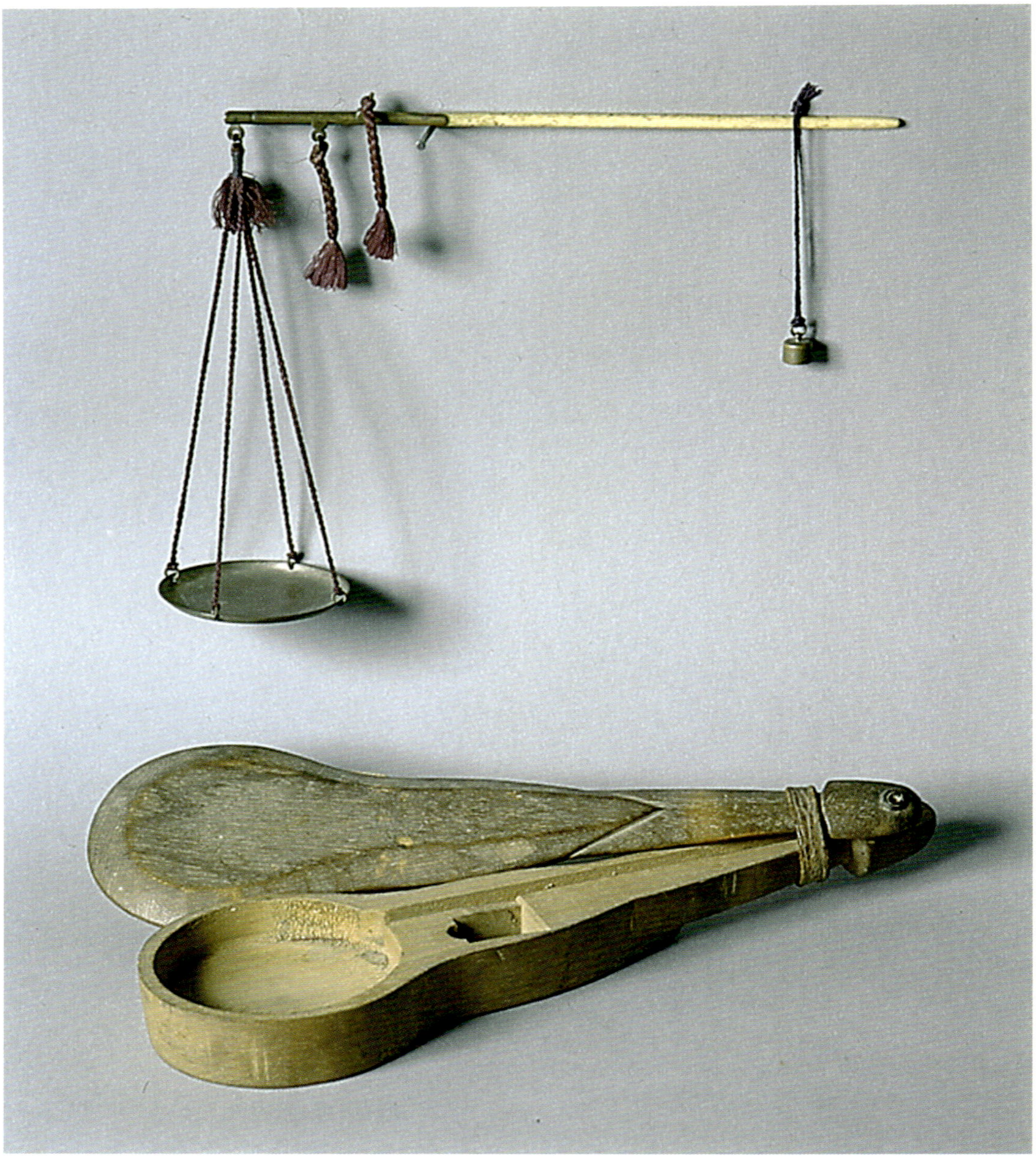

63. Pharmacy dispensing scale.
Bone, copper, wood (in gourd
shape), length 25.8 cm.

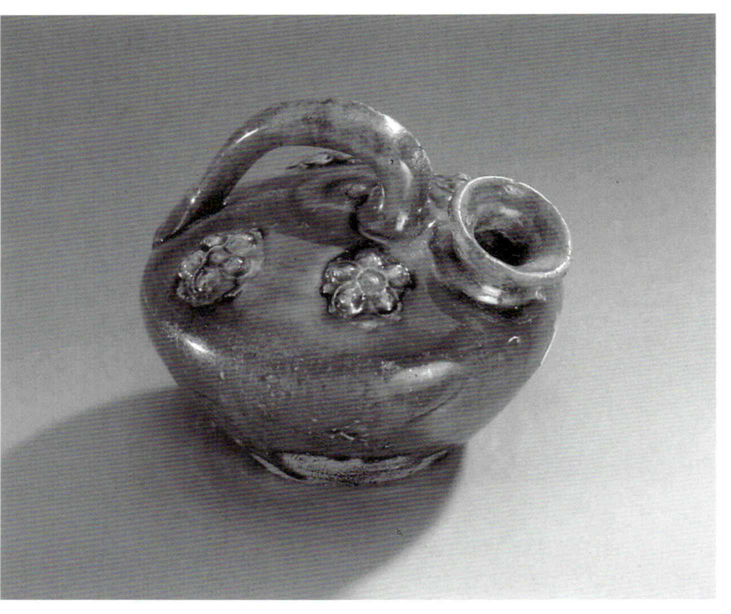

64. Collection container for boys'
urine (with handle) decorated
with reliefs of four blossoms.
Stoneware, golden brown glaze,
North China, seventeenth
century.

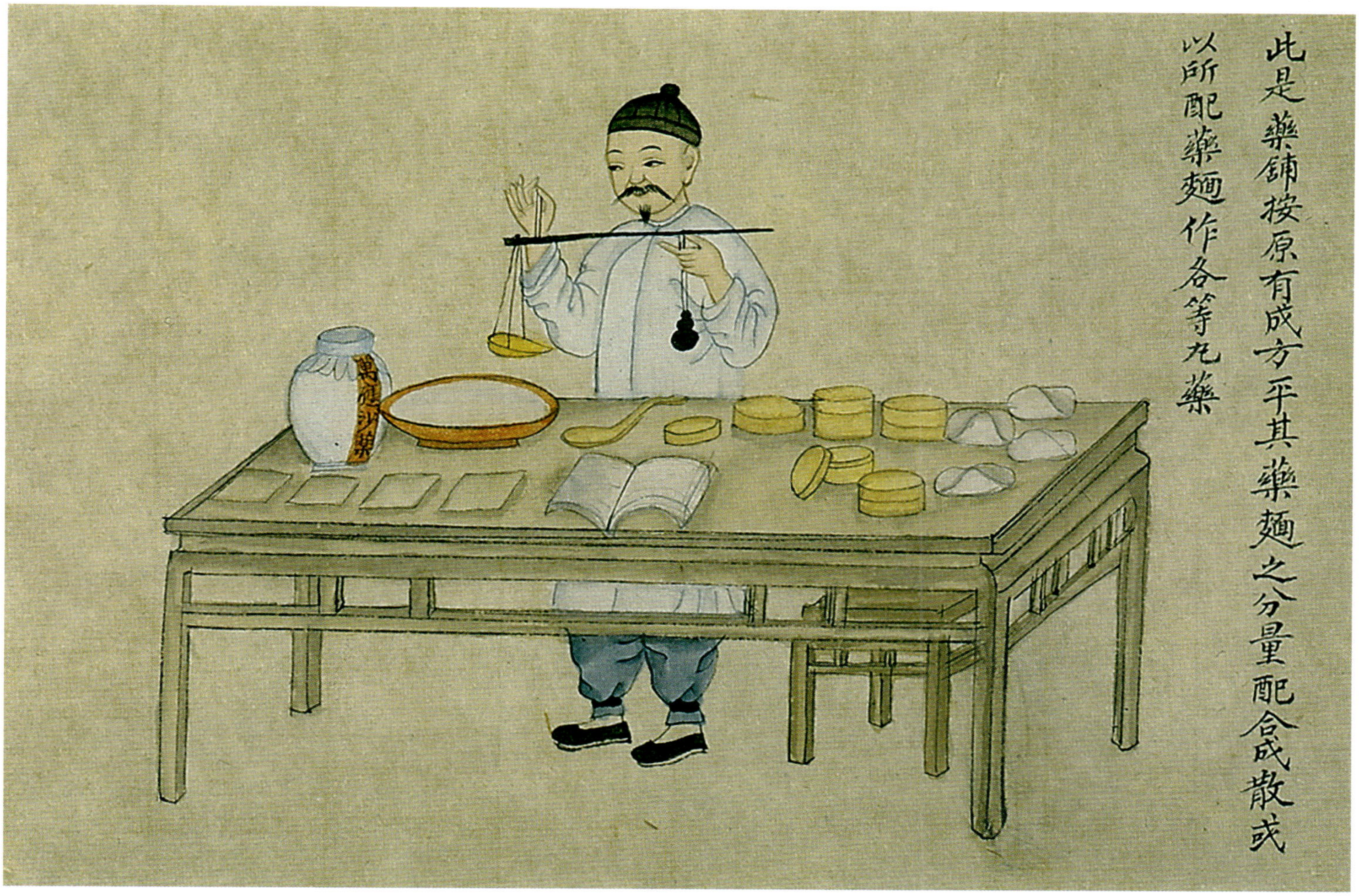

此是藥舖按原有成方平其藥麵之分量配合成散或
以所配藥麵作各等丸藥

65. "This illustration shows
the weighing of the primary
ingredients [of a prescription]
in powdered form for the
combination of [medicinal]
powders or for the manufacturing of all kinds of pills by way of
combining medicinal powders."
Gouache, second half of the
nineteenth century. Museum für
Völkerkunde, Berlin.

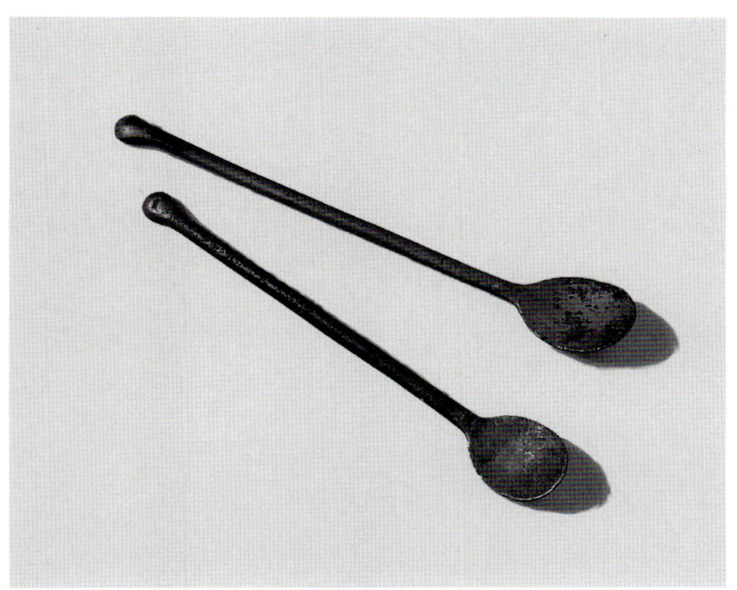

66. Two pharmacy dispensing
spoons. Brass, each 14/16 cm in
length

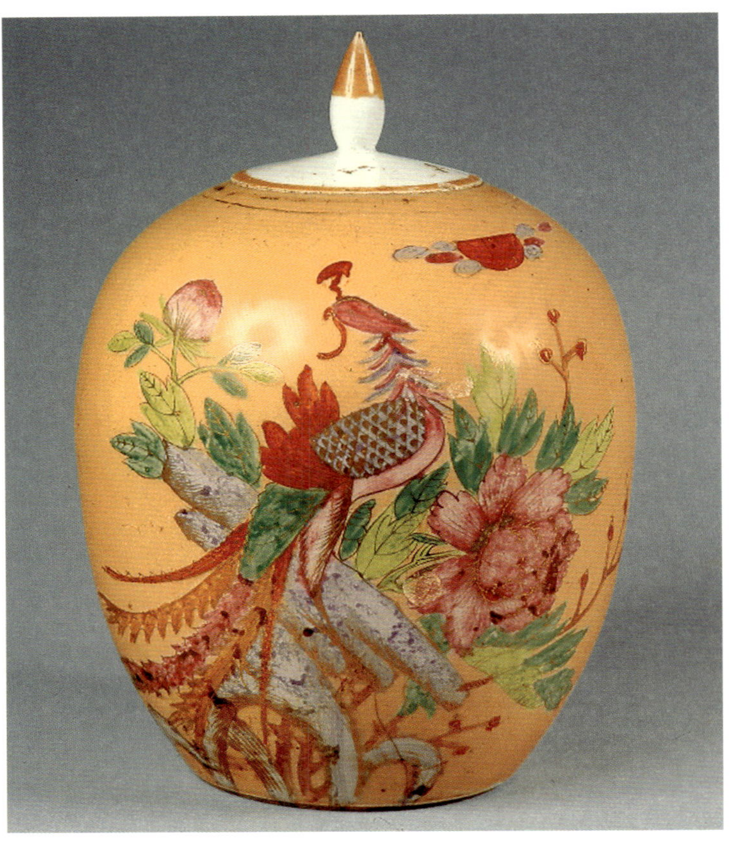

68. Pharmacy container and cover decorated with animals in a landscape. Porcelain, multicolored underglaze on white background, height 14.6 cm, South China.

67. Pharmacy container and cover decorated with a phoenix and blossoms. Porcelain, multicolored underglaze on light brown background, height 14.8 cm, South China.

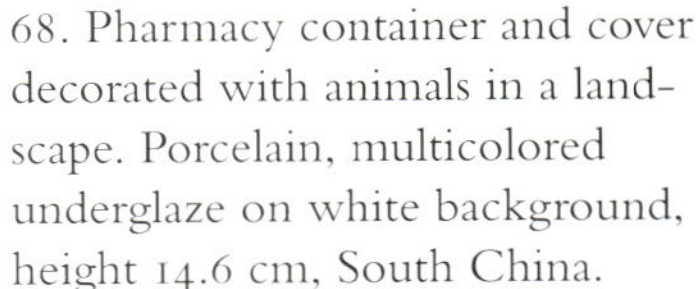

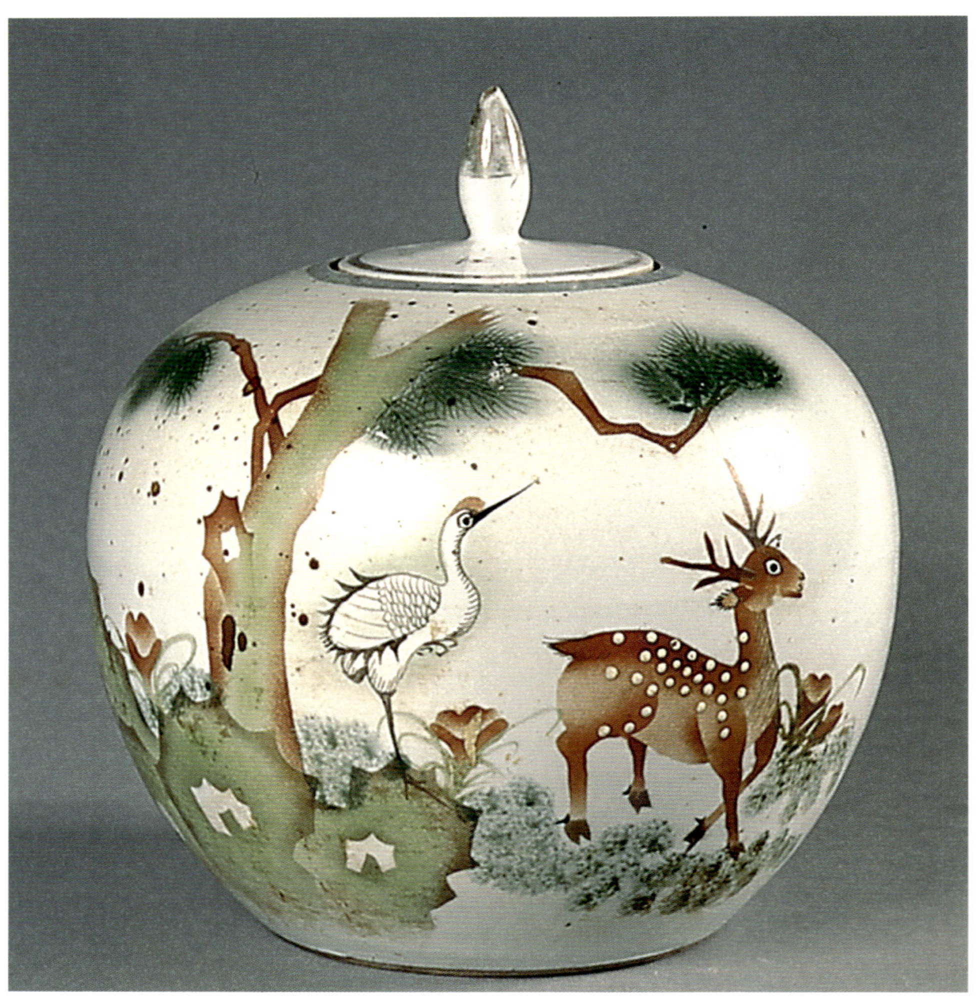

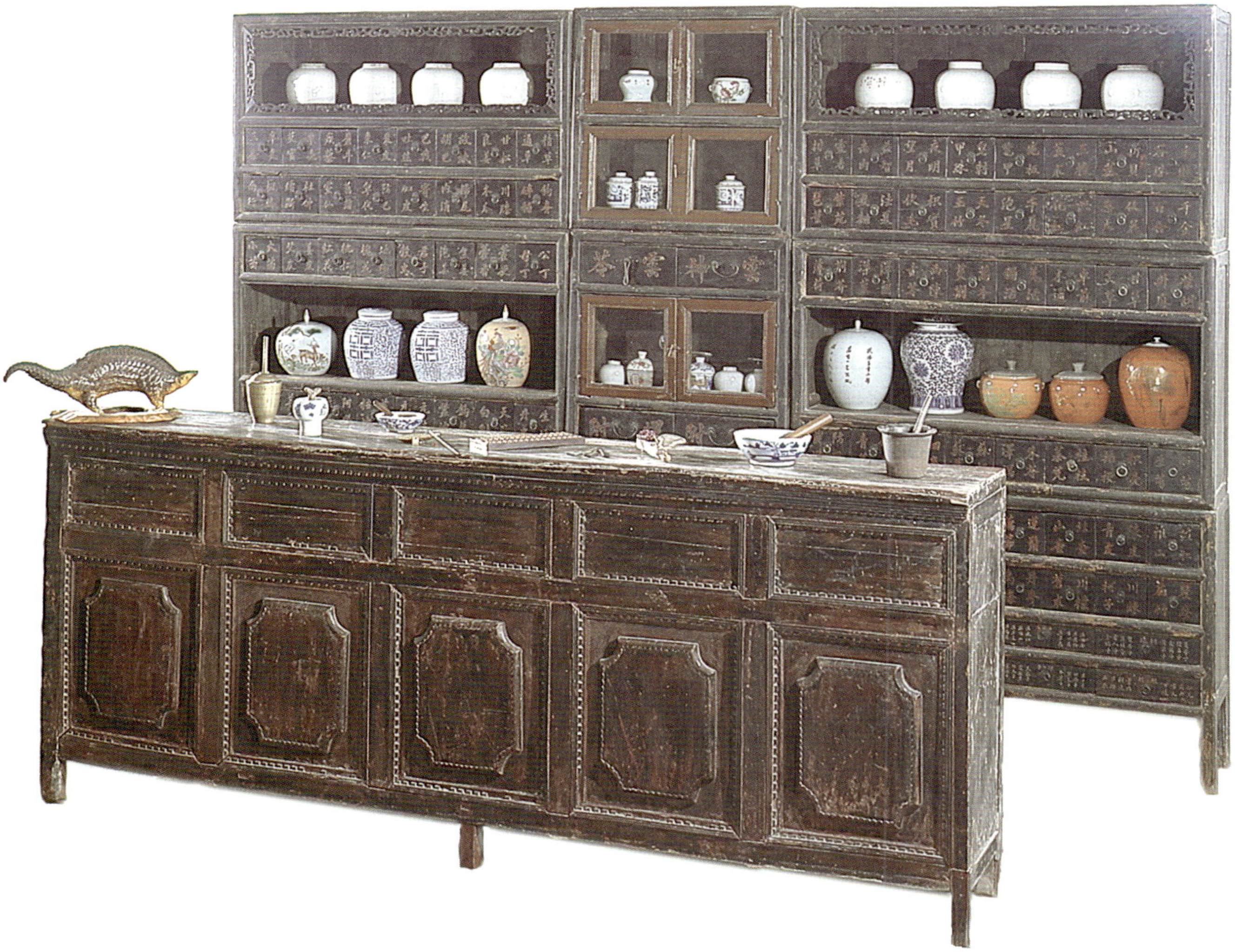

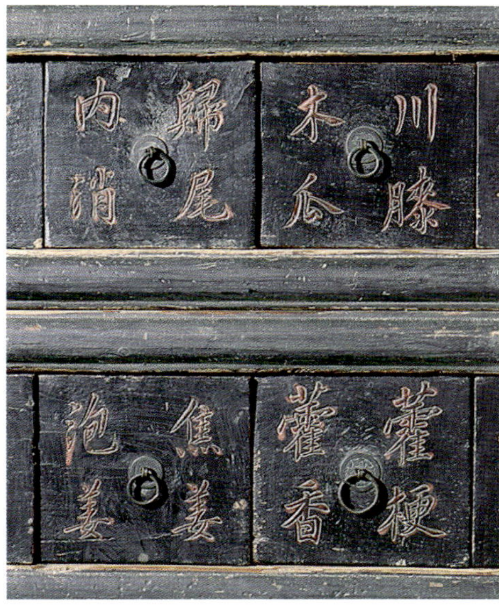

69. In the foreground is a retail table with hand scale, mortars, grinding bowls, and an ant-eater (pangolin). Behind it is a wall cabinet with drawers and open shelves (the glass doors installed later) for the storage of medicinal drugs. Pharmacy furnishings, mid–nineteenth century, Jiangxi.

70. Drawers with carved drug names.

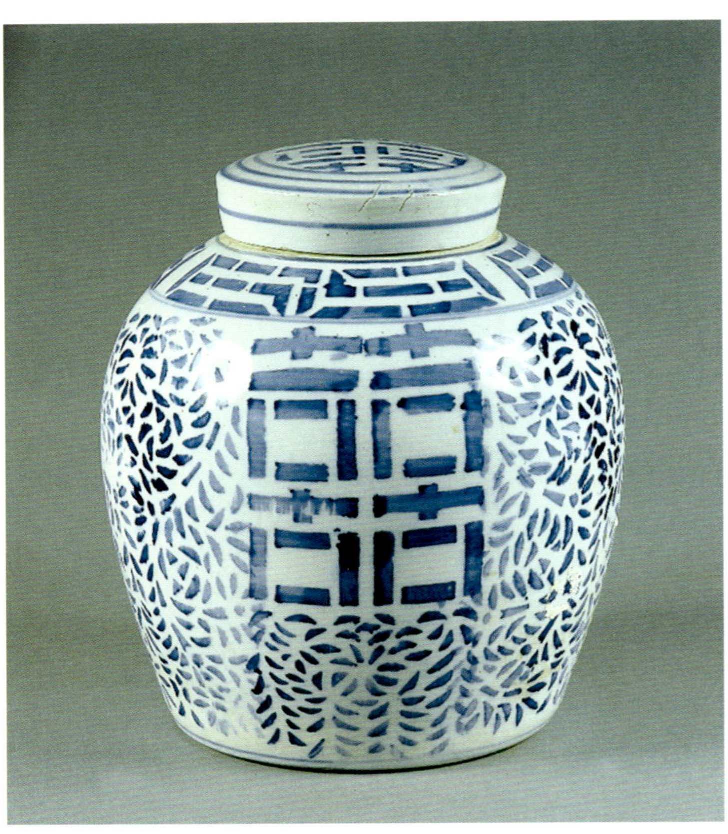

71. Pharmacy container and cover with the Double Fortune character and abstract decor. Porcelain, blue underglaze on white background, height 14.9 cm, South China.

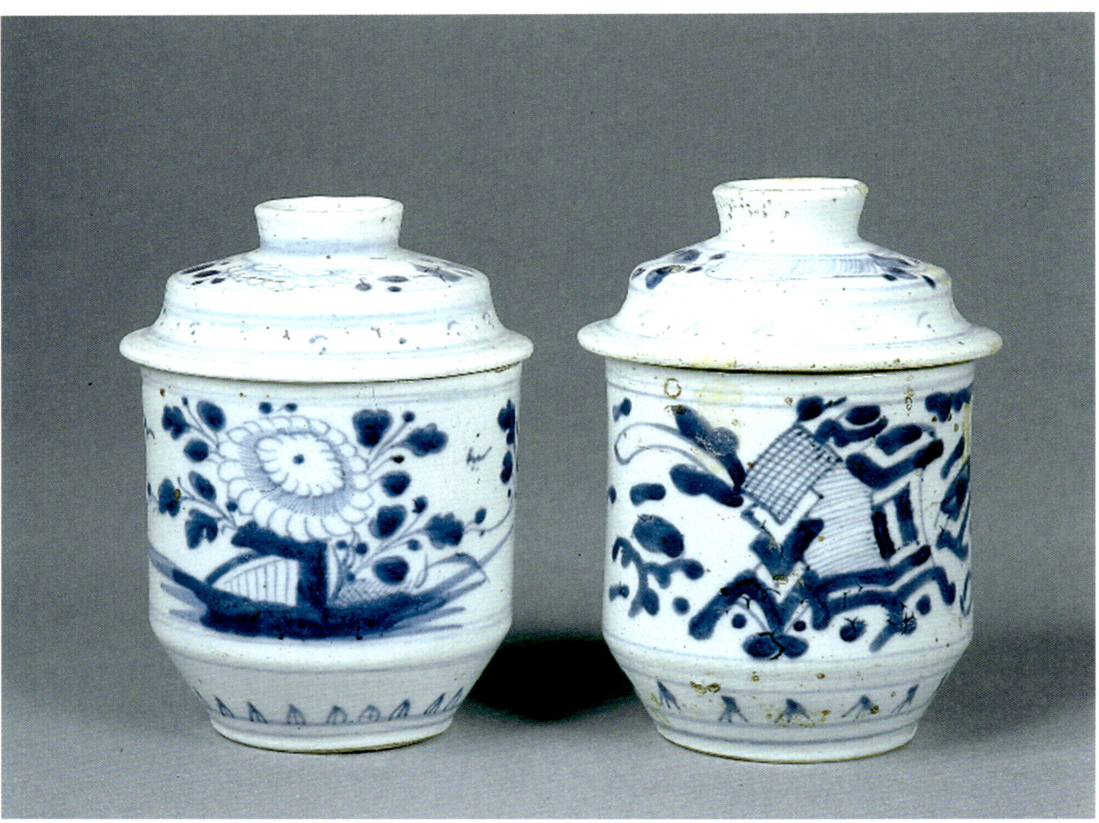

72. Two pharmacy containers with covers. Porcelain, blue underglaze on white background, height 14–14.3 cm, South China, late-nineteenth century.

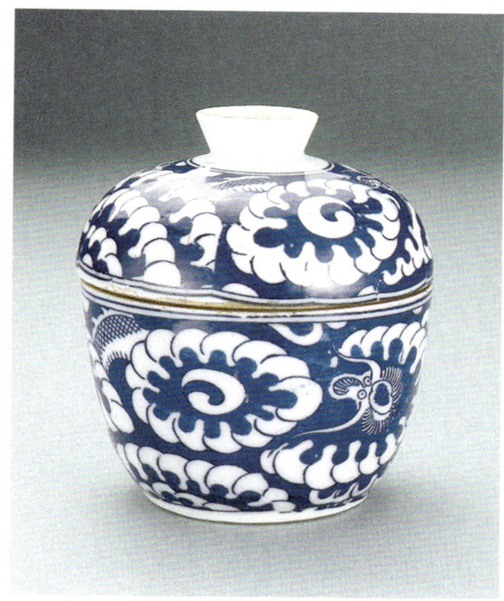

73. Pharmacy container and cover decorated with a dragon. Porcelain, blue underglaze on white background, height 13.2 cm, South China.

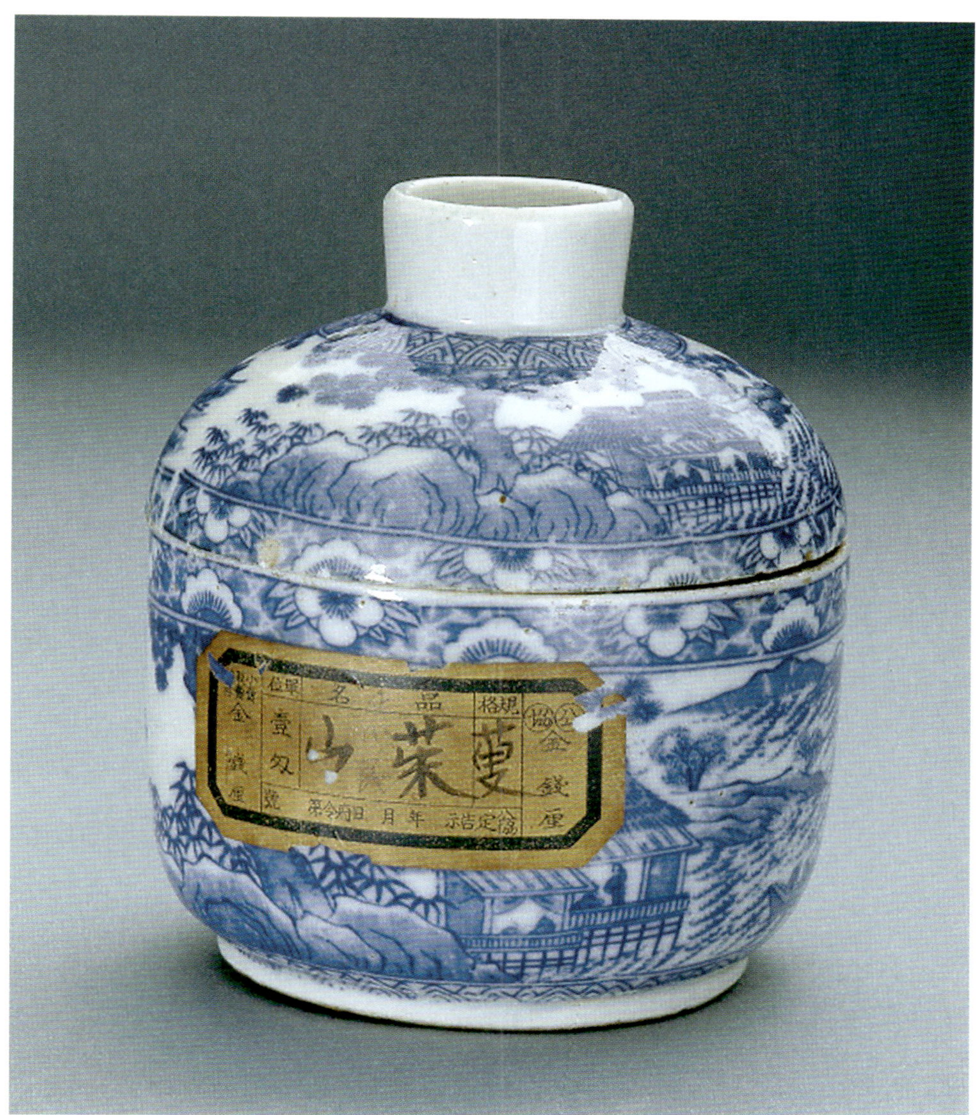


74. Pharmacy container and cover decorated with a landscape. Porcelain, blue underglaze on white background, height 13.8 cm, South China.

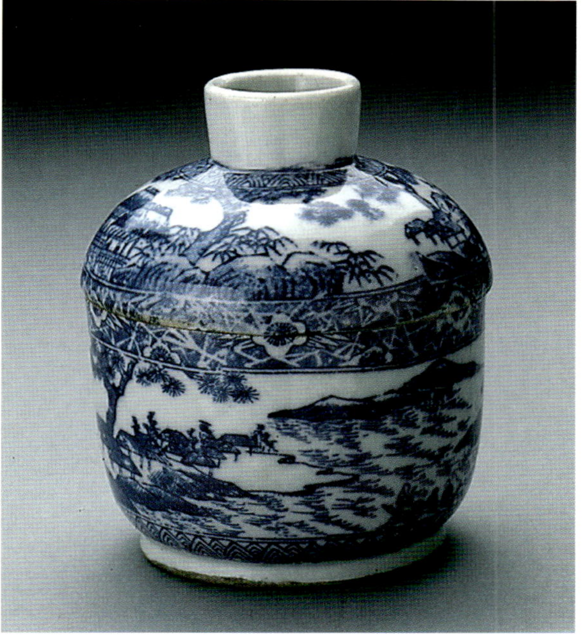

75. Pharmacy container and cover decorated with a landscape. Porcelain, blue underglaze on white background, height above cover 12 cm, South China.

In the centuries following the Song period, pharmaceutical producers in China developed remarkable sales strategies in order to encourage the ties between producers, their products, and their clientele.

Many famous medical formulae were produced generically, as it were, throughout the country and were marketed as ready-made preparations for very specific illnesses. Individual pharmacies were therefore forced to find ways to set themselves apart from their competitors. The design of delivery containers played a decisive role in this context. Pharmacies competed with each other to deliver their products in containers that would greatly appeal to the aesthetic sensibilities of their educated customers. Individual containers with representations of landscapes, figures, or animals as well as auspicious sayings or symbols served this purpose. Serial containers with changing historical or mythological scenes stimulated additional interest in their purchasers. Some pharmacies came up with characteristic designs which were unmistakable in their shape, calligraphy, and company trade-mark.

The strategy of secondary usage, which may have been common in China for centuries already, deserves particular attention. After fulfilling their pharmaceutical purposes, delivery containers often functioned as snuff bottles, tea tins, or flower vases—depending on their particular shapes.

Delivery containers were therefore not commonly recognized as medicine containers; information about their content and intended use was conveyed mostly on red labels, which could be removed after the container was empty. Famous pharmacies, however, did not refrain from adding their name, address, and even the intended medical content "under the glaze" on their containers.

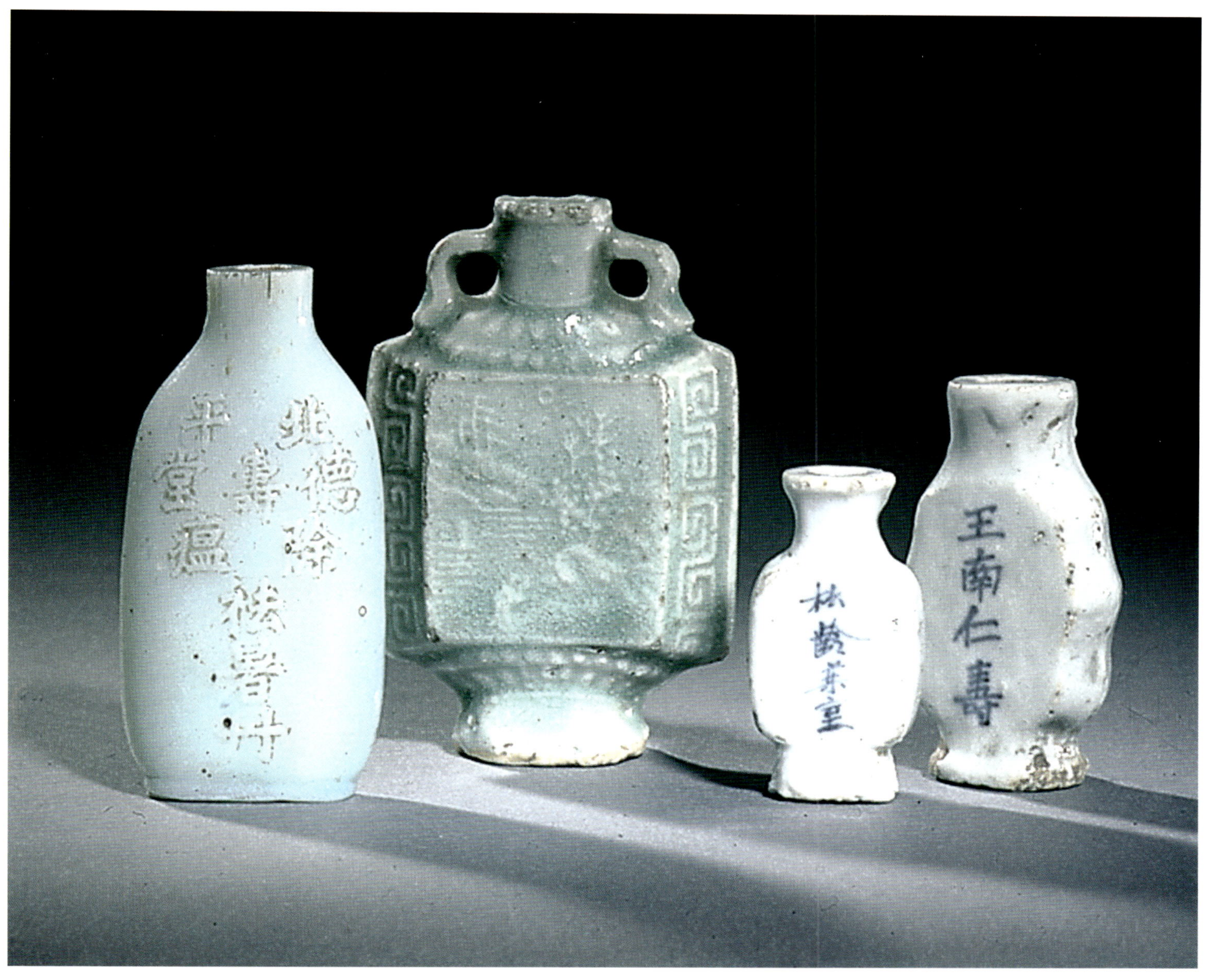

76. Four pharmacy delivery containers. (a) Front: 北平德壽堂除瘟祛暑丹 "Peping, Pharmacy Virtue and Longevity. Pills which expel heat epidemics and summer heat." Back: 除瘟祛暑丹居家旅行常備靈藥 "Pills which expel heat epidemics and summer heat. Whether at home or on the road, always keep a supply of miraculous medicine." (b) Amphora shape decorated with reliefs of a landscape and meander pattern. Stoneware, height 7.5 cm.
(c) Front: 松齡藥室 (Pharmacy Long Life). Back: 如意丸 "Pills which accord with one's wishes [in their effects]." Stoneware, height 4.3 cm.
(d) Front: 王南仁壽 ([Mr.] Wang Nan's [Pharmacy] Humaneness and Longevity). Back: 通州餘東場 "Yudongchang in Tongzhou." Stoneware, height 5.3 cm.

77. Pharmacy delivery container
decorated with plants. Lacquered
paper plug, porcelain, with blue
underglaze on white background,
height 5.2 cm.

78. Pharmacy delivery container
decorated with a dragon.
Porcelain, multicolored overglaze
on white background, height
7.5 cm.

79. Three pharmacy delivery
containers. (a) Front: 靈通萬應
丸 "Pills of miraculous pene-
tration and ten thousand results."
Porcelain with wooden plug,
height 5.8 cm.
(b) 漢鎮至德堂吳亮金,
(Hanzhen [= Hankou], Pharmacy
Utmost Virtue of [Mr.] Wu
Liangjin). Porcelain, blue underglaze on white background,
height 6.8 cm.
(c) Front: landscape. Porcelain,
height 6.1 cm.

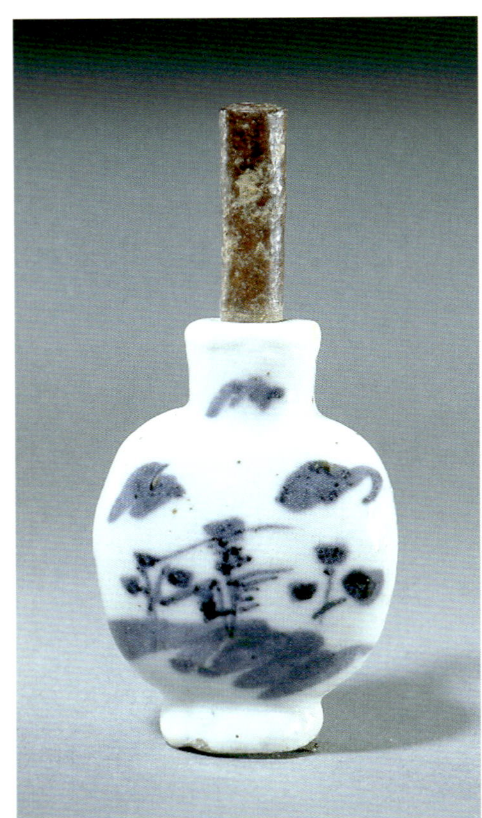

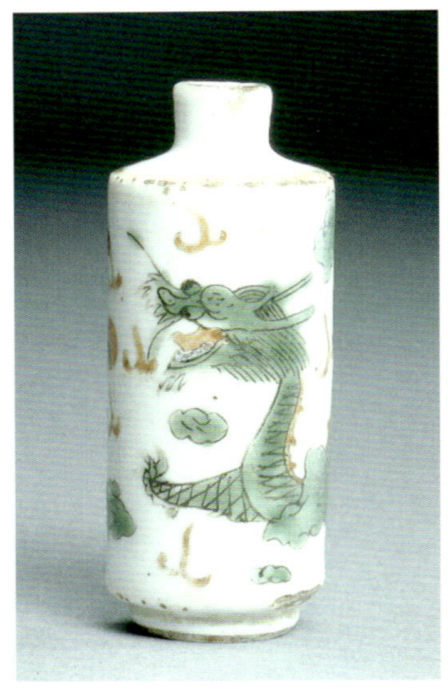

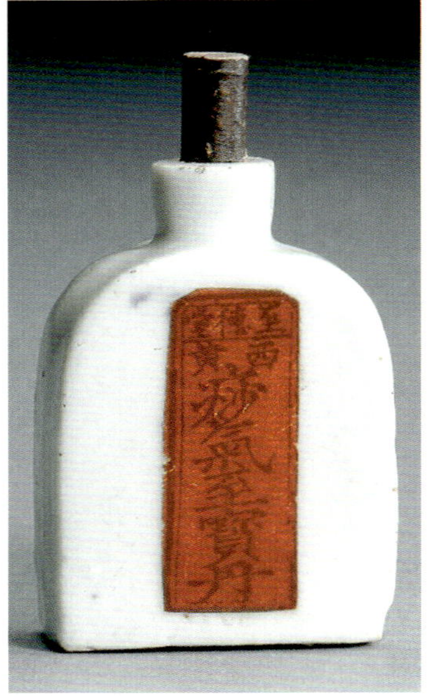

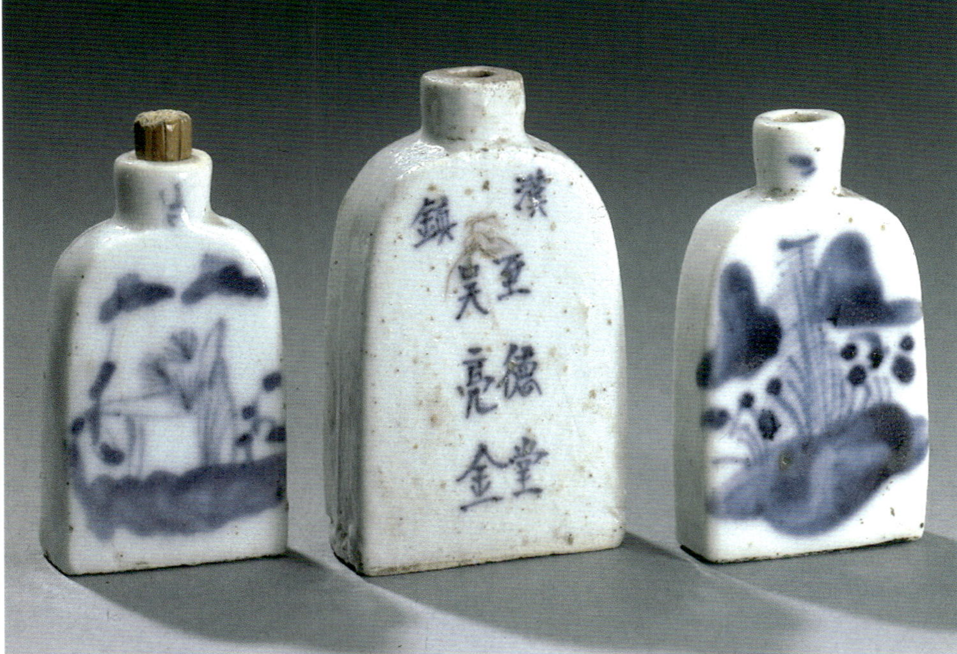

80. Pharmacy delivery container.
Front: 西黃痧氣至寶丹
"Pharmacy Utmost Virtue,
extremely efficacious pills with
western bovine bezoar for *sha*-
disorders." Back: 漢鎮至德堂
吳亮金, (Hanzhen, [=
Hankou], Pharmacy Utmost
Virtue of [Mr.] Wu Liangjin).
Porcelain, blue underglaze on
white background, height 5.5 cm.

81. Twenty pharmacy delivery
containers. Front: 誦芬堂雷
(Pharmacy Recitation and
Fragrance of [Mr.] Lei). Back:
姑蘇閶門內天庫前 "Gusu
[=Suzhou], within the palace
gates, in front of the Heavenly
Depot [of the palace]." Porcelain,
blue underglaze on white background, paper and crochet plugs,
heights vary 3.9–5.8 cm.

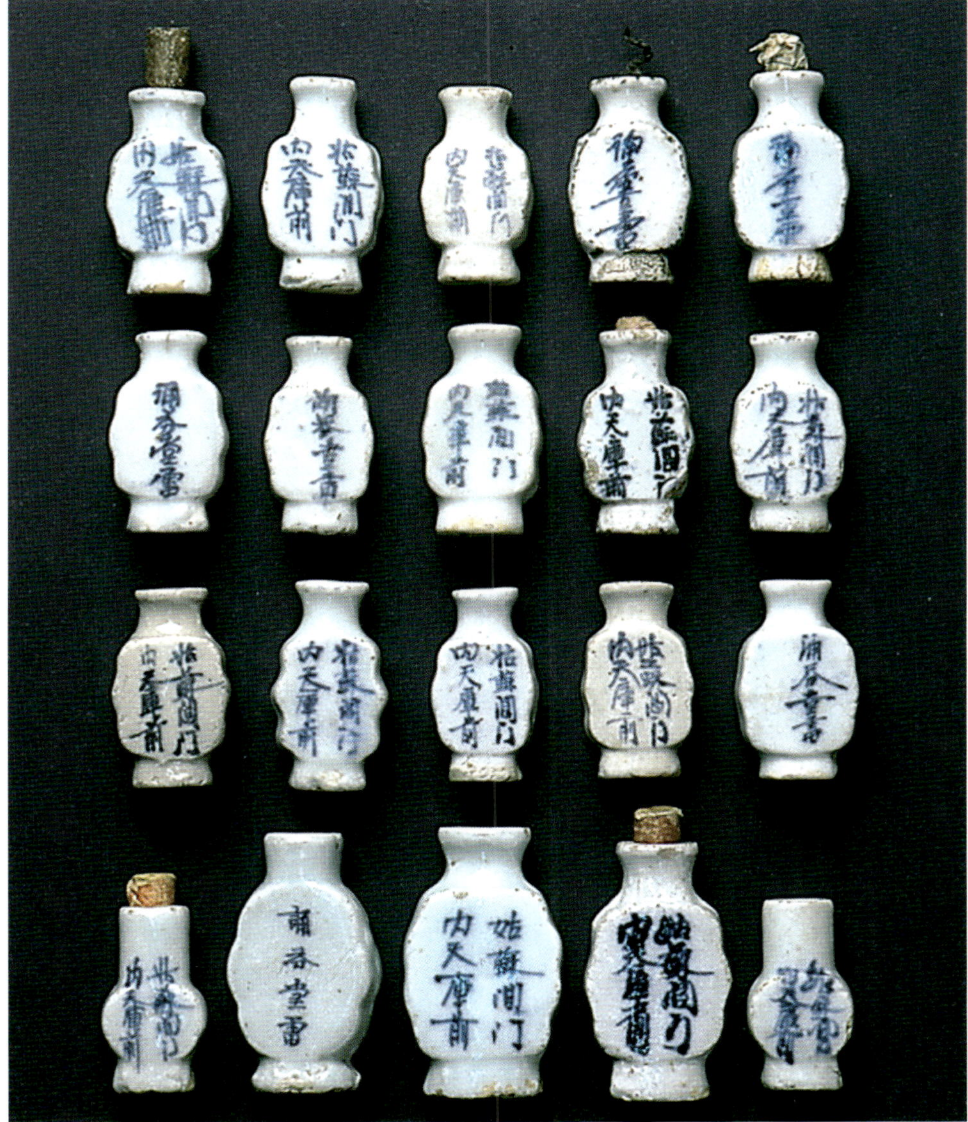

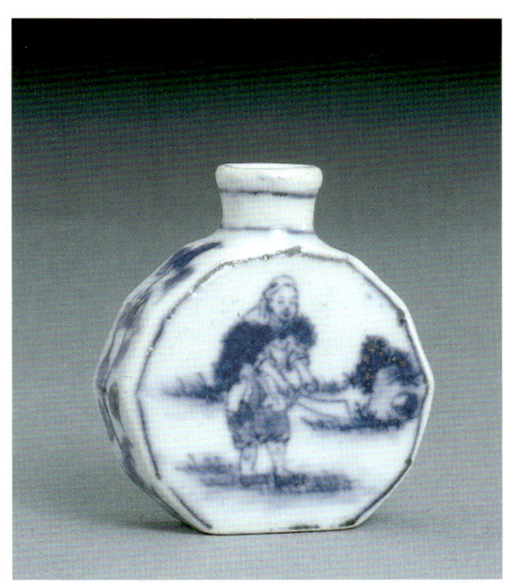

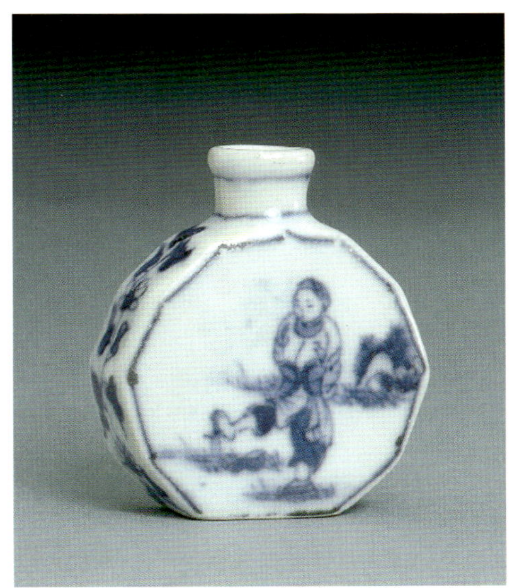

82. Octagonal pharmacy delivery
container. Front: warrior with
sword in hand. Back: armless man
with bare foot, reaching for a
sword stuck in the ground. Side
border: blossoms and leaves.
Porcelain, blue underglaze on
white background, height 4.5 cm.

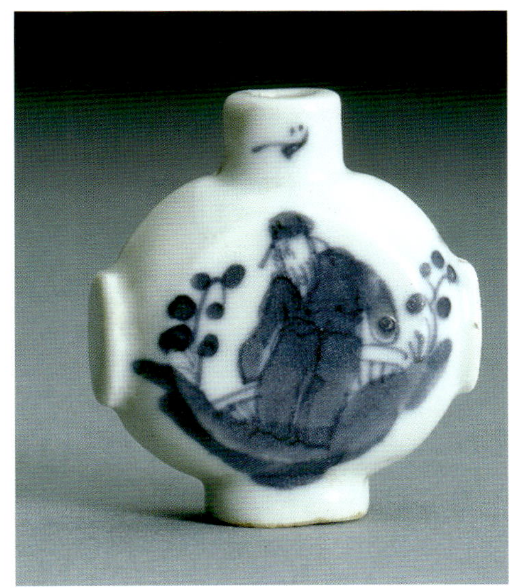

83. Pharmacy delivery container
decorated with an old man in
nature. Porcelain, blue underglaze
on white background, height
5.7 cm.

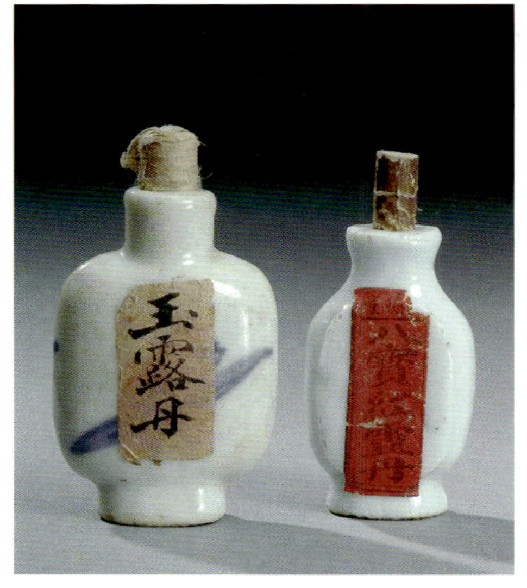

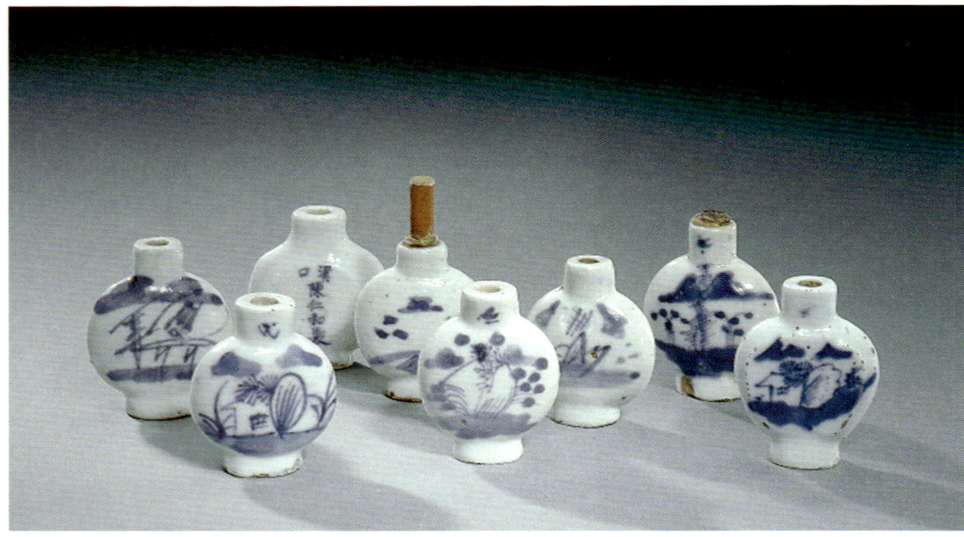

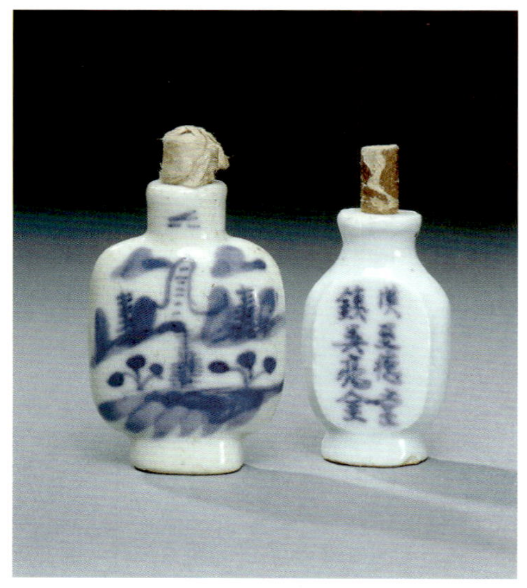

85. Eight pharmacy delivery containers decorated with plants, landscapes, and writing: 漢口陳仁和製 "Manufactured for Chen Renhe, Hankou." Porcelain, height 5–5.3 cm.

86. Pharmacy delivery container decorated front and back with a grasshopper. Underside: 慎德堂 (Pharmacy of Careful Attention to Virtue). Porcelain, multicolored underglaze on white base, height 6.5 cm.

87. Pharmacy delivery container decorated with lines and text oval. Front: 同仁堂 (Pharmacy which Lets Everybody Partake in its Humaneness). Back: 痧氣丹 "pills for *sha*-disorder." Porcelain, blue underglaze on white base, height 5 cm.

84. Two pharmacy delivery containers. (a) Front: 至德堂八寶紅靈丹 (Pharmacy Utmost Virtue, Red Miracle Pills with the Eight Precious [Ingredients]). Back: 漢鎮至德堂吳亮金 (Hanzhen [=Hankou], Pharmacy Utmost Virtue of [Mr.] Wu Liangjin). Porcelain, height 5 cm. (b) Front: 玉露丹 "Jade Dew Pills." Base: 玉露丹 "Jade Dew Pills." Porcelain, blue underglaze on white background, height 5.7 cm.

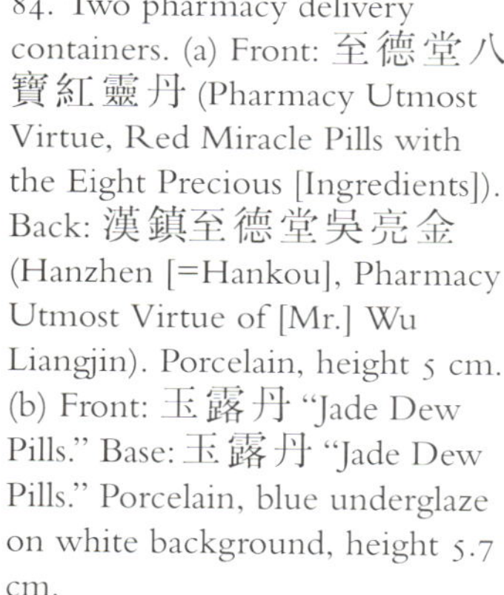

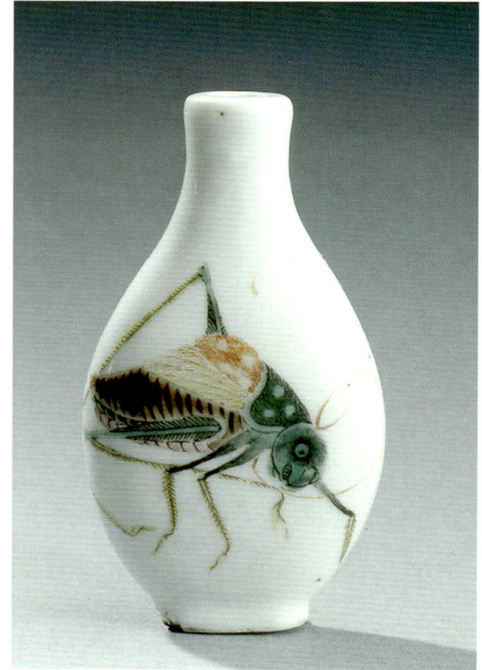

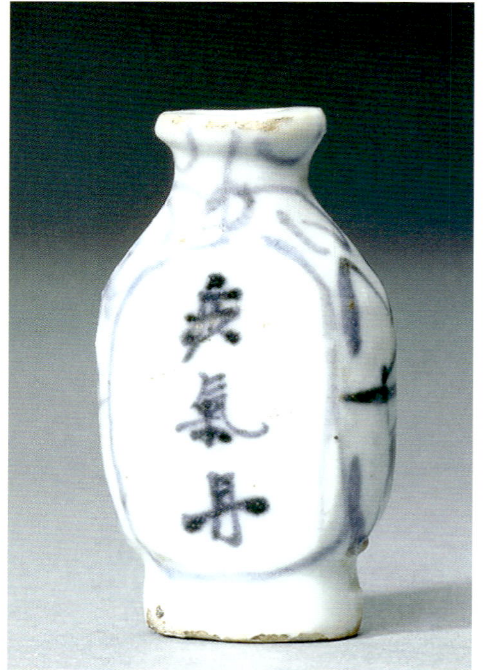

88. Pharmacy delivery containers shaped like amphoras. Front and back: pharmacy name, location, and content. For example: 江右洗馬池濟春堂如意丹 "Jiangyou [Province] [=Jiangxi], Horse Washing Pond [=district in Nanchang], Pharmacy Help [for a Return to] Spring; pills [whose effects] comply with one's desires." Porcelain, partial blue underglaze on partially overglazed white base, height 2.5–5.4 cm.

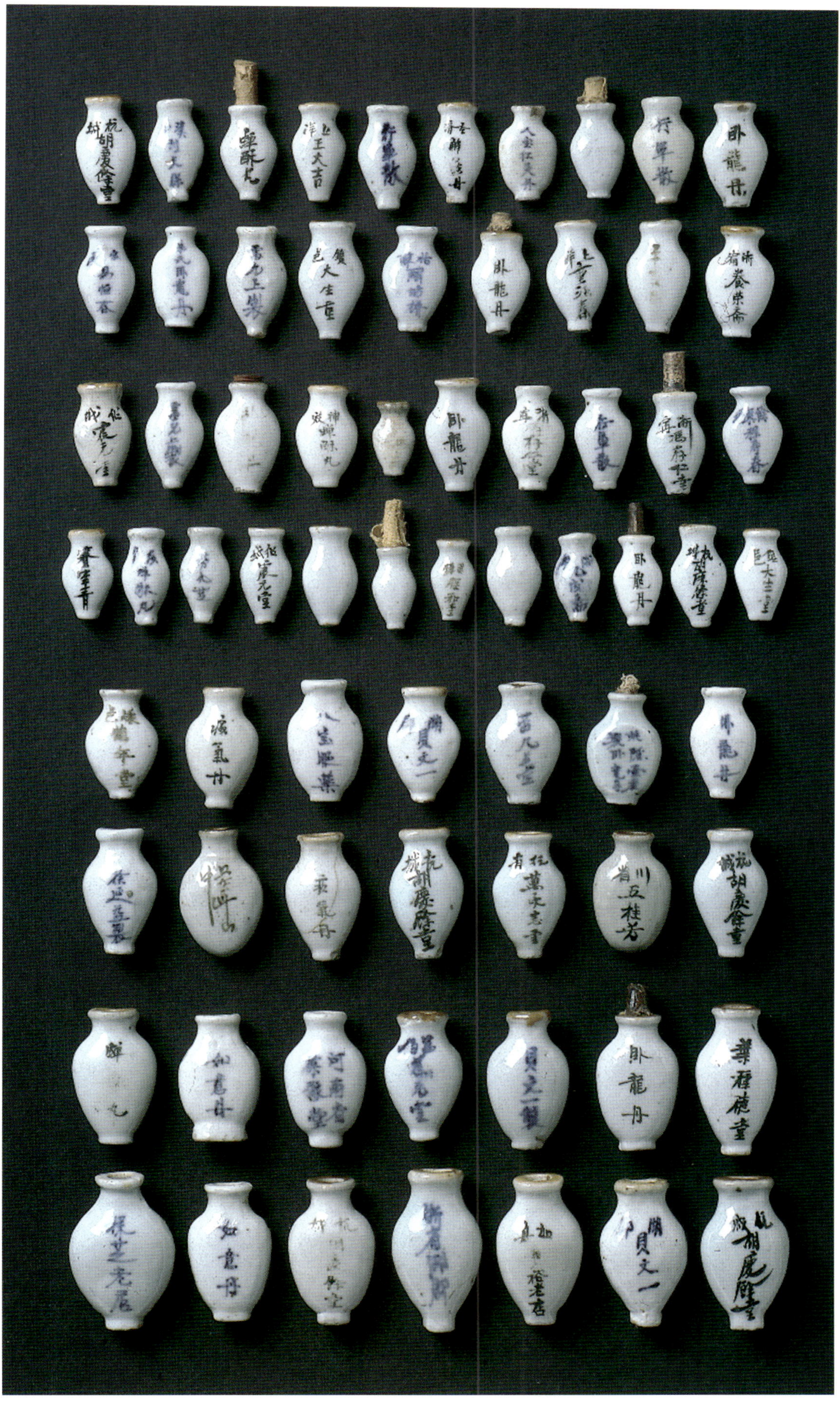

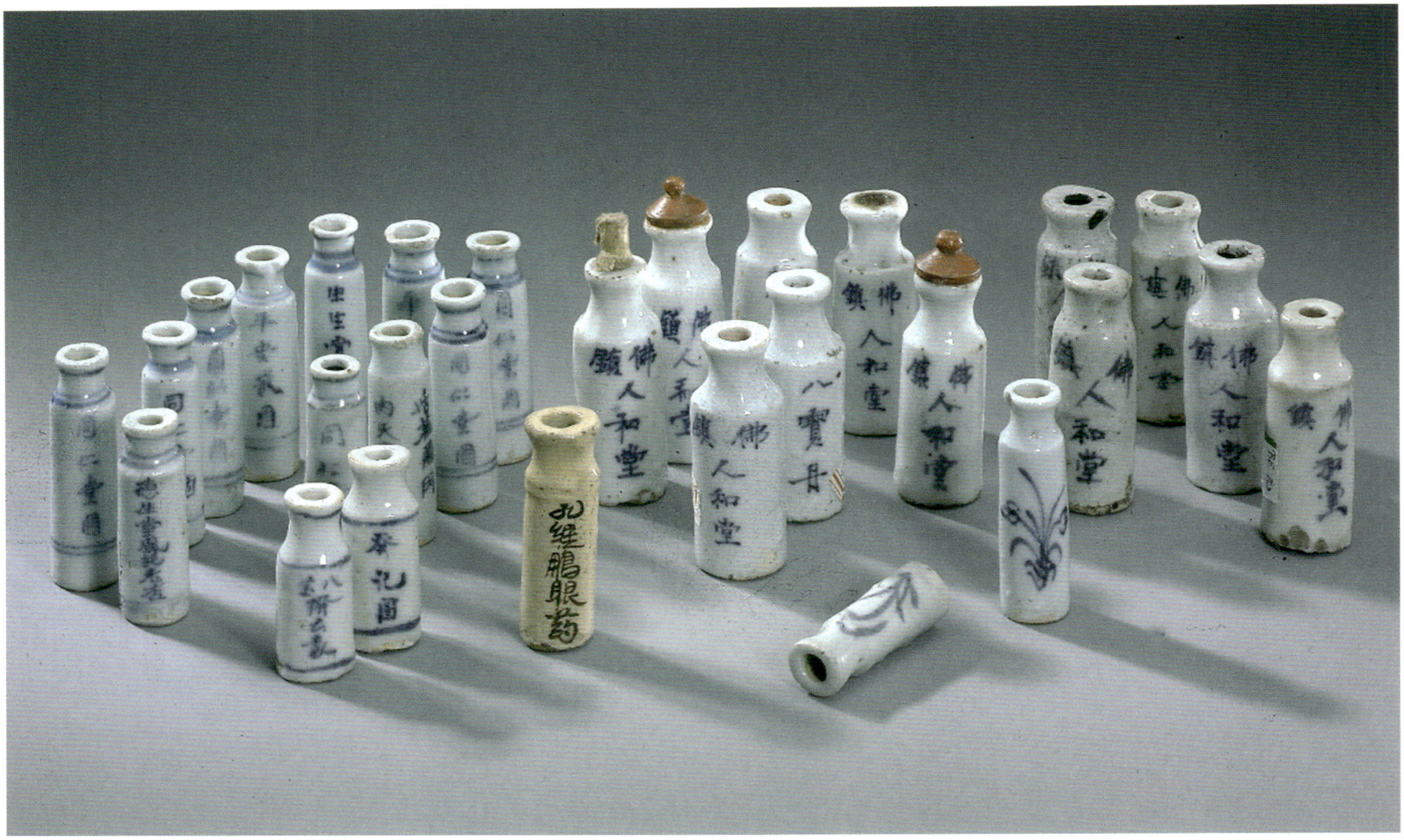

89. Pharmacy delivery containers
shaped like cylinders. Front and
back: pharmacy name, location,
and content. Porcelain and
stoneware, blue underglaze on
white base, some wooden plugs
with measuring spoon, height
4.4–6.4 cm.

90. Pharmacy delivery container
decorated with figure and plants.
Porcelain, blue underglaze on
white base, height 6 cm.

91. Three pharmacy delivery containers. (a) Rectangular, decorated
with a man in a landscape, height
6 cm. (b) Rectangular, decorated
with a man in a landscape, height
6.4 cm. (c) Hexagonal, decorated
with a landscape, height 5.7 cm.
All porcelain, blue underglaze on
white base.

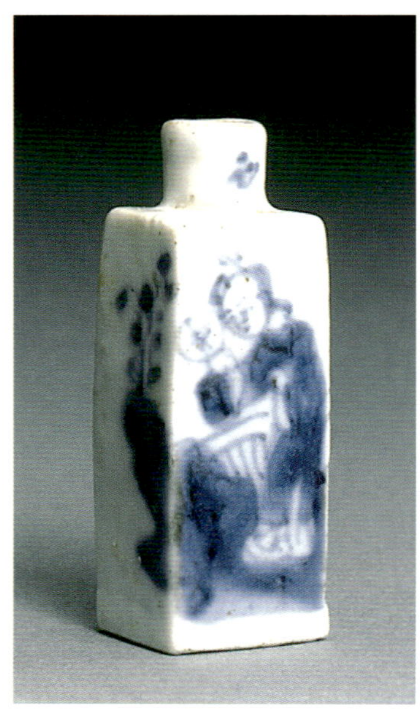

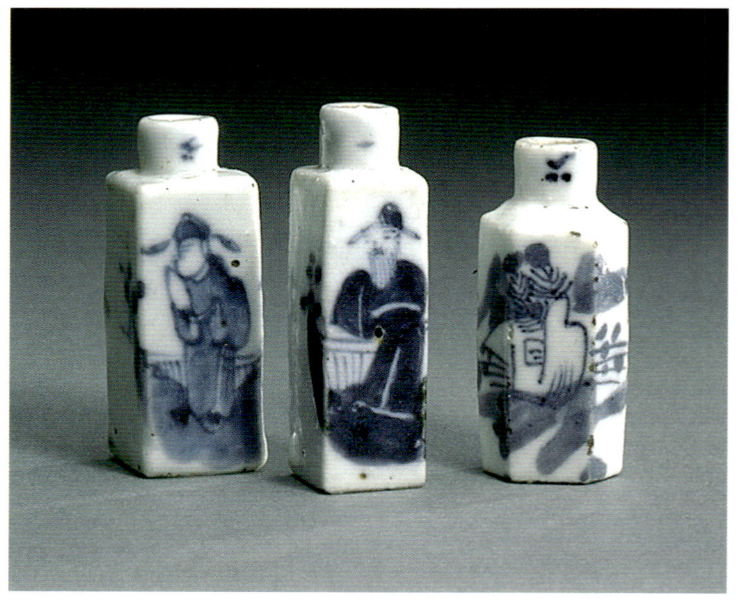

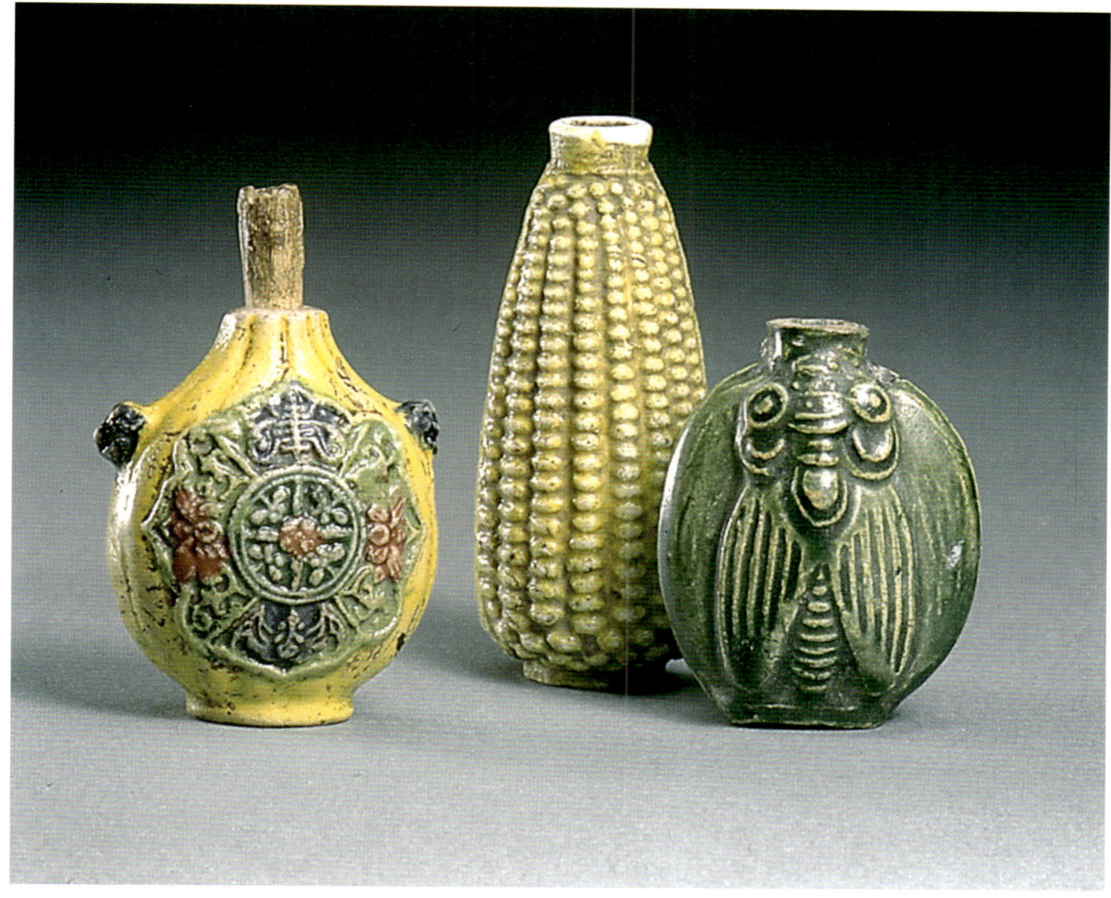

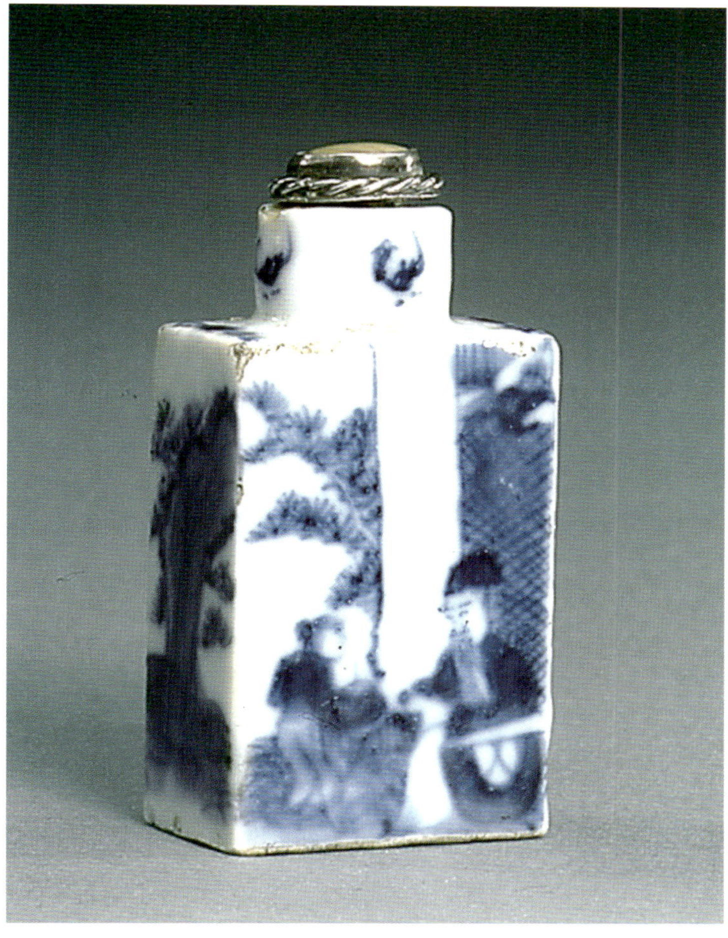

93. Pharmacy delivery container
decorated with a servant presenting a container to a gentleman, rock, pine, and bats.
Porcelain, blue underglaze on
white base, silver plug with semi-
precious stone, height 4.8 cm.

169

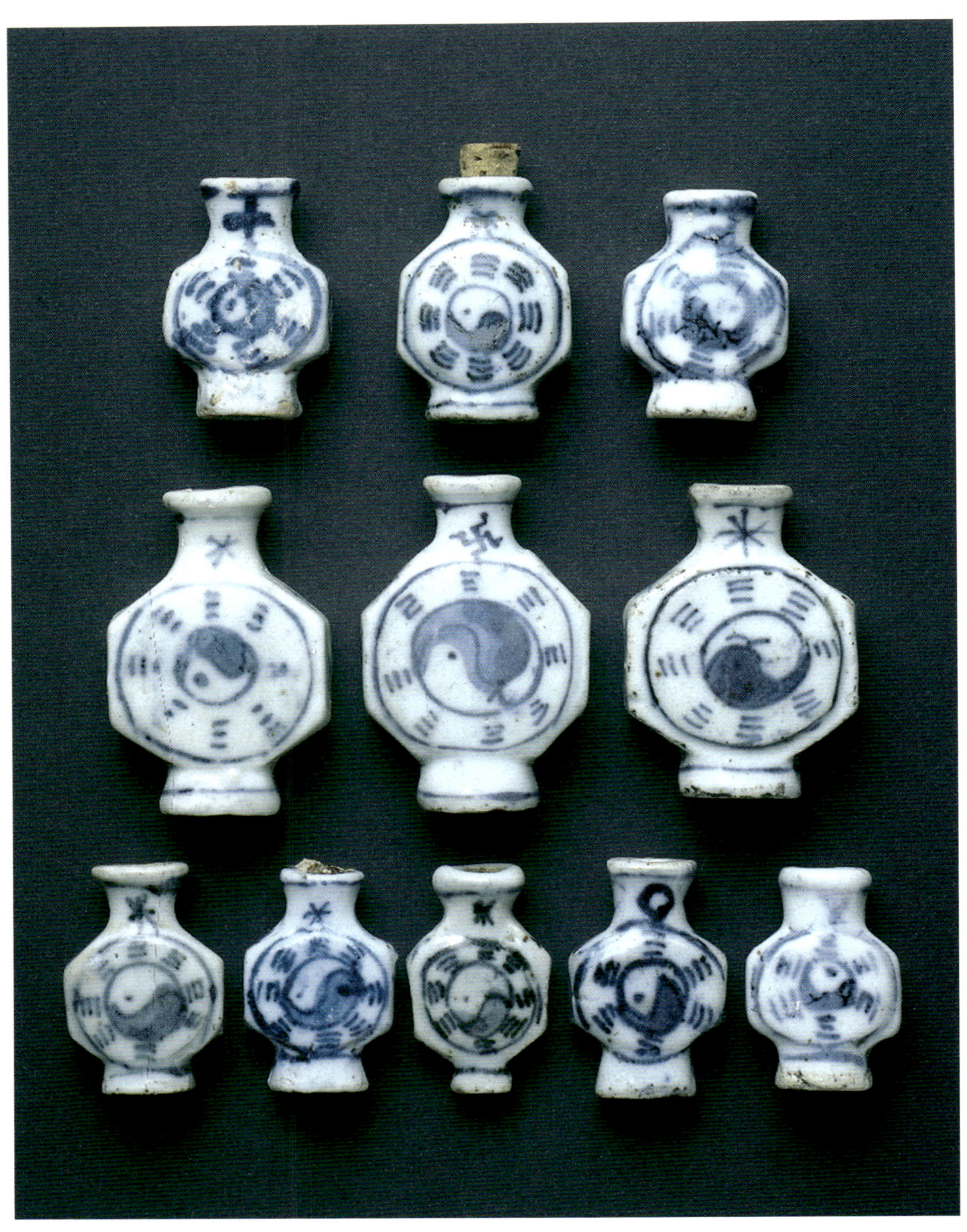

94. Eleven pharmacy delivery containers. Front and back: Yin-yang symbol, framed by *Yijing* trigrams. Porcelain, blue under-glaze on white base, with paper and cork plugs, height 3.6–5.3 cm.

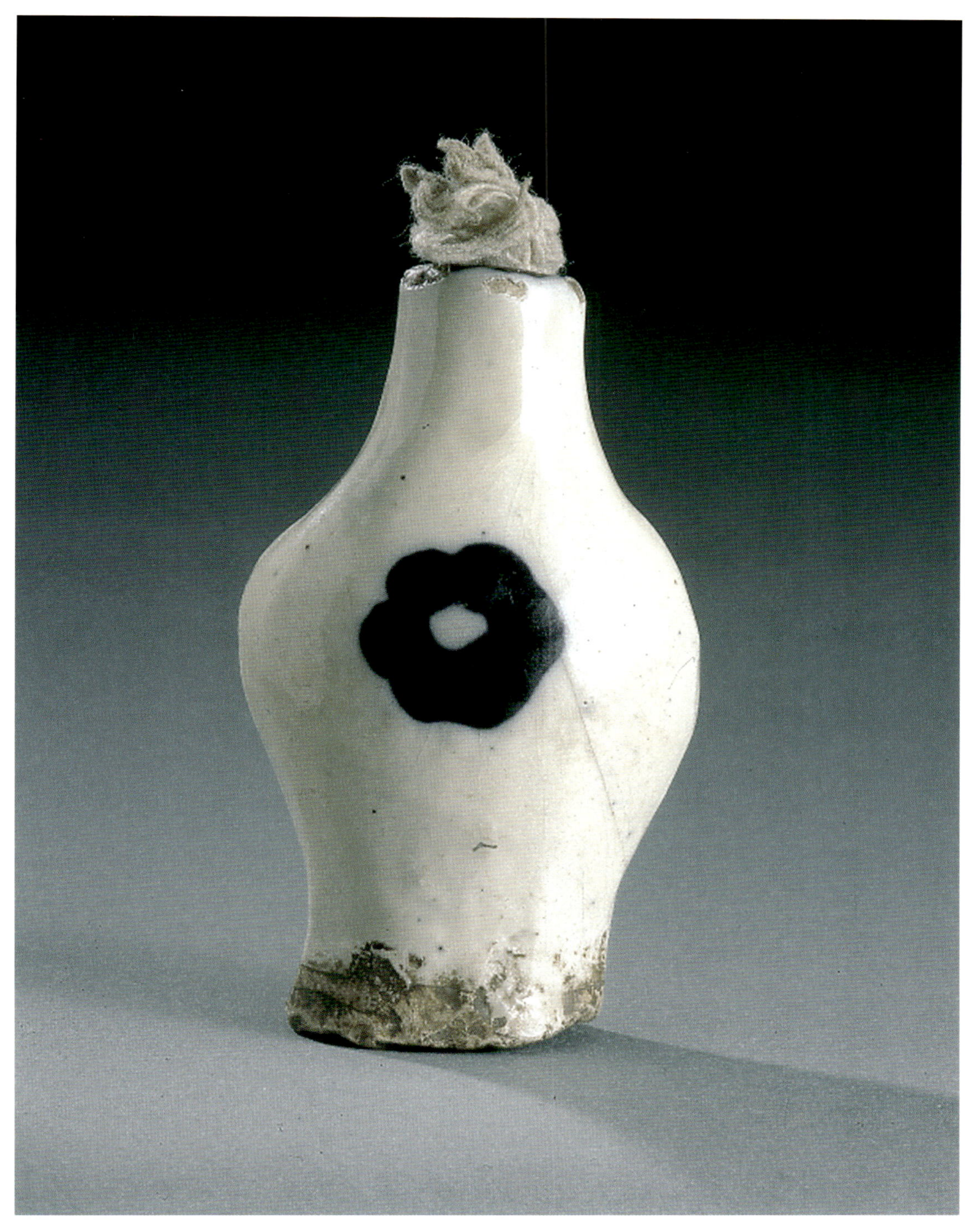

95. Pharmacy delivery container decorated, front and back, with flowers. Underside: 吹喉散 "Powder to be blown into the throat." Stoneware, dark blue underglaze on white base, paper plug, height 6.5 cm.

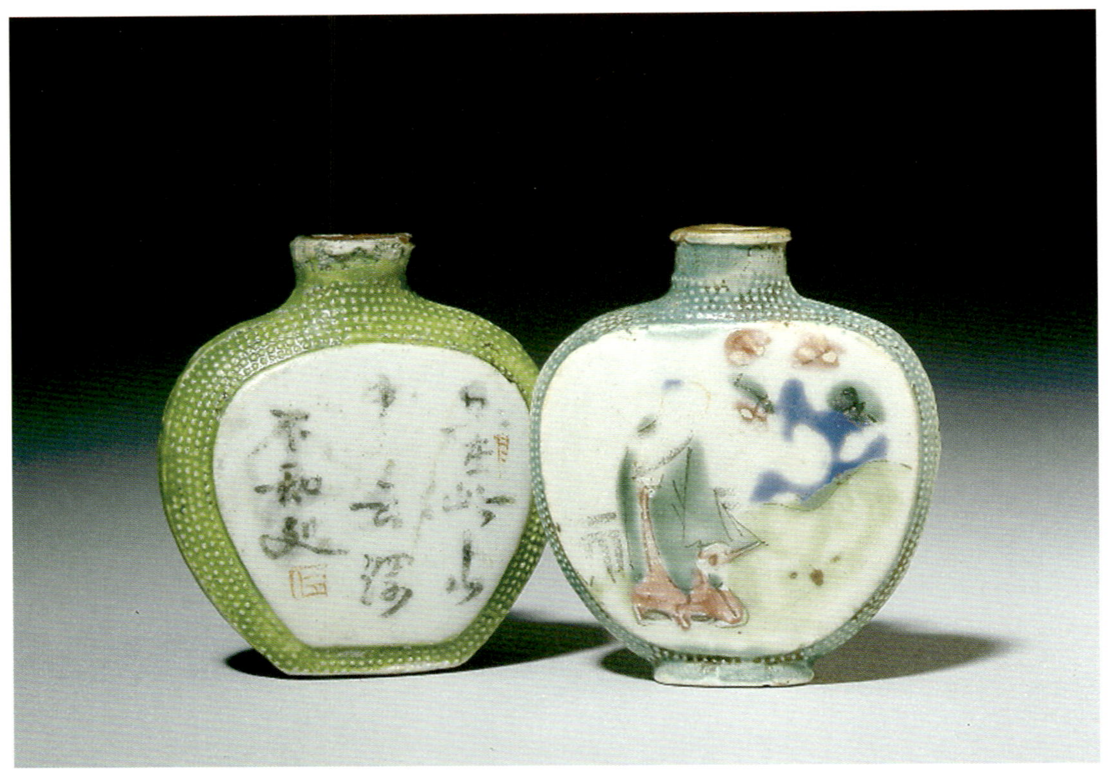

96. Two pharmacy delivery containers, each carrying half of a Tang-period four-line expression. (a) Heart-shaped container decorated front and back; with a figure in a landscape and text. Right (back): 松下問童子言師授藥去 "Under the pine, I asked the child [where the master was]. He responded: The master went to gather medicines." Left: 只在此山中雲深不知處 "[I] only [know] that he is in the mountains. The clouds are hanging low; I don't know his exact location." Porcelain, multicolored overglaze drawing on smooth white base in goose-skin frame, height 5.4 cm. See also plate 130.

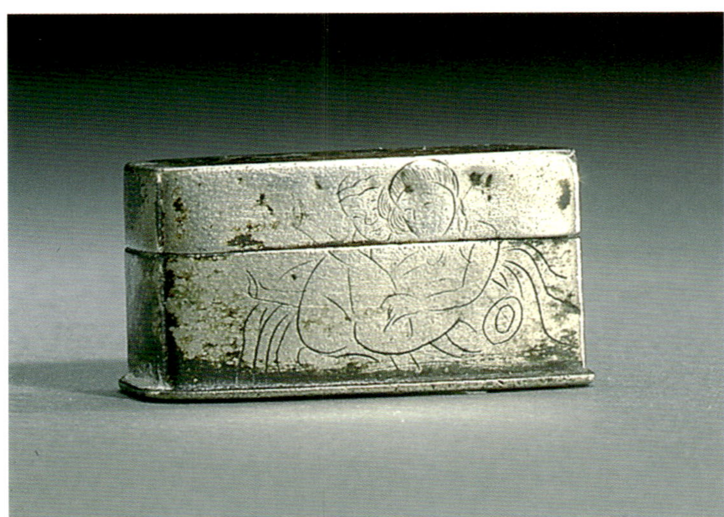

97. Opium container decorated, front and back, with love scenes. Tin-plate, lined with copper, height 2 cm, nineteenth century.

98. Pharmacy delivery container decorated with flowers, frame, man, and plant. Porcelain, blue underglaze on white base, multicolored overglaze, height 7 cm.

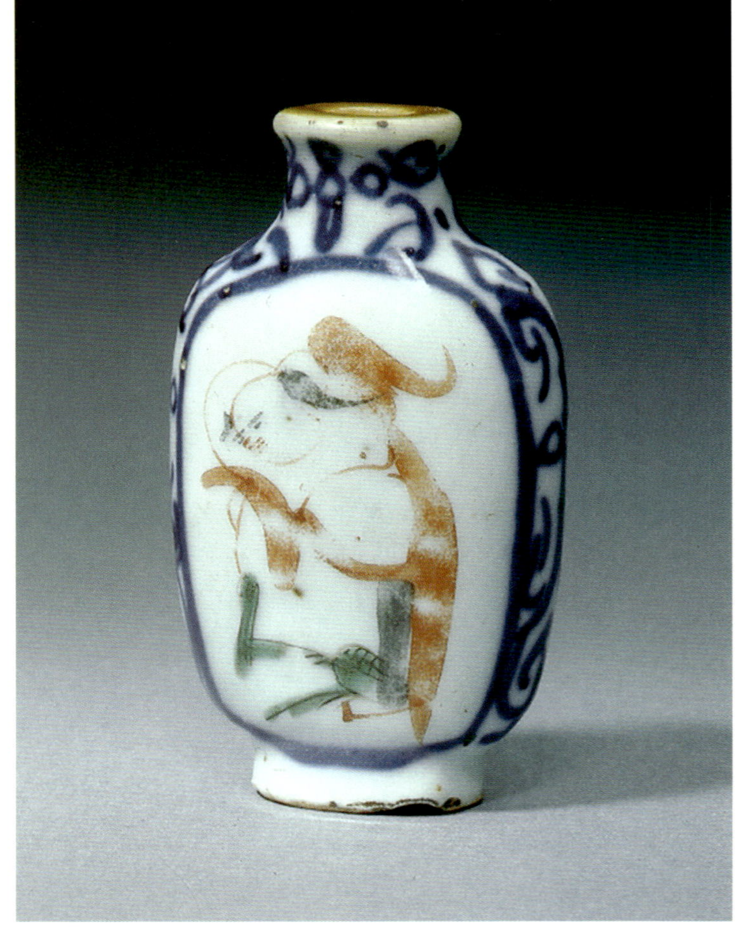

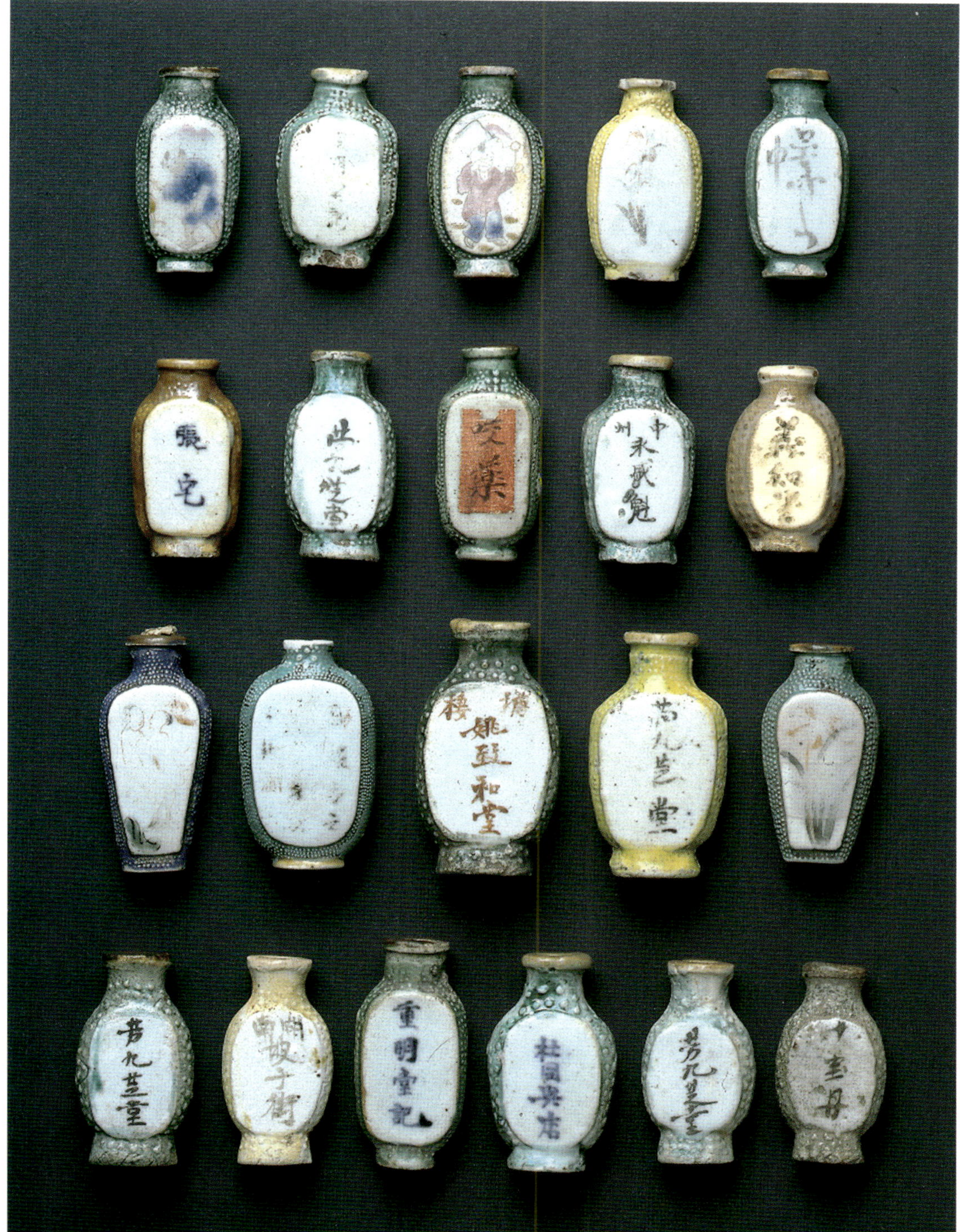

99. Pharmacy delivery containers with green, yellow, blue, or brown goose-skin exteriors and smooth white ovals for inscriptions or paintings. Marked with pharmacy name, location, and contents and decorated with figures in a landscape, love scenes, or flowers. Porcelain and stoneware, partial underglaze on white base, mostly multicolored overglaze painting, height 4.4–6 cm.

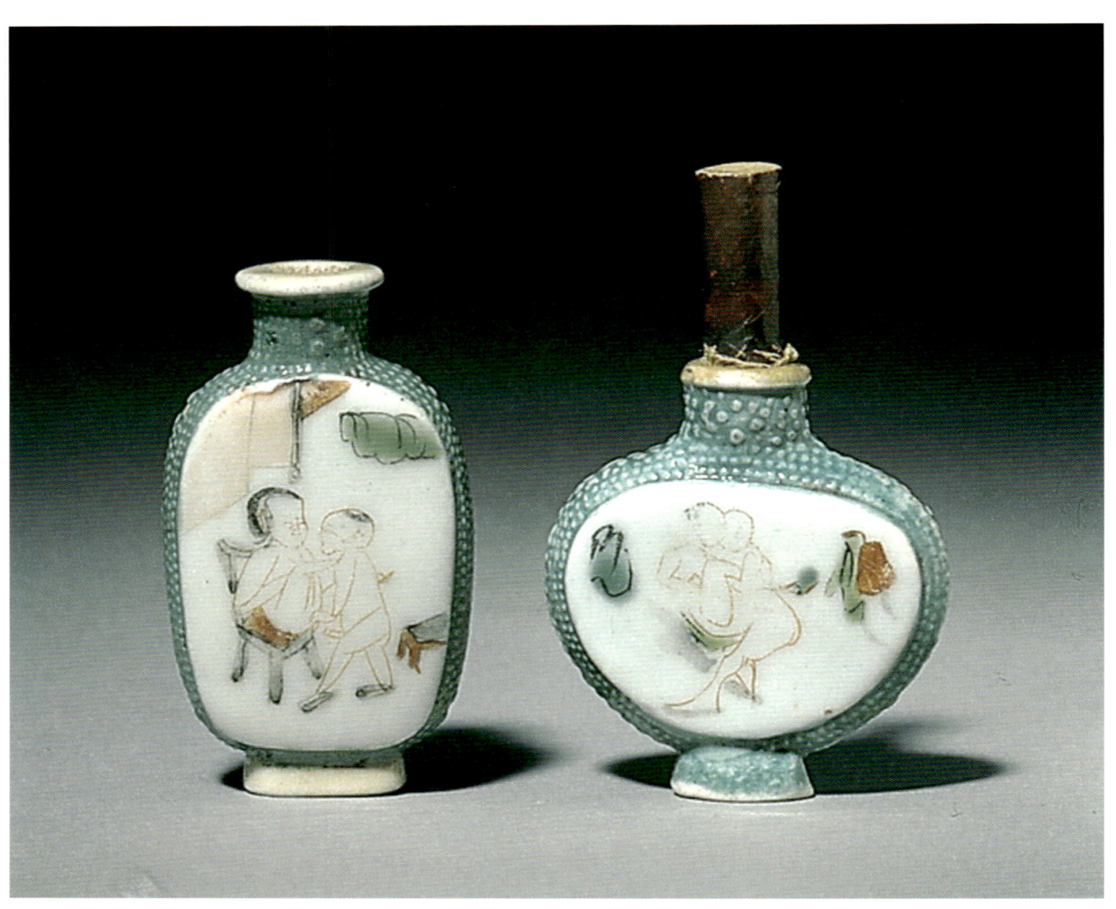

100. Two pharmacy delivery
containers. Front: love scenes.
Back: 夜來明去到有天長地
久 "Night is coming and the light
disappearing for as long as Heaven
and Earth exist," a two-line
expression which is frequently
found on containers for aphrodisiacs. Porcelain, multicolored
overglaze drawing on smooth
white base in goose-skin frame,
height 4.8–5.4 cm.

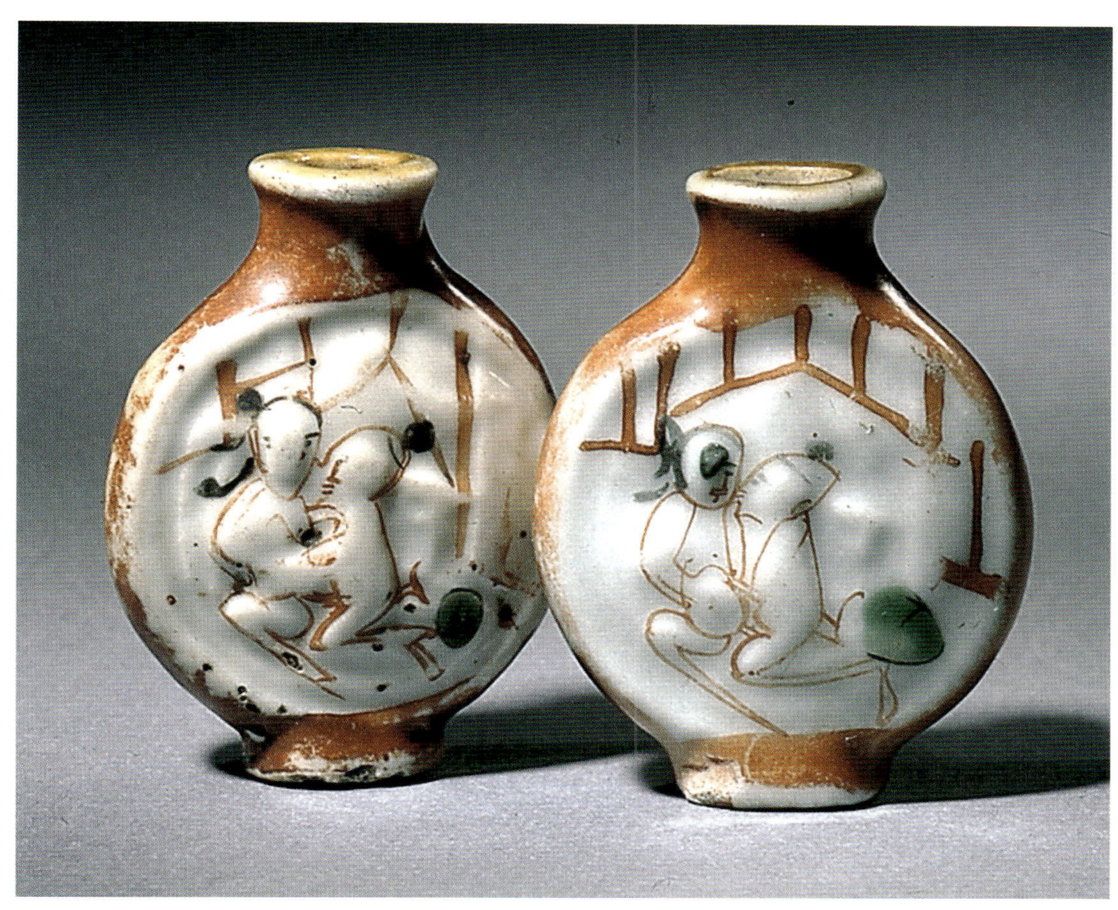

101. Two pharmacy delivery
containers decorated, front and
back, with figures and love scenes
in relief. Porcelain, multicolored
overglaze drawings on white
round in red frame, height 5 cm.

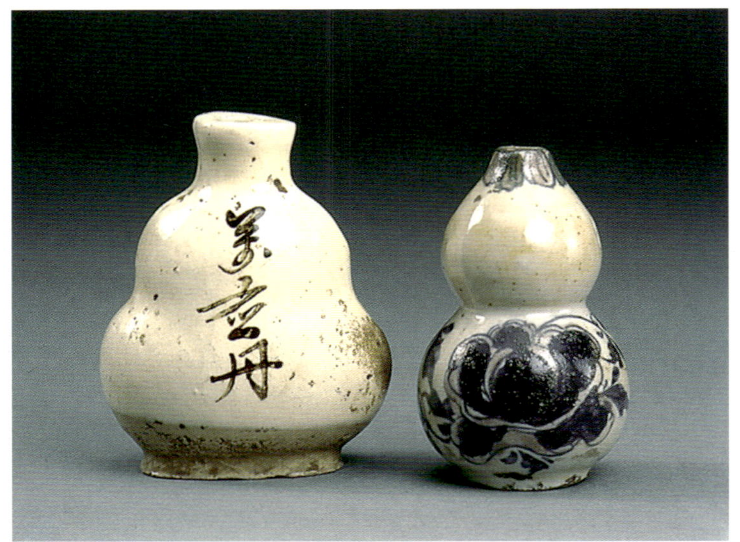

102. Two pharmacy delivery containers shaped like gourds. (a) Text 萬應丹 "pills with myriad results." Porcelain, brown underglaze on tan background, height 7.8 cm. (b) Front: flower with tendrils. Porcelain, green-blue-pink underglaze on gray-white base, height 7.2 cm.

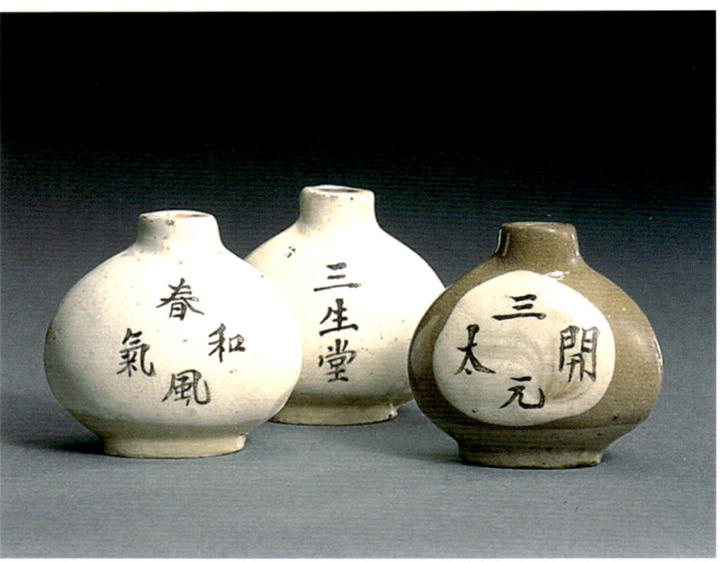

103. Three pharmacy delivery containers. (a) Front: 春風和氣 "Spring wind, harmonious qi." Bottom: 紅升丹 "red sublimation pills." (b) Front: 三元汲第 "The three best examination graduates of the third degree." Back: 三生堂 "Pharmacy of Triple Life." Bottom: 白降丹 "white fall-out pills." (c) Front: 一元復始 "New Year's Day is starting anew." Back: 三元開太 "The triple beginning [of year, month, day] on New Year's Day." All porcelain, black-and-blue underglaze on white base, ink, height 5 cm.

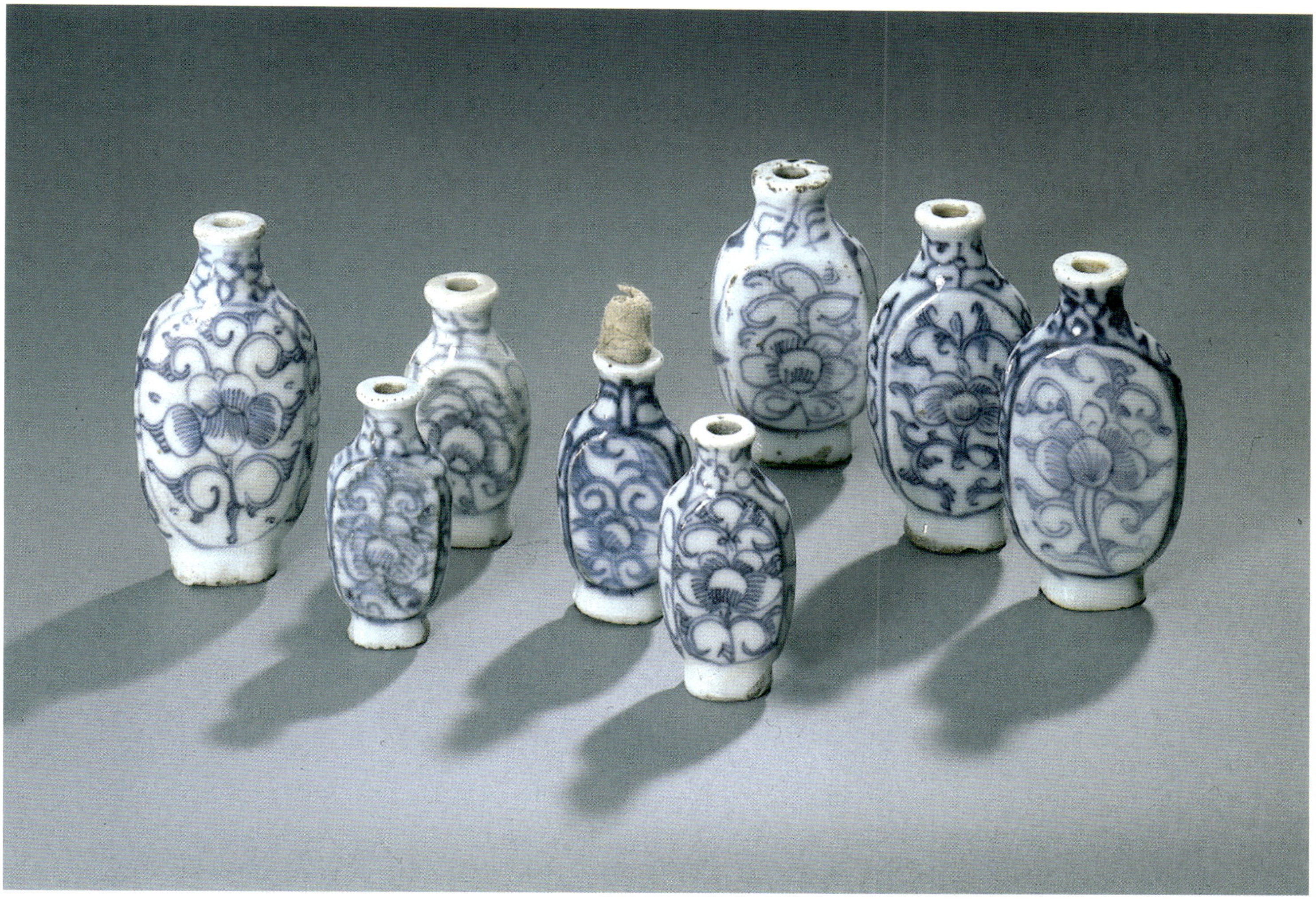

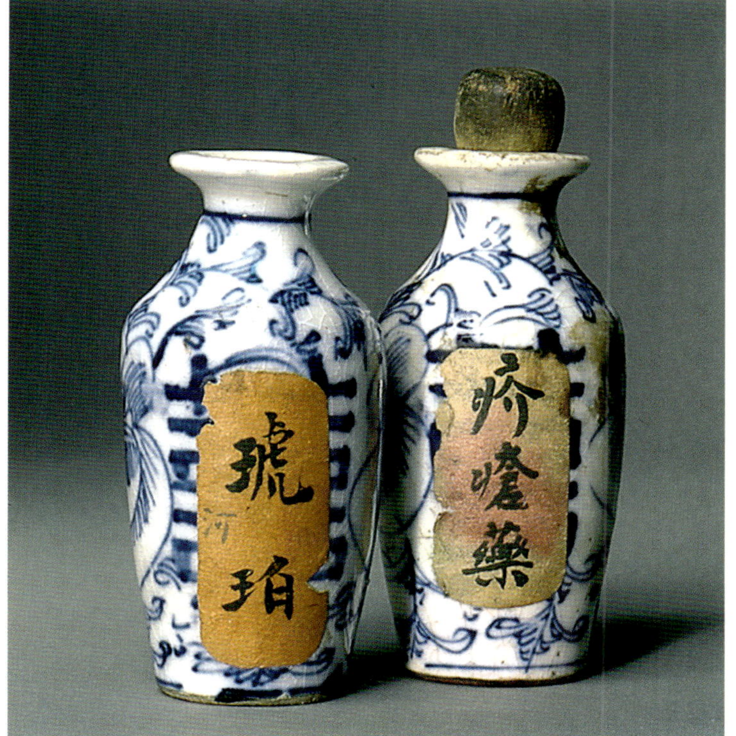

104. Eight pharmacy delivery containers shaped like vases and decorated with peonies. Porcelain, blue underglaze on white base, height varies 5–7.2 cm.

105. Two pharmacy delivery containers shaped like vases and decorated with peonies and double fortune characters.
(a) Red paper label indicating the content: 琥珀 "amber." Porcelain, height 10 cm. (b) Red paper label indicating the content: 雄黄散 "realgar powder," arsenic disulfide, and the indication 疥瘡藥 "medicine for scabious sores." Porcelain with wooden plug, height 10 cm. Both blue underglaze on white base.

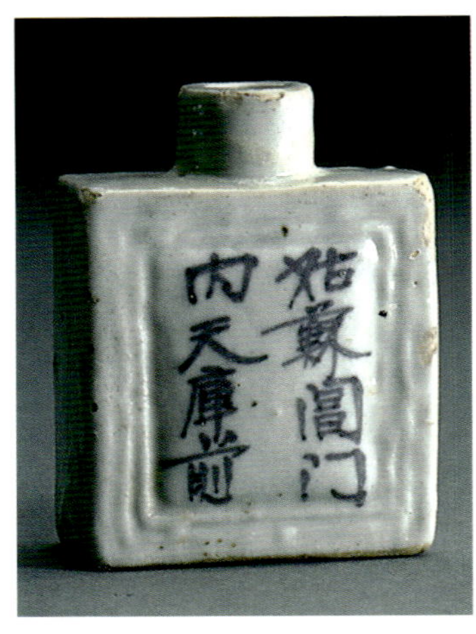

106. Pharmacy delivery container. Front: 誦芬堂雷 "Pharmacy Recitation and Fragrance of [Mr.] Lei." Back: 姑蘇閶門內天庫前 "Gusu [=Suzhou], inside the palace gate, in front of the Heavenly Depot [of the palace]." Stoneware, blue underglaze on white base, height 7.3 cm.

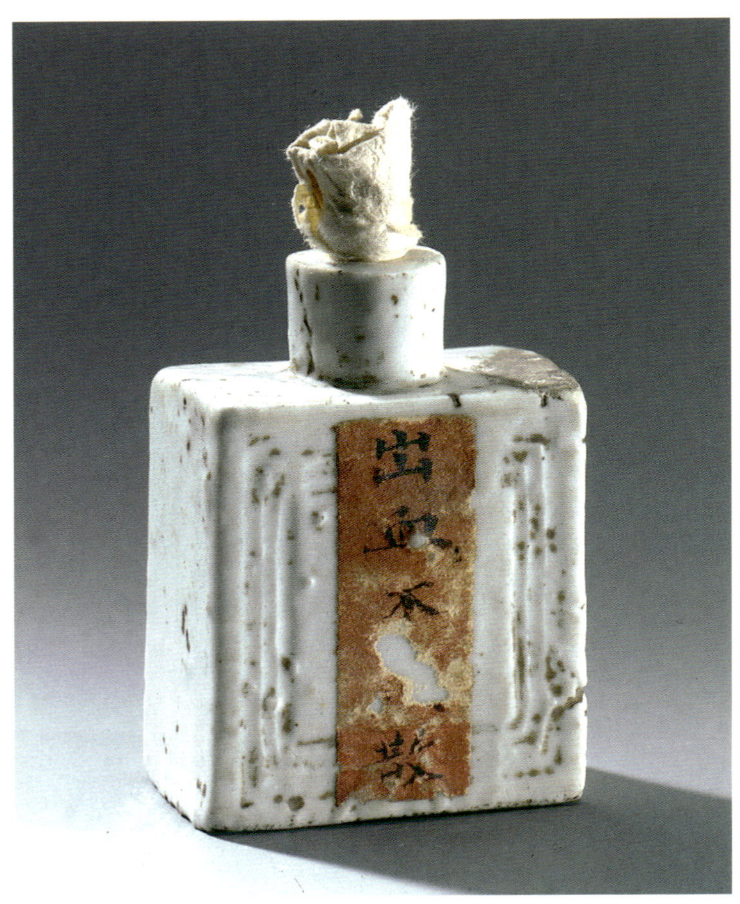

107. Pharmacy delivery container in the shape of a small tea-caddy. Front: 漢鎮至德堂吳亮金 "Hanzhen [=Hankou], Pharmacy Utmost Virtue of [Mr.] Wu Liangjin." Red paper label explaining the indication: 出血不止散 "powder for bleeding which will not stop." Porcelain, blue underglaze on white base, paper plug.

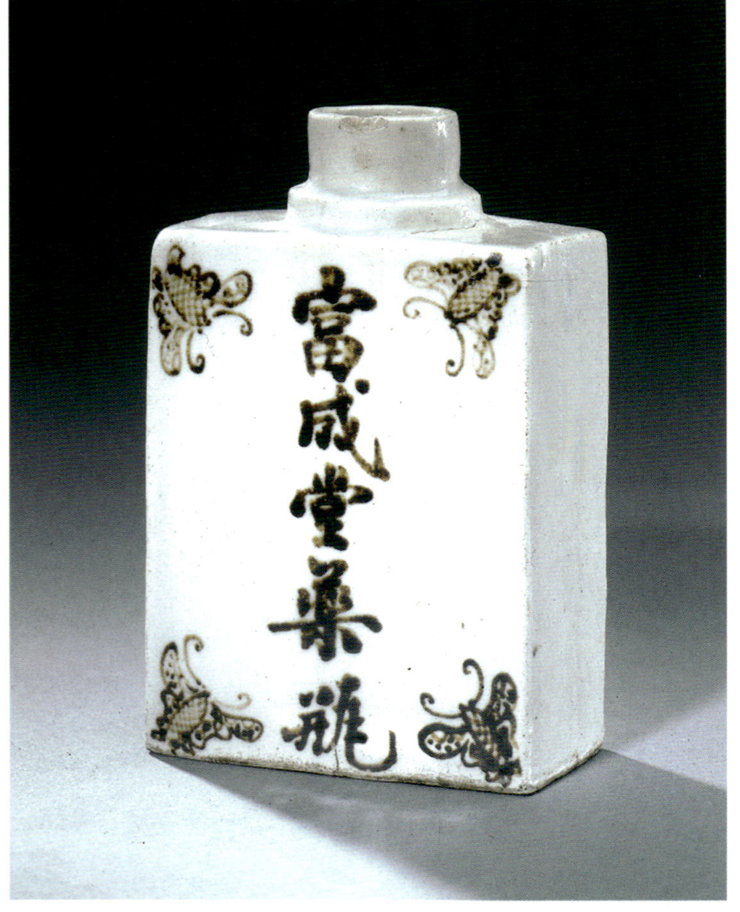

108. Pharmacy delivery container in the shape of a tea-caddy and decorated with butterflies. Front: 富成堂藥瓶 "Medicine container of the Wealth and Perfection Pharmacy." Stoneware, height 15.3 cm.

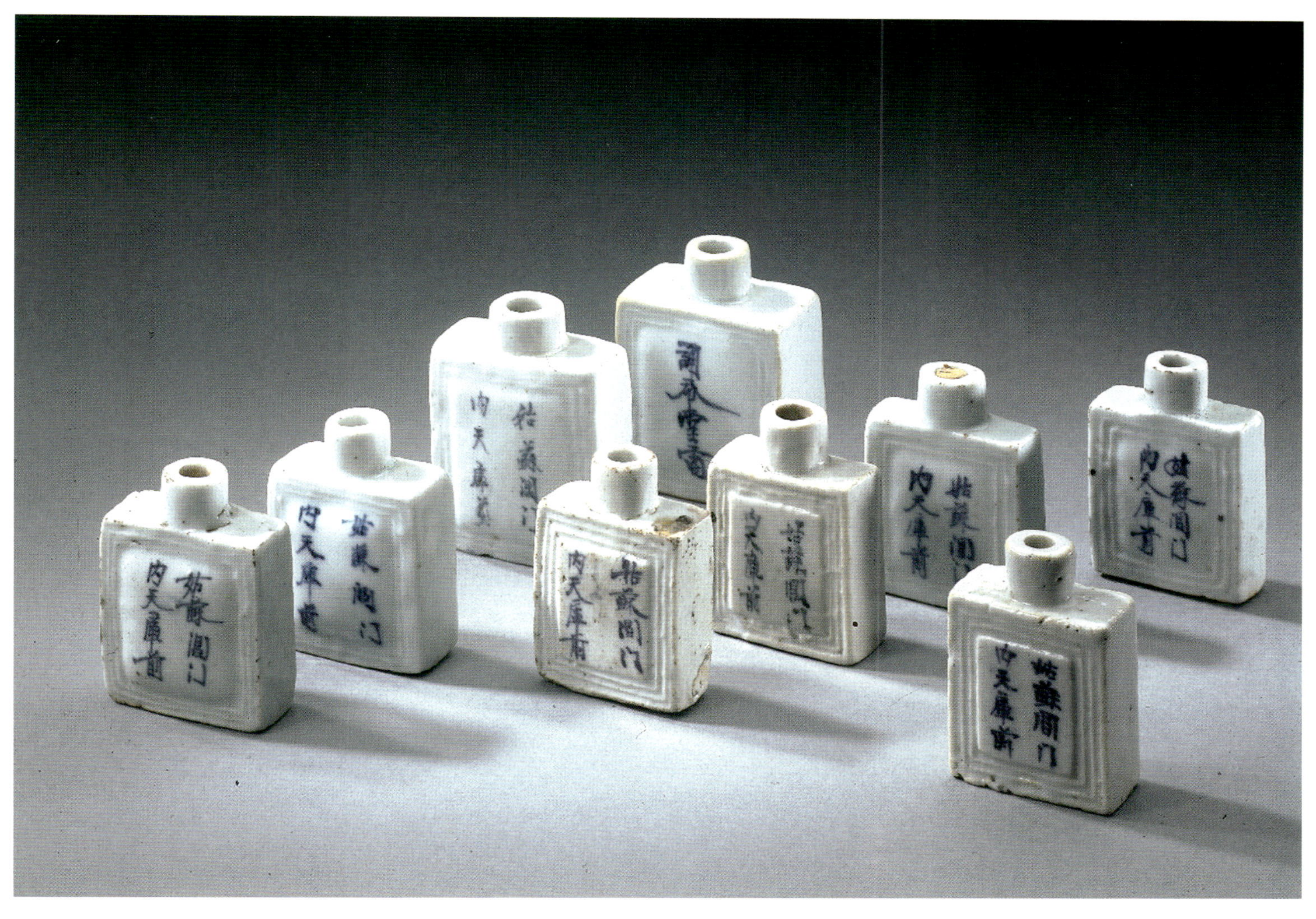

109. Nine pharmacy delivery containers shaped like small tea-caddies. Front: 誦芬堂雷 "Pharmacy Recitation and Fragrance of [Mr.] Lei." Back: 姑蘇閶門內天庫前 "Gusu [=Suzhou], inside the palace gate, in front of the Heavenly Depot [of the palace]." Porcelain, blue underglaze on white, height 6.2–7.3 cm.

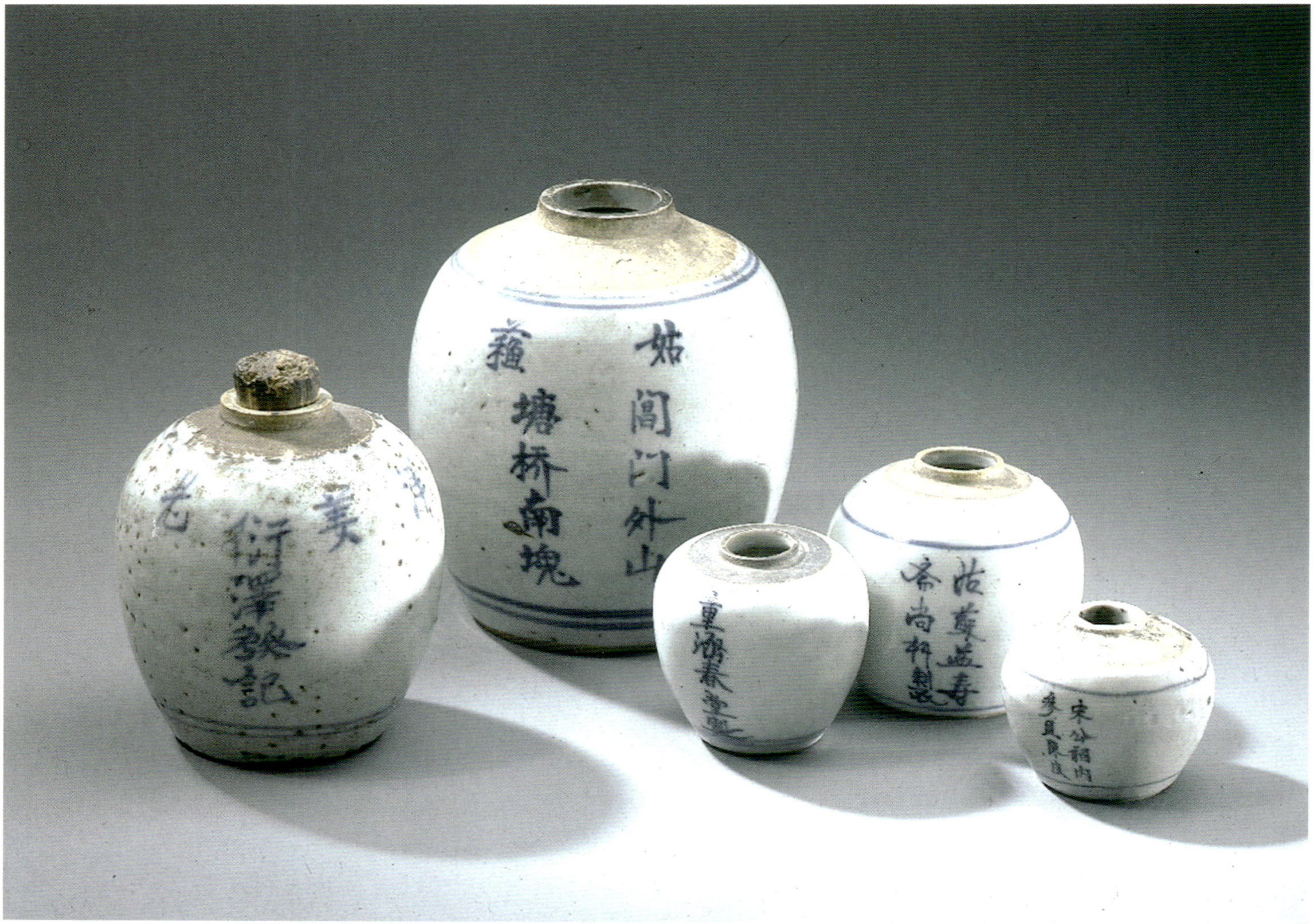

110. Five sphere-shaped pharmacy delivery containers. (a) height 10 cm. "Shanyang. Outside of the Small Southern Gate. Original [Pharmacy] Distributing the Welfare of Jiang [Bingyuan]. Flower dew container." The Jiangyanzetang 姜衍澤堂 was founded in 1668 and is the oldest pharmacy still in operation in Shanghai. Porcelain, height 10 cm. (b) 姑蘇閶門外山塘橋南塊 (=塊)太乙堂發兌 "Wholesaler of the Pharmacy Supreme One at the Southern End of the Mountain Lake Bridge outside the palace gate in Gusu [=Suzhou]." Porcelain, height 14.3 cm. (c) 上洋小東門内童涵春堂製 "Product of the Pharmacy Magnanimity and Spring of [Mr.] Tong inside the Small Eastern Gate in Shangyang [=Shanghai]." Porcelain, height 6 cm. (d) 益壽堂選製宋公祠内參貝陳皮 "Selected preparation for the Pharmacy Benefiting Longevity inside the ancestral temple of Mr. Song. [Ren]shen (ginseng); bei[mu] (flowers of *Fritillaria thunbergii Miq*); chenpi (fruit skin of *Citrus retuculata Blanco*)." Porcelain, height 7.2 cm. (e) 姑蘇益壽齋尚扦 (=監)製老宋公祠參貝陳皮 "Produced under government supervision: *renshen, beimu, chenpi* of the Pharmacy Benefiting Longevity [inside the] ancestral temple of the old Mr. Song in Gusu [=Suzhou]." Porcelain, height 5 cm.

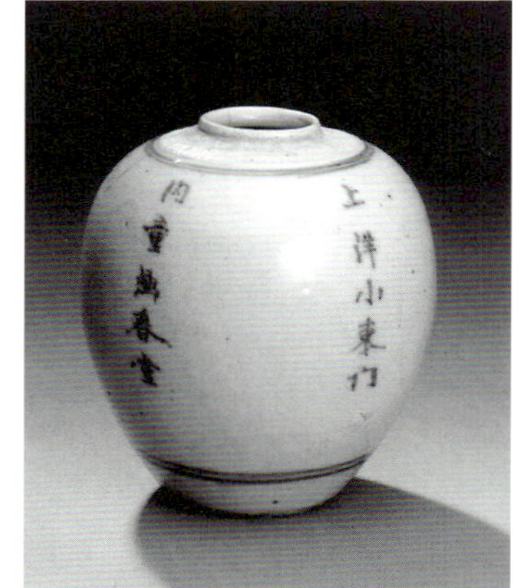

111. Sphere-shaped pharmacy delivery container. 上洋小東門内童涵春堂 "Shangyang. Inside the Small Eastern Gate. Pharmacy Magnanimity and Spring of [Mr.] Tong [Shanchang] 童[善長]." Founded as Pharmacy of the Magnanimity and Spring of [Mr.] Zhu in 1783, this pharmacy developed into one of the four largest pharmacies in Shanghai. Porcelain, height 14 cm.

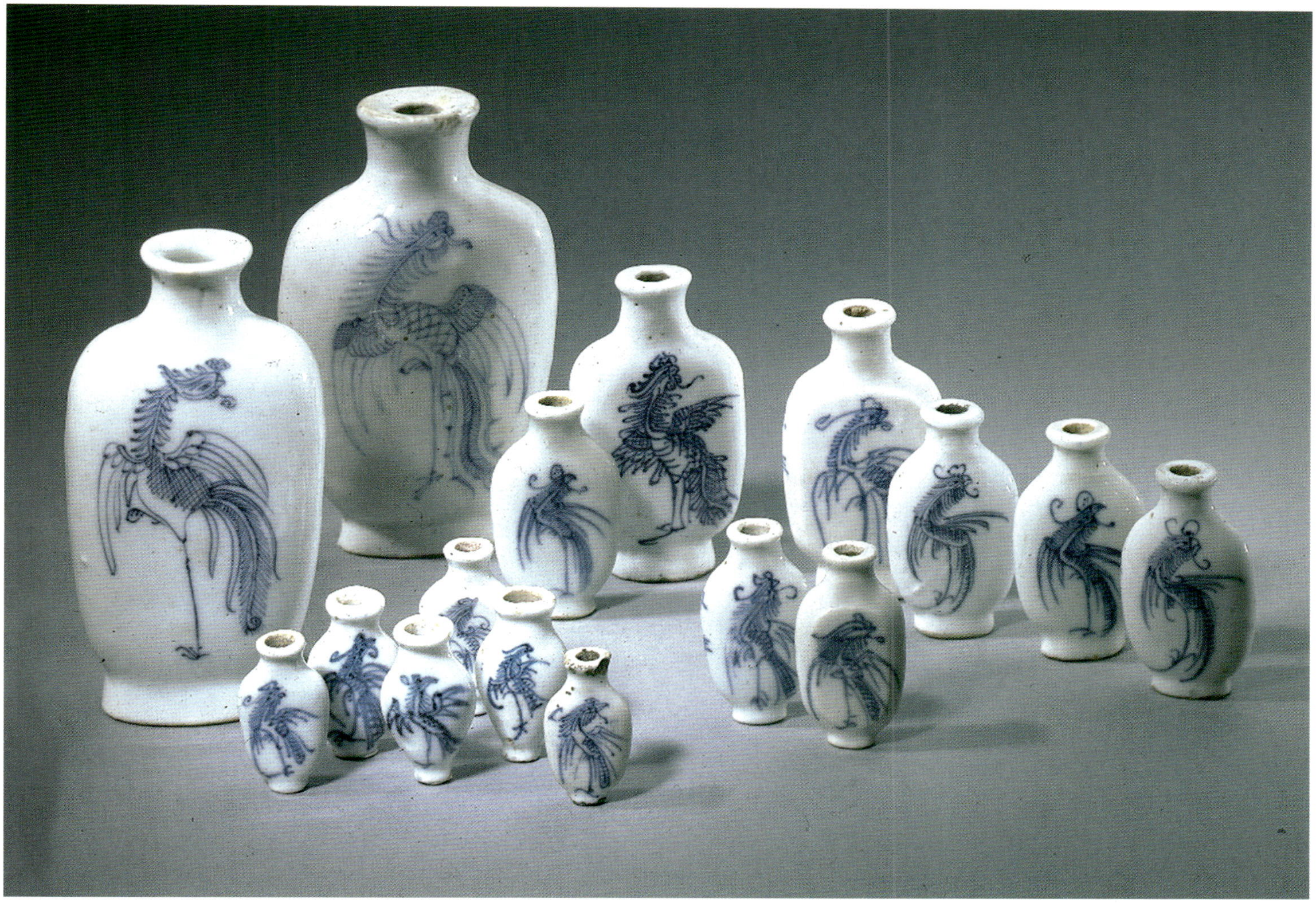

112. Sixteen pharmacy delivery containers shaped like amphoras, by the "original Desheng Pharmacy" west of the New Bridge in the market-town of Chang'an 長安鎮, County Haining 海寧縣, near Hangzhou 杭州 in Zhejiang 浙江. Text: 卜年朱德生堂鳳記老店 "Pharmacy Virtue and Life of [Mr.] Zhu Bunian; original store with the phoenix trademark." Porcelain, blue underglaze on white base, heights vary 3.7–12.2 cm.

113. Pharmacy delivery container decorated with a phoenix. Text: "The original store of the pharmacy Virtue and Life of [Mr.] Zhu Bunian with the phoenix trademark west of the New Bridge in the market town Chang'an in Haining [County] near Hang[zhou] in Zhe[jiang]." Porcelain, blue underglaze on white base, height 12 cm.

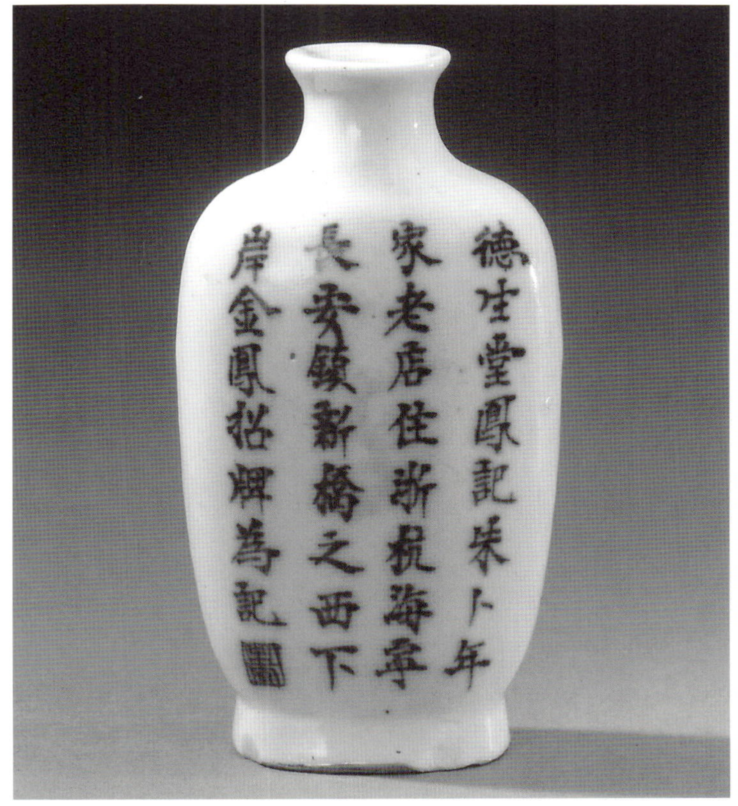

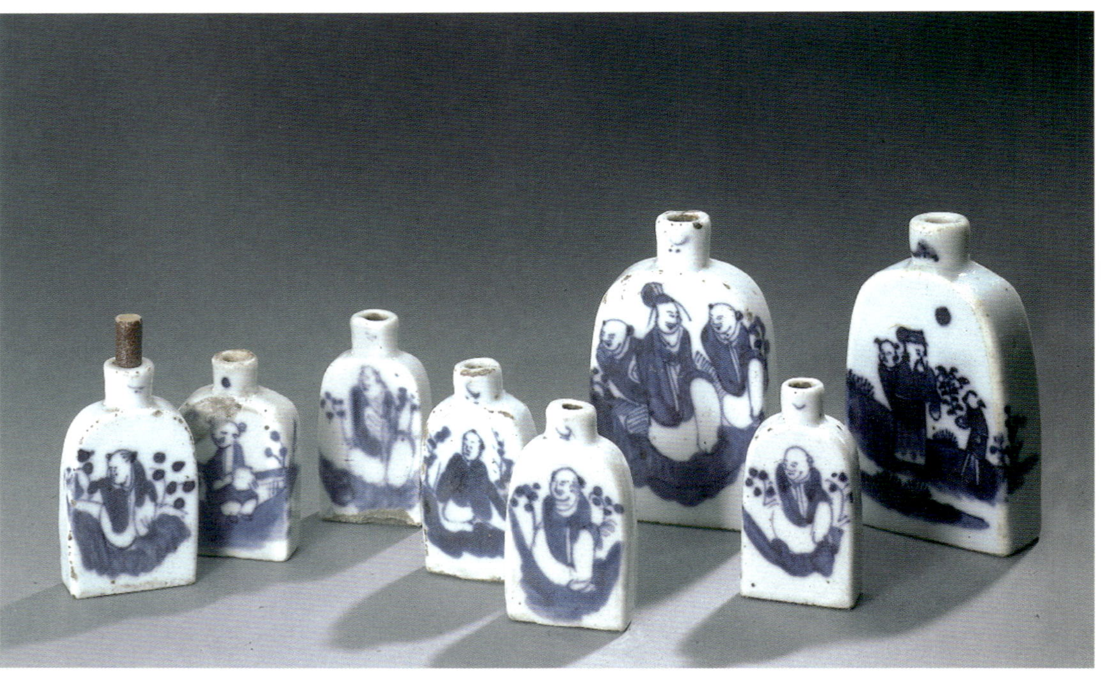

114. Eight pharmacy delivery containers decorated with figures in a landscape. Porcelain, blue underglaze on white base, heights vary 5.8–9 cm.

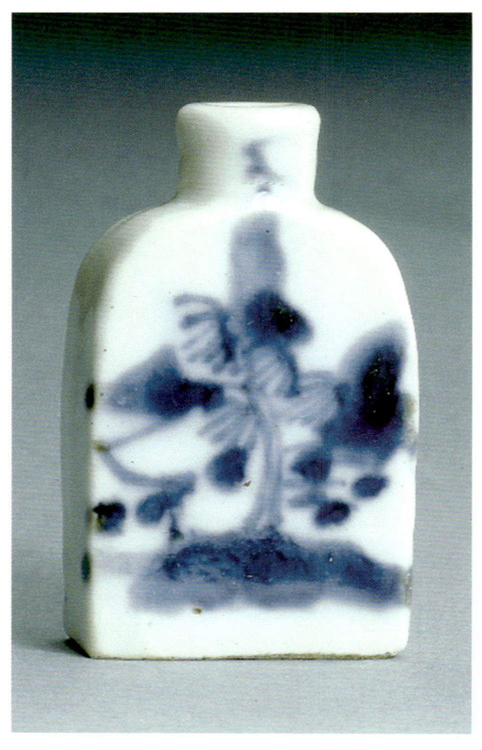

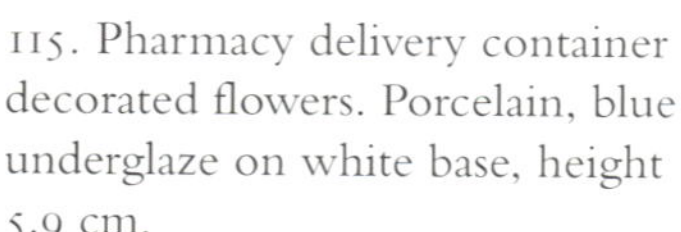

115. Pharmacy delivery container decorated flowers. Porcelain, blue underglaze on white base, height 5.9 cm.

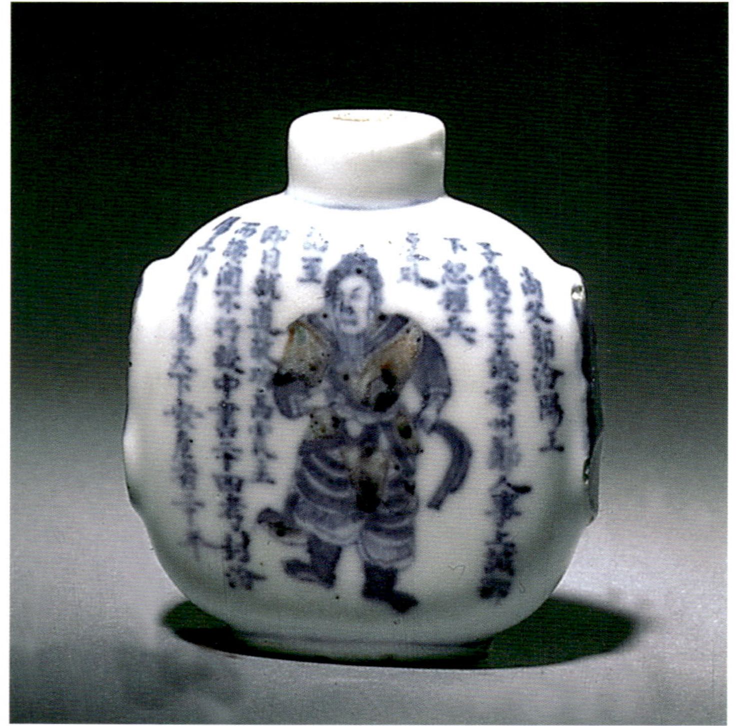

116. Pharmacy delivery container decorated on all sides with illustrations and text about the life and history of general Guo Ziyi 郭子儀 (697–781), famous for his military successes and long life. Bottom: 慎德堂製 "Product of the Pharmacy Careful Attention to Virtue." Porcelain, blue underglaze on white base, height 6.5 cm.

117. Six pharmacy delivery containers from the series of the baxian 八仙 "Eight Immortals." Front: Each of the eight immortals. Back: the corresponding symbols. Left: 範子燗作 "By Fan Zinan." Right: 萬病回春 "Returns one from myriad illnesses back to spring." Porcelain, multicolored underglaze on white base, partial paper plugs, height 7 cm.

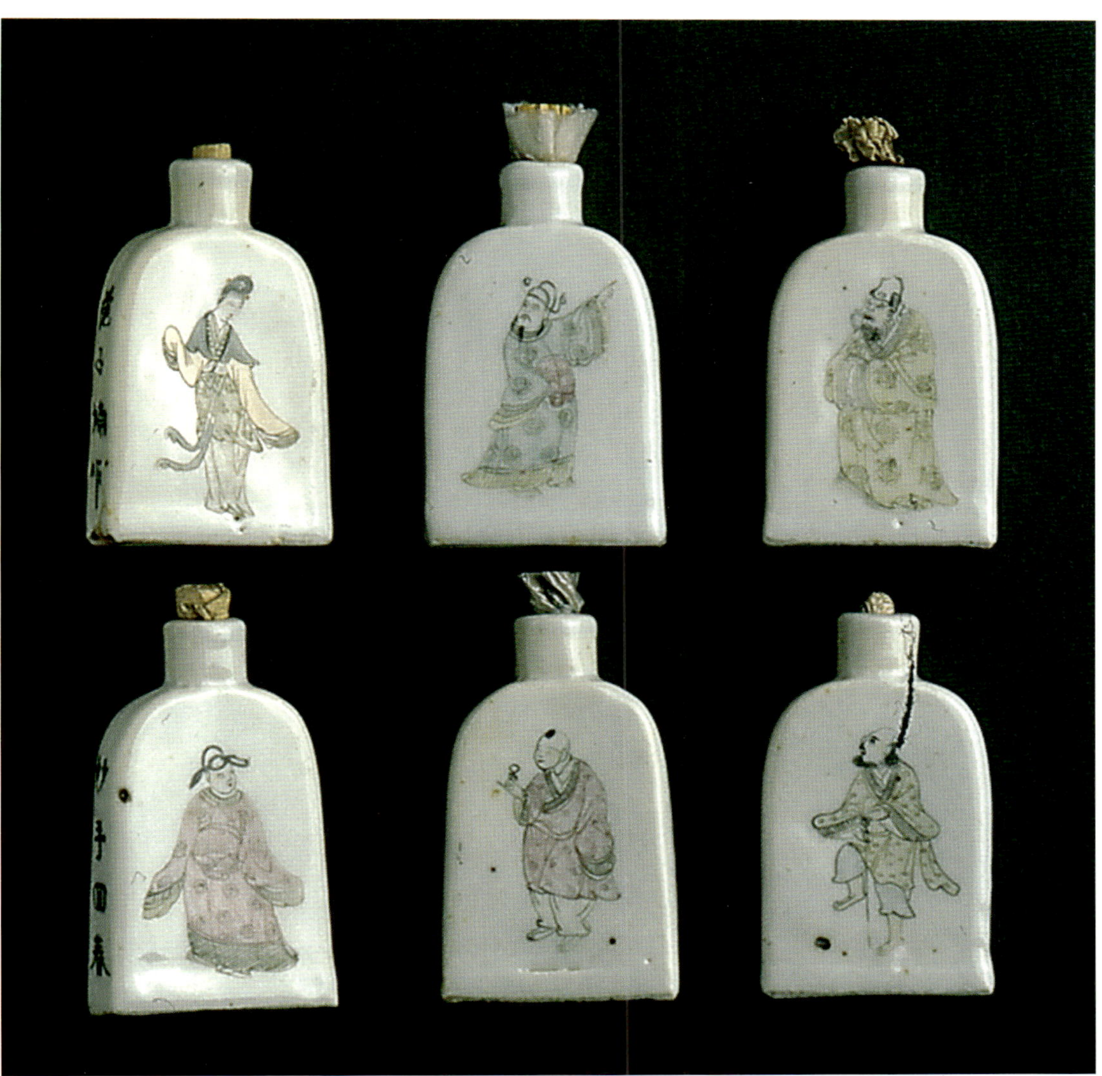

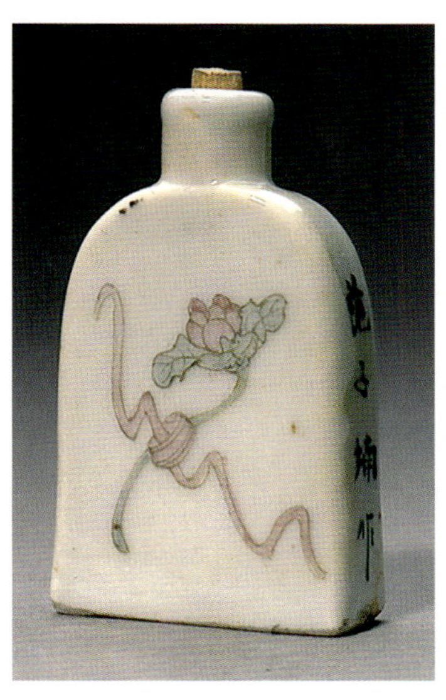

118. Pharmacy delivery container from the series of the "Eight Immortals." The back of the container depicts a water-lily, the symbol of the only woman, He Xiangu 何仙姑, among the eight immortals. Porcelain, multicolored underglaze on white base.

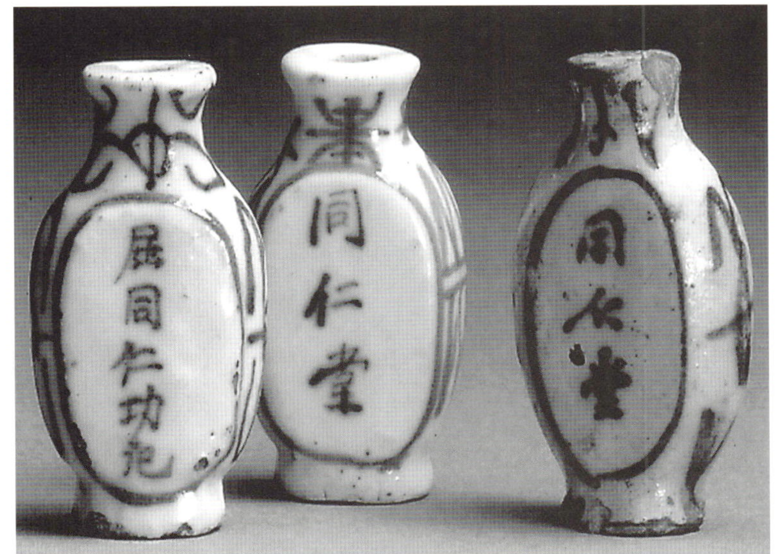

119. Three pharmacy delivery containers decorated with lines and text ovals. Front (a) and (b): 同仁堂 "Pharmacy Letting Everybody Partake in Humaneness." Front (c): 屈同仁功記 "[Mr.] Qu Tongren's [Pharmacy] record of merits. Back (a), (b), (c): 痧氣丹 "pills for sha disorder." Stoneware, blue underglaze on white, heights vary 5.3–5.5 cm.

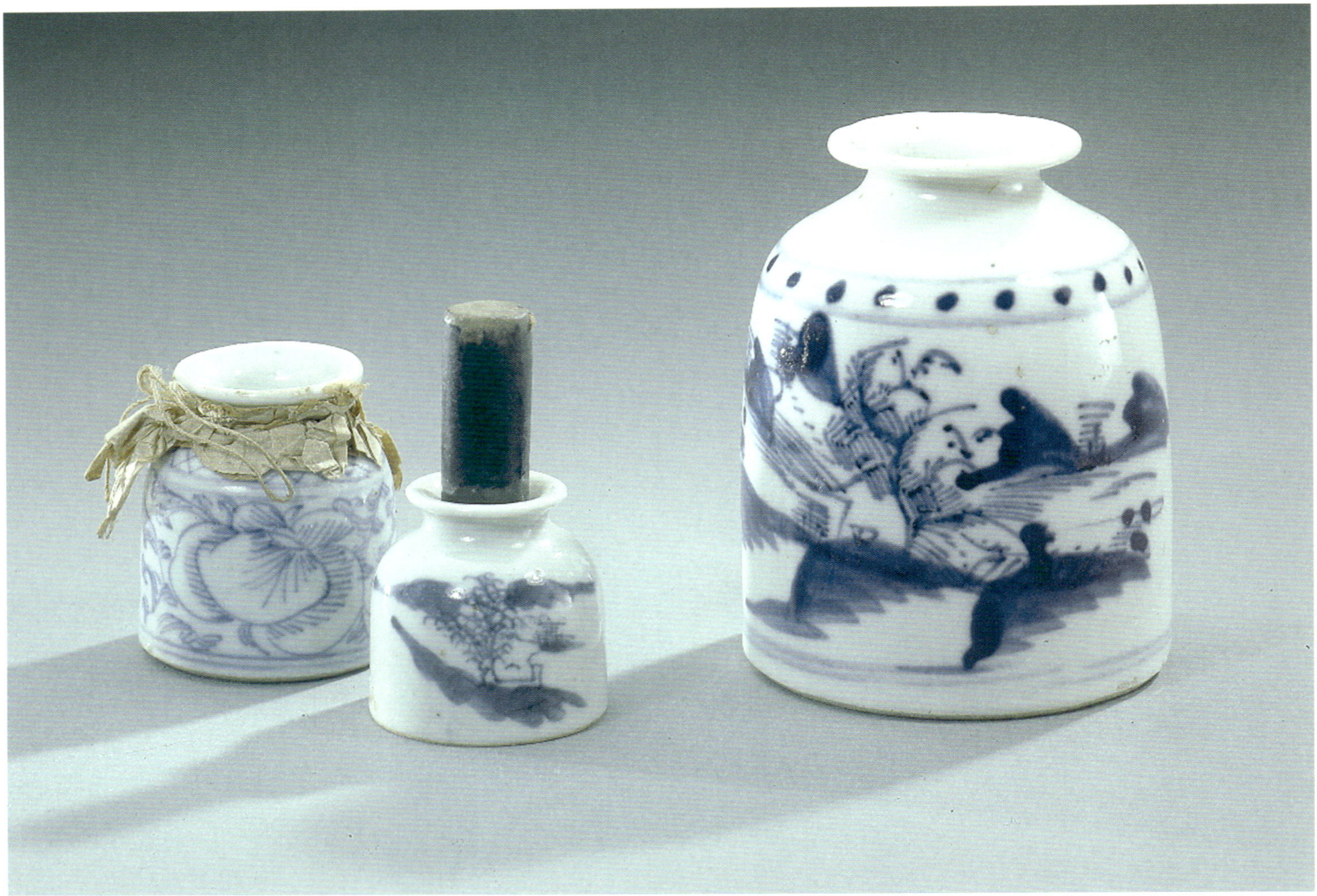

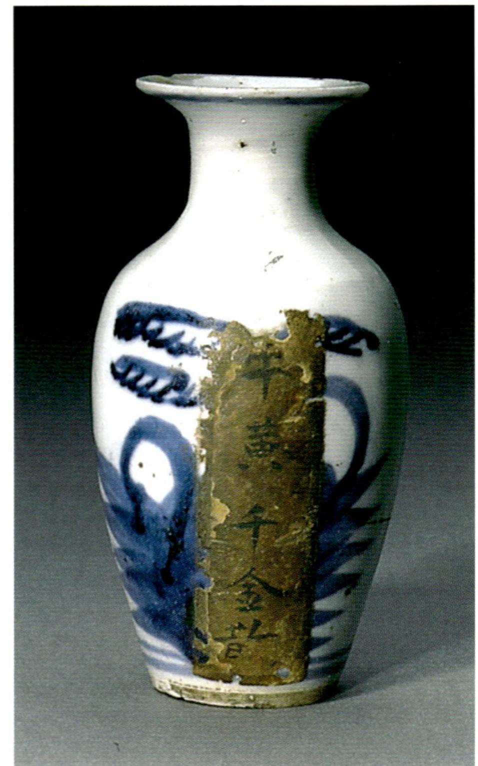

120. Three pharmacy bottle-neck jars, nineteenth–twentieth centuries.
(a) Peony decoration. Tecture residues. Porcelain, blue under-glaze on white base, plug lacquered paper roll, height 6 cm.
(b) Landscape and text: 吳榮泰香粉局選製 "Selected preparation for the Pharmacy Fragrant Powder of [Mr.] Wu Rongtai." Porcelain, height 4.4 cm.
(c) Landscape. Porcelain, height 10.5 cm.

121. Pharmacy delivery container in the shape of a vase and decorated with flowers. Paper label: 牛黃千金散 "powder with bovine bezoar worth a thousand pieces of gold." Porcelain, blue underglaze on white base, height 11.8 cm.

123. Two pharmacy containers shaped like vases. (a) Red paper label: 瘡毒散 "powder for ulcer poison." Stoneware, height 9.2 cm. (b) Red paper label: 黃水散 "powder for Yellow Water [edema]." Stoneware, height 8 cm, North China.

124. Three pharmacy delivery containers shaped like vases.
(a) Red paper label: 通耳散 "powder to make the ear open." Brown-black stoneware, height 6.5 cm.
(b) Red paper label: 消疳散 "powder for the dispersal of *gan* disorders." Brown stoneware, height 5.1 cm.
(c) Red paper label: 三白散 "powder with the three [medicinal drugs which contain the character for the color] white [in their names]." Stoneware, height 6.5 cm.

122. Two pharmacy delivery
containers shaped like vases. (a)
Front red paper label indicating
the content: 萬靈丹 "pills with
a myriad powers." Back: red paper
label indicating method of
ingestion: 每用四五丹將葱
白咬如泥男左女右吐手心
包藥在內黃[]皮或汗瀉俱
好 "The single dose consists of
four or five pills. Chew onion
cores into a pulp. For men, spit it
into the left [palm], for women,
into the right palm and coat the
medicine [i.e. the pills] with it.
Sweating, diarrhea. All is cured."
Bottom: red label: 飛龍奪命丹
"Pills of the flying dragon snatch-
ing life [from death]." Stoneware,
paper plug, height 9.9 cm.
(b) Front red paper label: 四妙
散走馬牙疳先用淘米水漱
淨口再搽之萬世不漱帖藥
"Powder with the four
miraculous [ingredients] [for the
treatment of] gan disorder in the
teeth which progresses as rapidly
as a running horse. First rinse the
mouth clean with rice rinsing
water. Then rub in repeatedly.
Firmly adhering medicine which
cannot be rinsed off in ten
thousand generations." Back red
paper label: faded writing.
Brown–black stoneware, paper
plug, height 9.2 cm.

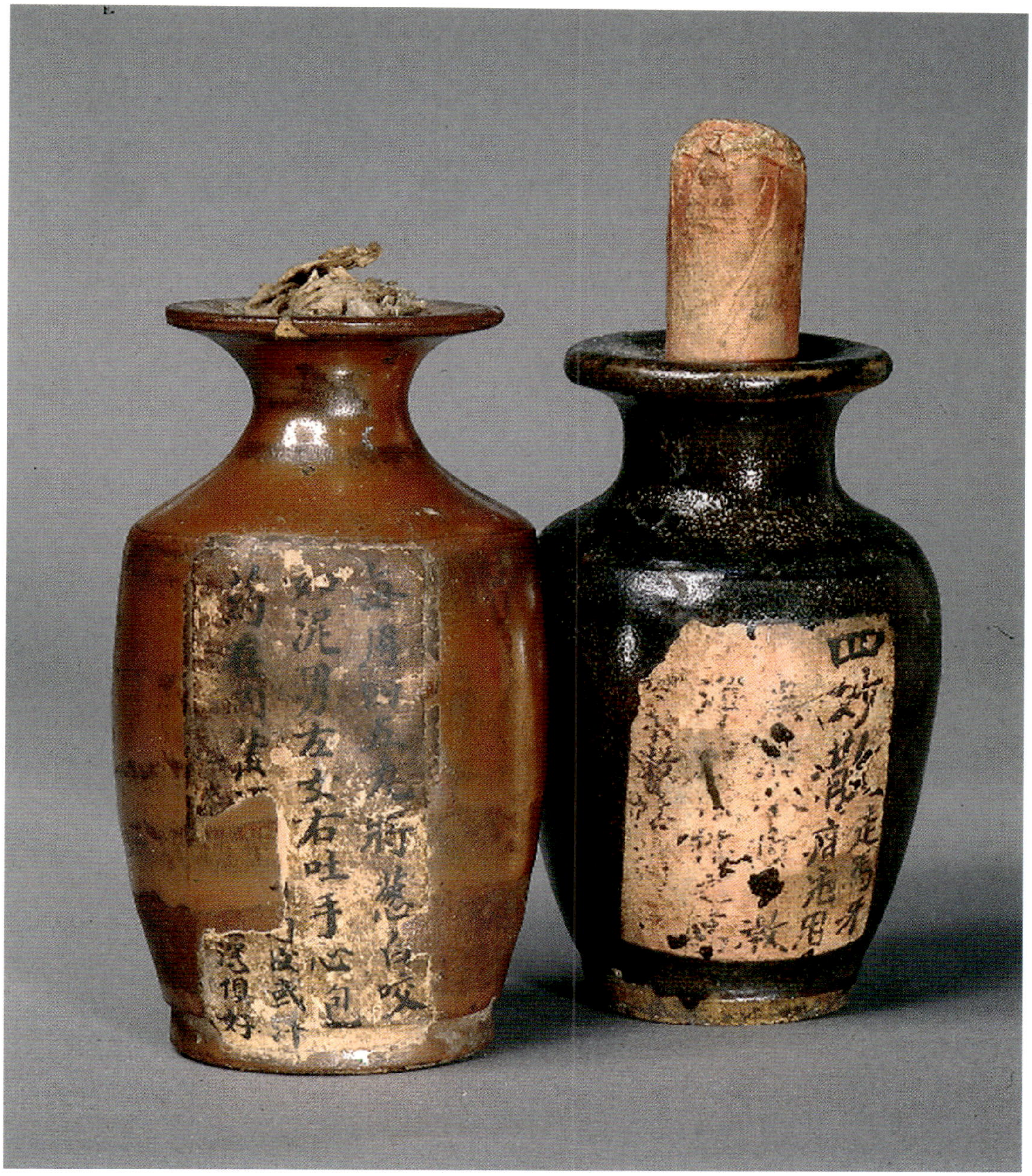

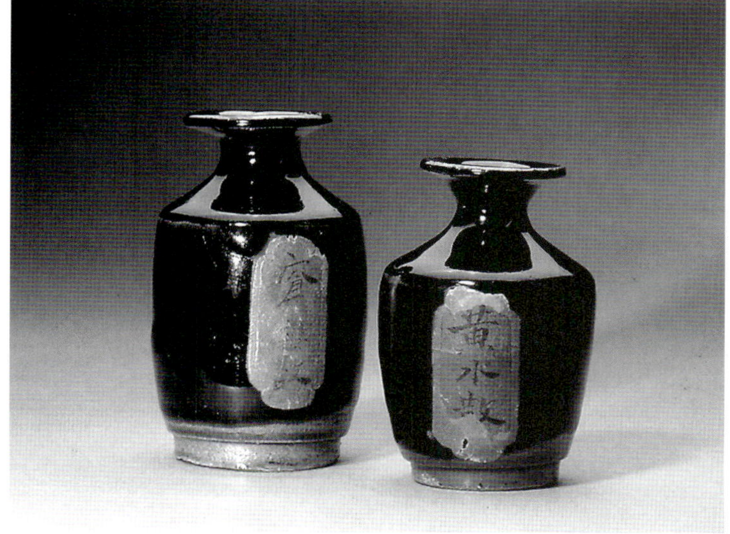

123

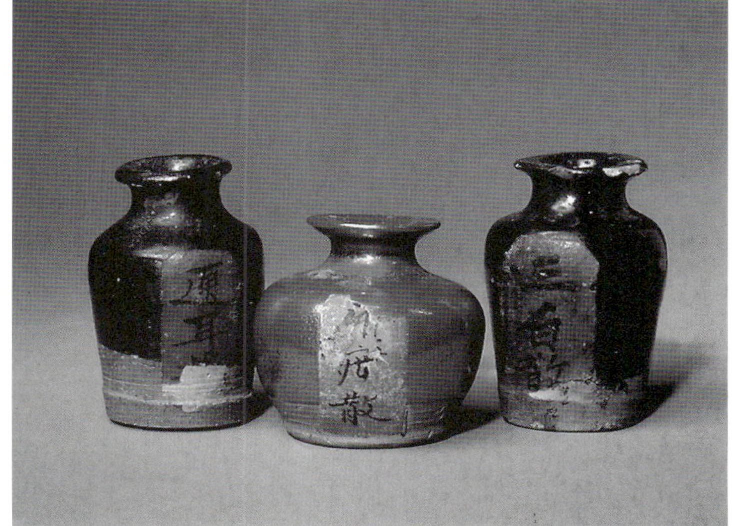

124

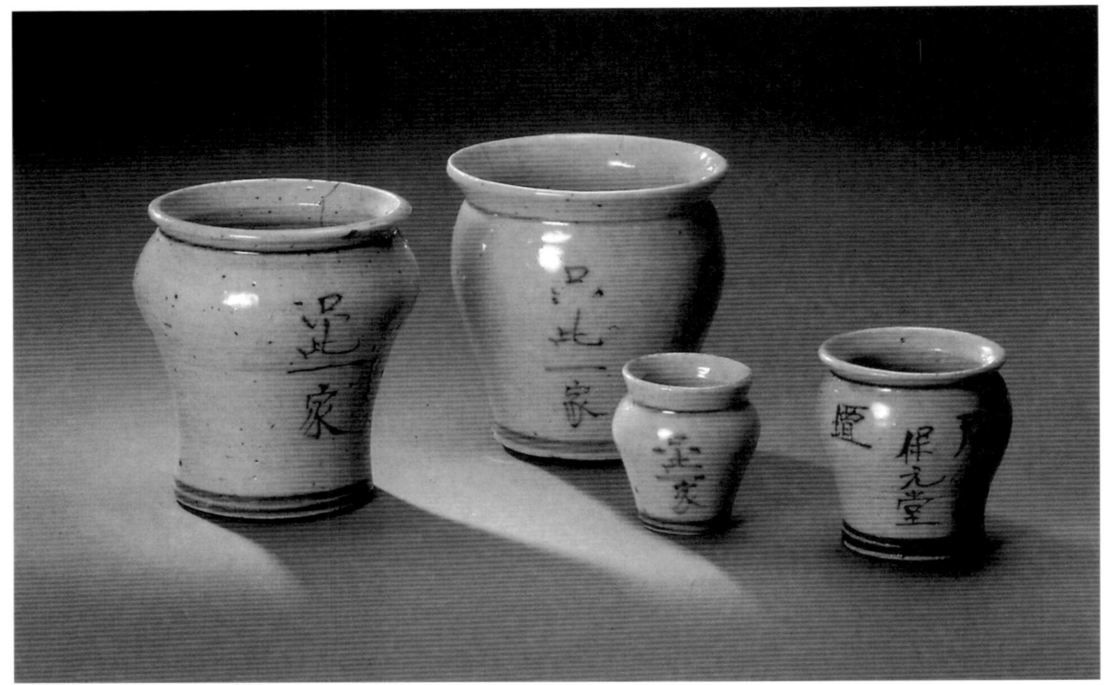

125. Four wide-neck jars from two Peking pharmacies. (a) 天坛保元堂只此一家 "Altar of Heaven. Pharmacy Preserving the Original State. Only this one establishment." (b) 天坛天德堂只此一家 "Altar of Heaven. Pharmacy Heavenly Virtue. Only this one establishment." Each porcelain, heights 6.3–12 cm, nineteenth–early twentieth centuries.

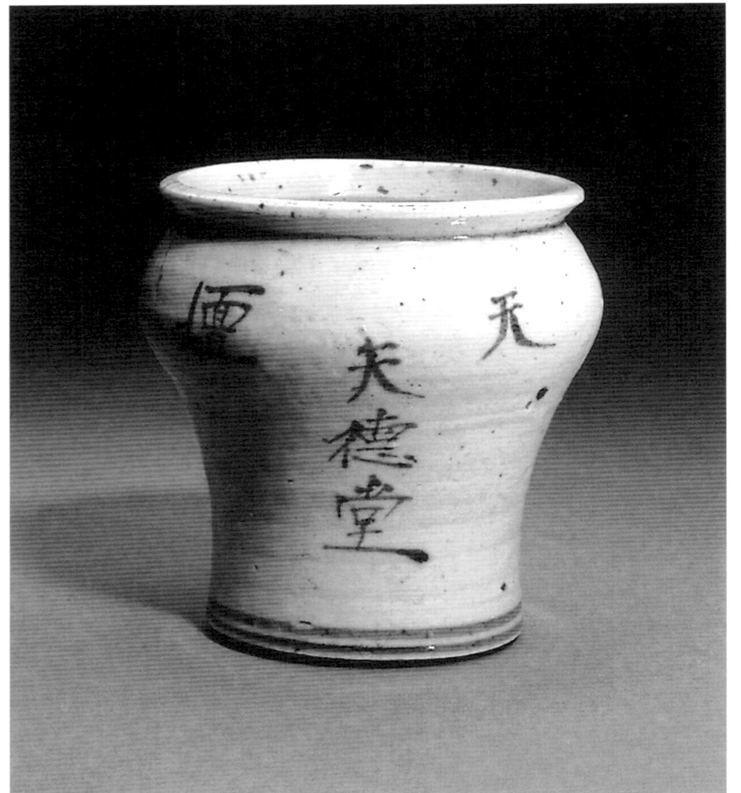

126. Pharmacy wide-neck jar. Front: 天坛天德堂只此一家 "Altar of Heaven. Pharmacy Heavenly Virtue. Only this one establishment." Porcelain, height 12 cm, Peking.

127. Three pharmacy delivery containers. (a) Engraving on front indicating the content: 如意丸 "pills that bring the desired effect" and 卧龍丹 "pills [with the strength of] a sleeping dragon." Back: Landscape. White brass with two parts connected by a hinge, screw top, height 4.5 cm. (b) Engraving on front indicating the content: 砂藥丹 "pills with drugs for *sha* [disorder]." Back: Plants. White brass, one piece, screw top, height 4.4 cm. (c) Engraving on front indicating the content (right to left): 南沙藥 "southern drug for *sha* [disorder]", 紅靈丹 "red miracle pills," 平安散 "calming powder." Back: Figure drawings. Side border: Turtle shell decoration. Silver with three parts connected by hinge, three screw tops, two with added measuring spoon, height 4.2 cm.

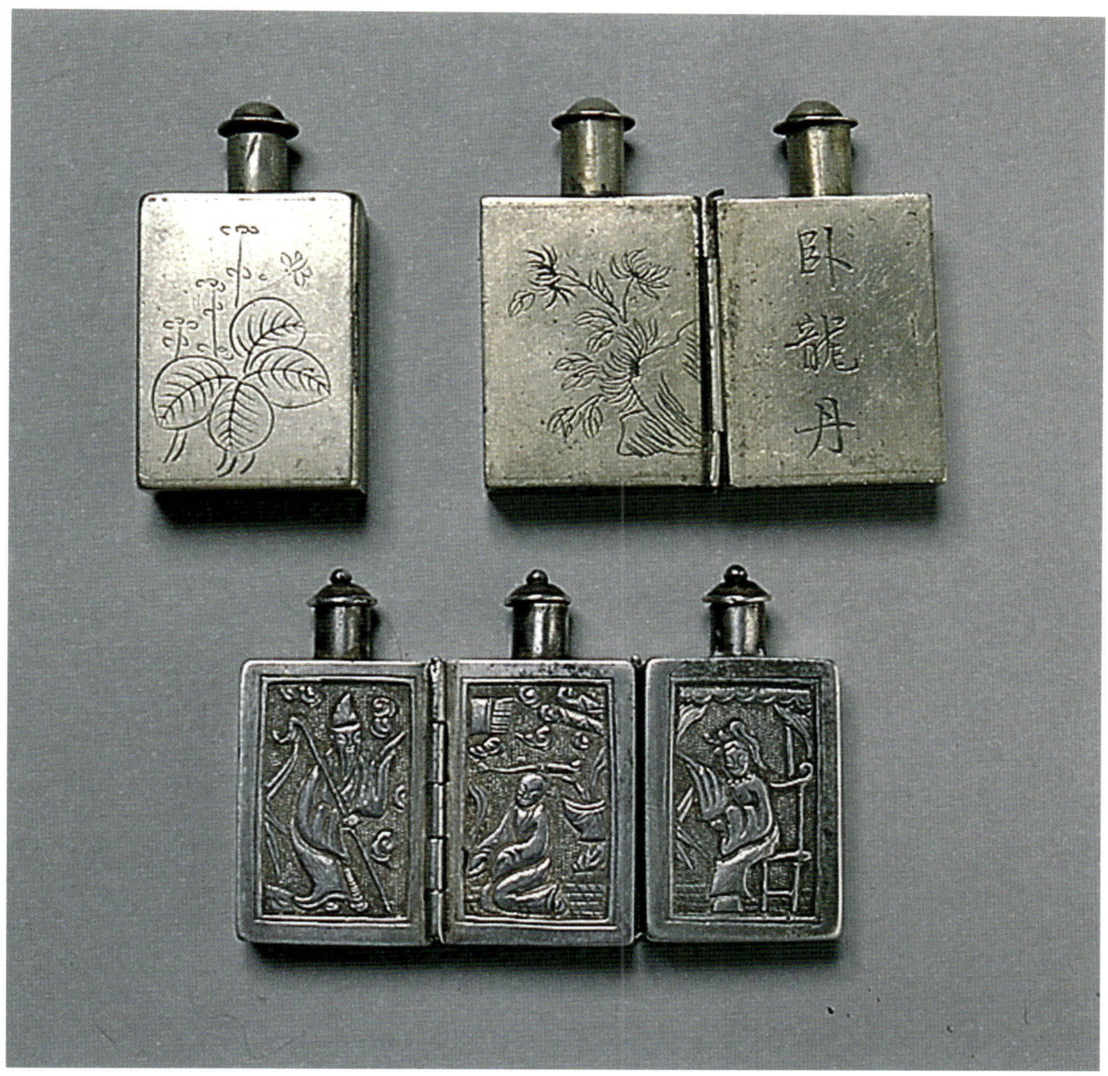

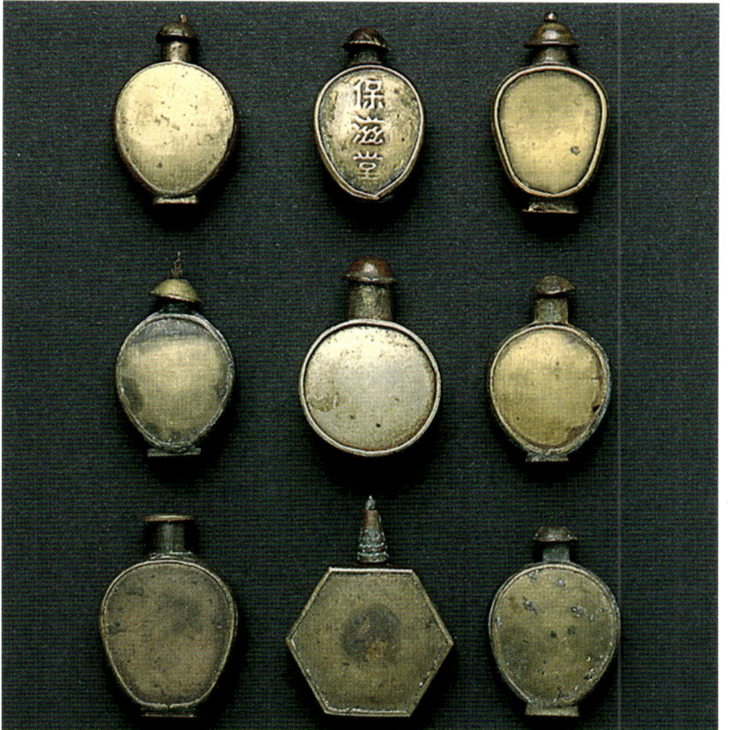

128. Nine pharmacy delivery containers, one front with relief inscription: 保滋堂 "Pharmacy Protection and Nurturing." Back: 通關散 "powder which breaks through gates." Bubble-shaped powder tin, brass, screw tops and plugs, heights vary 3.1–3.8 cm.

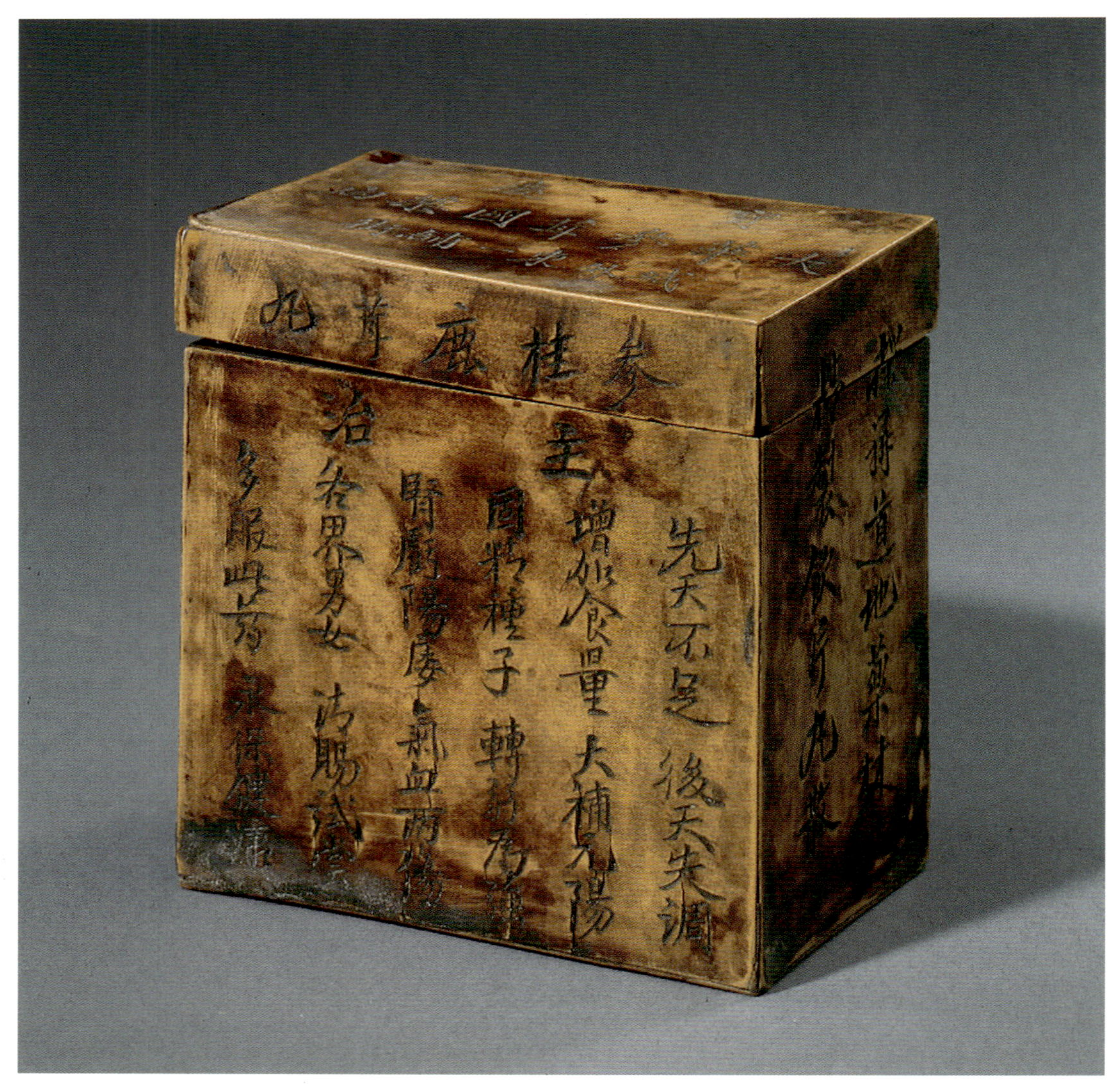

129. Pharmacy delivery container. Front text in verse form:

參桂皮茸丸主治
先天不足後天失調
增加食量大補元陽
固精種子轉弱為強
腎虧陽痿氣血兩傷
各界男女請賜試嘗
多服此藥永保建康

"Powder with ginseng, cinnamon bark, and deer antlers. Main indications: When the constitution has been problematic since birth, when the nutrition was unbalanced in later life, [these pills] supplement the diet and replenish the original yang [qi]. They solidify the seed for procreation and turn weakness into strength when the kidneys are exhausted and the yang [i.e. the penis] tires, when qi and blood are harmed. Men and women of all regions, please try them out and take a lot of this medicine. Your health will be protected forever!" Left: 發揚國藥精華保障人群健康 "These pills spread the spirit and glamor of national medicines. They protect the health of humanity." Right: 授辦道地藥材精製飲片丸散 "[This pharmacy] gathers and prepares unadulterated drug products and exercises care in the manufacture of [herbal] tablets for [the preparation of] potable [decoctions], pills, and powders." Back: Medical sage with gourd on top of a deer in front of a pine. 壽鹿商標 "Trademark: Deer of long life.". Top: 寶慶大華參茸國藥局 "[Government district] Baoqing. Pharmacy Great China for ginseng, deer antlers, [and other] national medicinal drugs. Outside the city walls, Eastern Shopstreet One." Wood, height 10.3 cm. Before 1913 since the term Baoqing for the modern Shaoyang District in Hunan Province was abolished in that year.

130. Home and traveling pharmacy, nineteenth- or early twentieth century. Three-piece lacquered wooden box with lid, tray, and base. Contents: Thirteen porcelain medicine bottles partially decorated with flowers and figures. Inscription: (a) 行軍散 "powder which causes soldiers to run," (b) 只此山中 "Only in these mountains." This inscription is found on numerous medicine containers for aphrodisiacs, sometimes with the complete four-line verse: 松下問童子言師授藥去只在此山中雲深不知處 "Under the pine I asked the boy where [the master was]. He replied: The master has gone to gather medicines. [I only know] that he is in these mountains. The clouds are hanging low; I don't know his exact location." It is unclear why this particular Tang poem was inscribed on medicine containers for aphrodisiacs.

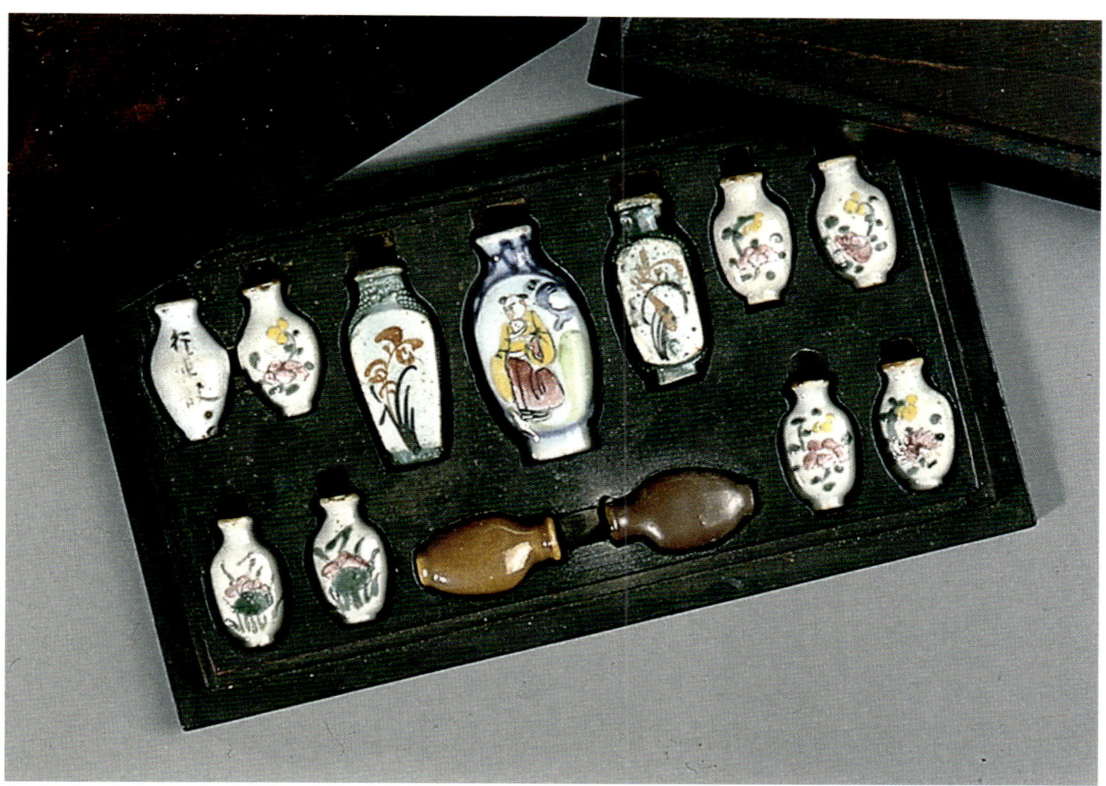

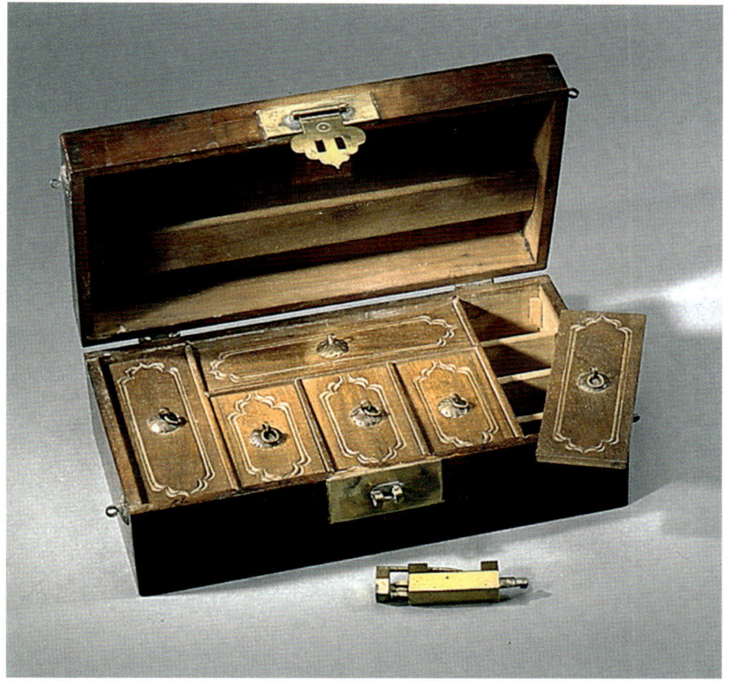

131. Home and traveling pharmacy, nineteenth or early twentieth century. Six large compartments with inside partitions for twenty medicinal drugs. Six cover plates with brass knobs and carved line decorations. Inside of lid: label indicating the manufacturer of the box. Underside of cover plates: names of medicinal drugs written in ink. From right to left: 肉桂 rougui (bark drug of *Cinnamon cassia Presl.*), 南星 nanxing (rhizome drug of *Arisaema consanguineum Schott*), 黑付子 heifuzi (bulb drug of *Aconitum carmichaeli Debx.*), 白付子 baifuzi (rhizome drug of *Typhonium giganteum Engl.*), 乳香 ruxiang (resin of *Boswellia carterii Birdw.*), 沒藥 moyao (myrtle), 龍骨 longgu (dragon bones), 血竭 xuejie (resin of *Draemonorops draco Bl*), 蒼术 cangshu (rhizome drug of *Atractylodes lancea [Thunb.] DC.*), 同祿 tonglü (copper dust), 白芷 baizhi (root drug of *Angelica anomala Lallem.*), 防風 fangfeng (root drug of *Saposhnikovia divaricata [Turcz.] Schischk.*), 廣木香 guangmuxiang (root drug of *Saussurea sinensis Lam.*), 自然同 zirantong (natural copper), 川烏 chuanwu (bulb drug of *Aconitum carmichaeli Debx.*), 蒿本 gaoben (root drug of *Ligusticum sinense Oliv.* and other types of L.), 泡姜 paojiang (soaked ginger), 良姜 liangjiang (rhizome drug of *Alpinia officinarum Hance*), 馬前子 maqianzi (seed drug of *Strychnus nux-vomica L.*), 半夏 banxia (rhizome drug of *Pinellia ternata [Thunb.]*). Wood, wide outside brass lock, height 5 cm.

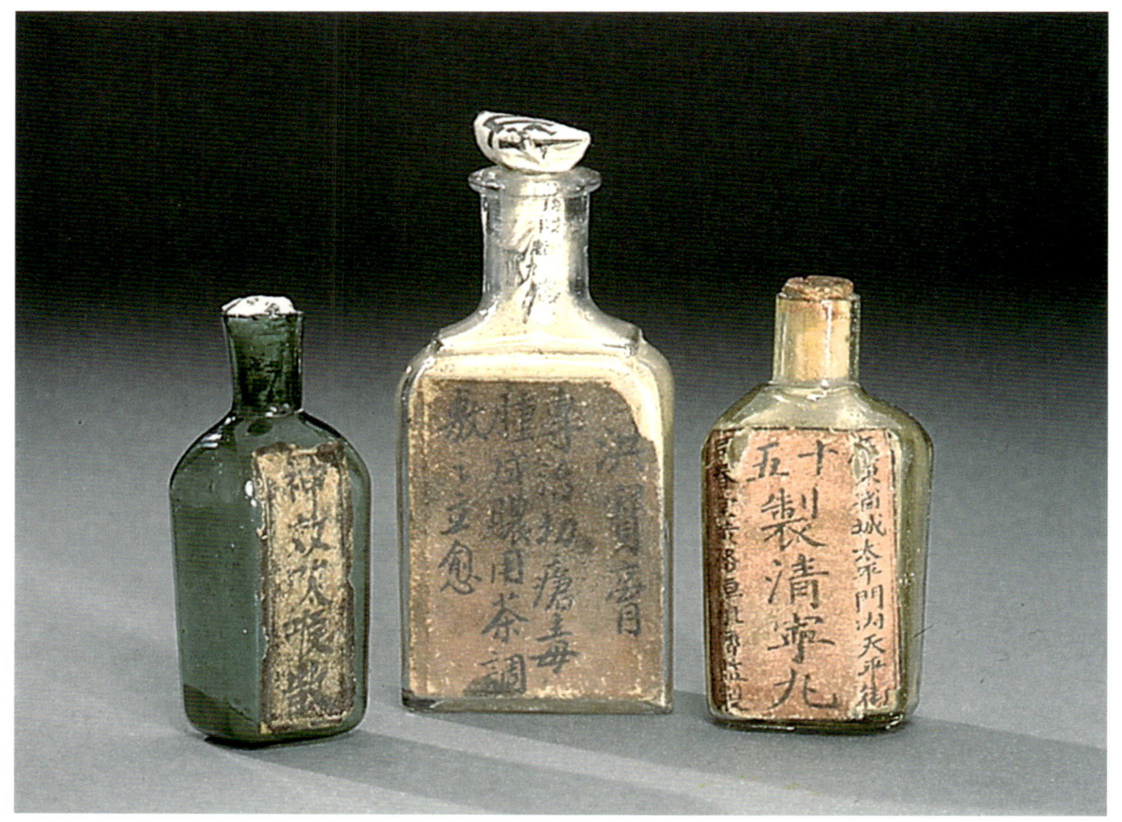

132. Three pharmacy delivery containers. (a) Front: "Shanghai Rose Scented Glycerin." Back red paper label: 洪寶膏專治切瘡毒種成膿用茶調敷之立愈 "Extensive treasure ointment. Particularly [suited] for the treatment of all ulcer poisons and swellings with suppuration. When applied mixed with tea it will cause immediate healing." Glass, height 9.5 cm. (b) Front label: 神效吹喉散 "Powder of divine efficacy, to be blown into the throat." Glass, height 7.3 cm. (c) Front red paper label: 製清寧丸廣東省城太平門內天平街十五同春堂廣務恆祖傳監製 "Provincial capital of Guangdong, inside the Taiping Gate. 15 Taiping Street. Pharmacy which lets everybody partake in spring. [Owner]: Tong Wuheng. Pills for creating calm peace, transmitted from the ancestors and manufactured under government supervision." Glass, wooden plug sealed with wax, height 7.5 cm.

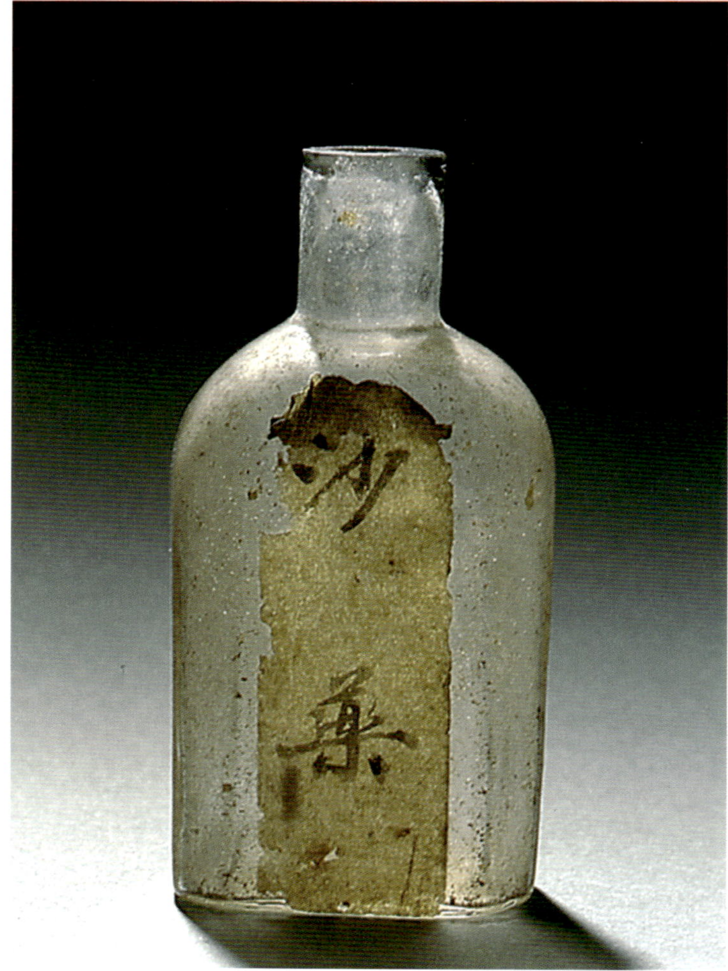

133. Pharmacy delivery container. Front white paper label: 沙藥 "Medicine for *sha* [disorder]." Glass, height 7.2 cm.

The technical equipment of a doctor of traditional Chinese medicine was modest. Until the recent past, the doctor required no instruments for a diagnosis; it has only been towards the end of the twentieth century that many doctors of traditional Chinese medicine have learned to combine the technical and diagnostic procedures of Western medicine with traditional methods of treatment.

Only the wrist support, for feeling a patient's pulse, has been part of a doctor's standard equipment in China for many centuries. Pulse pillows preserved from earlier times are made of stoneware; modern wrist supports are made only of wicker or fabric.

Medical therapy also required only minor technical expenditures. Since surgery remained limited to small external operations it was never forced to develop the same kind of implements which, until the Modern period, constituted the most extensive and important part of medical technology in Europe. Due to this, only the classical methods of therapy—cupping, massage, and acupuncture—provided a reason to develop certain material techniques. The support-and-pull technique in orthopedics, the cataract depression in ophthalmology, and other small invasions, on the other hand, were performed with implements from daily life, so no specific material evidence is available.

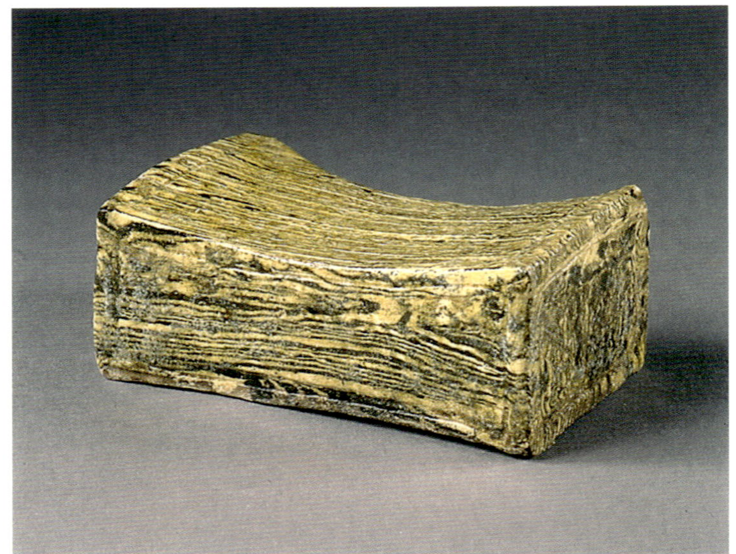

134. Wrist support for feeling the pulse. Stoneware, green glaze on white-red shard, height 5.8 cm, North China, Hunan Province, thirteenth–fourteenth centuries.

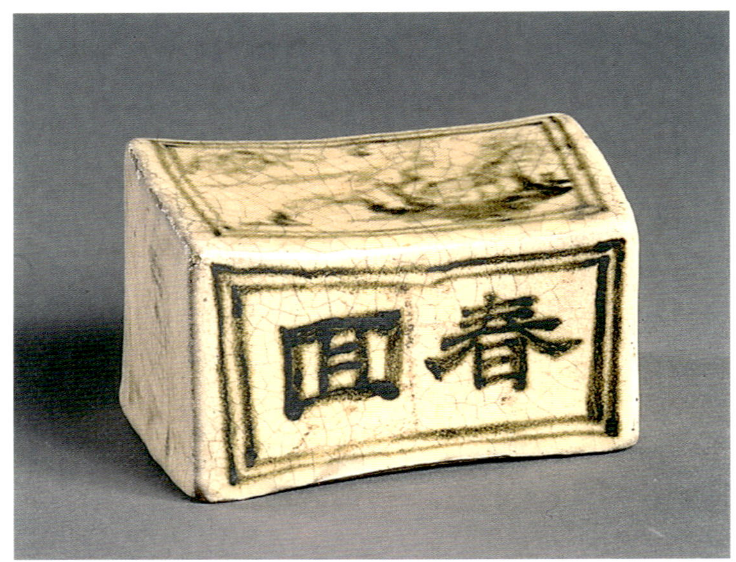

135. Wrist support for feeling the pulse decorated with a line border and writing: *huichun* 回春 (return to spring). Stoneware, dark brown underglaze on broken white crackle, height 5.4 cm.

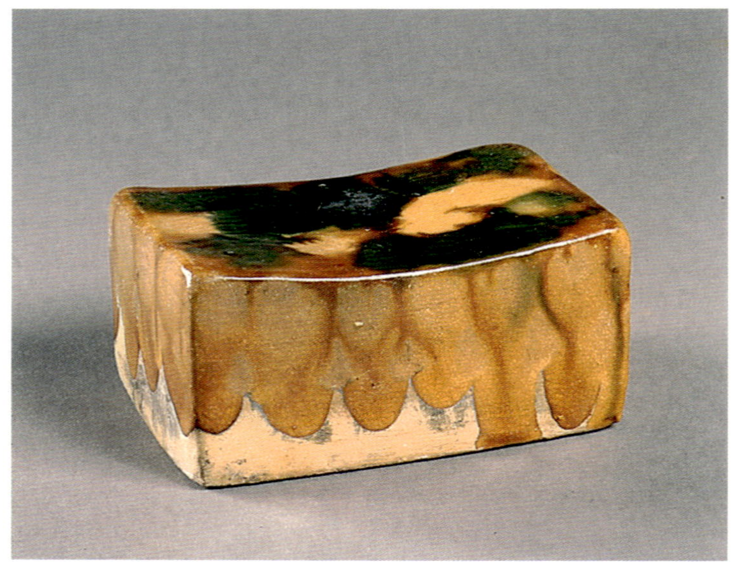

136. Wrist support for feeling the pulse. Stoneware, three-color glaze, height 5.3 cm, tenth–eleventh centuries.

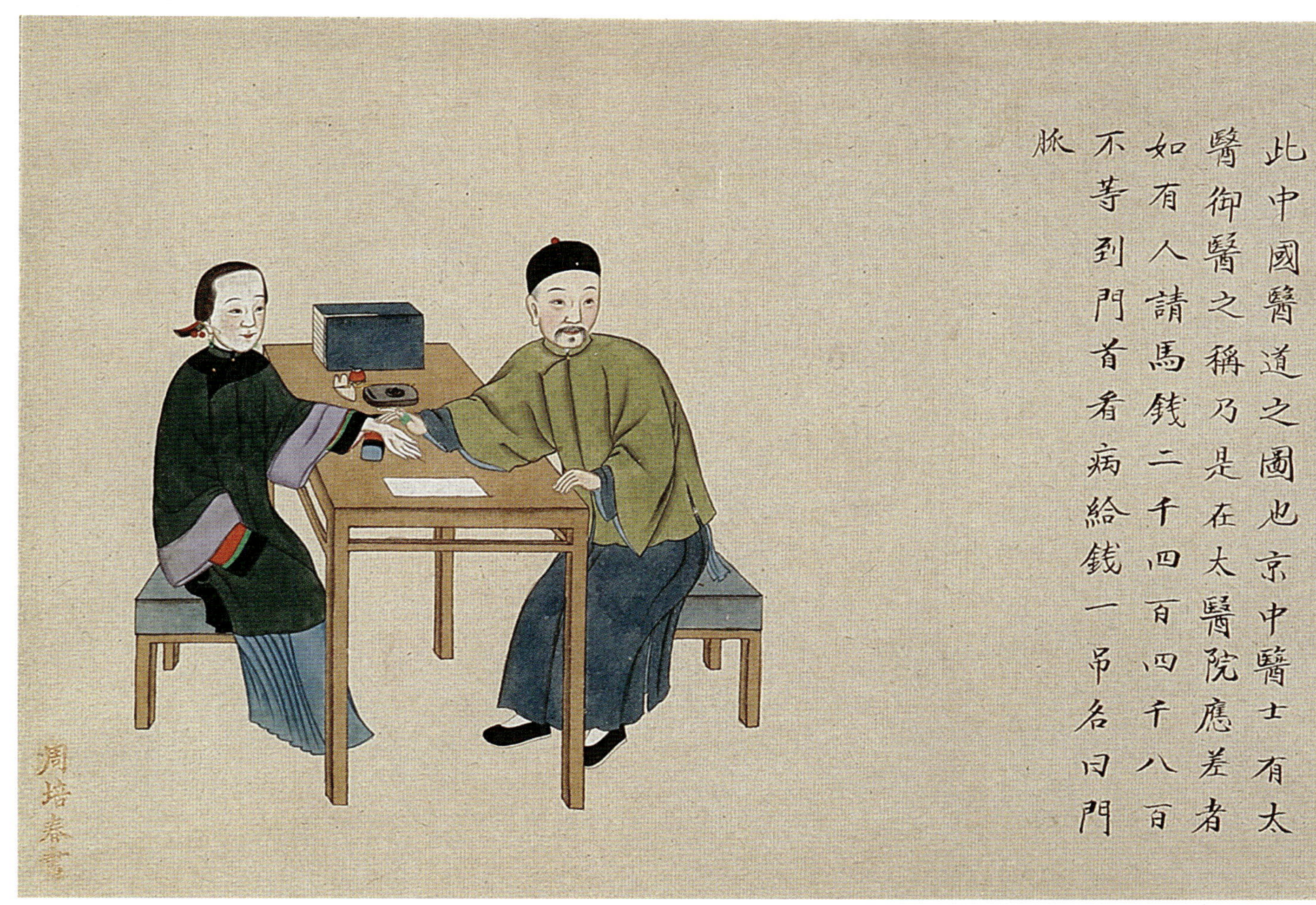

此中國醫道之圖也京中醫士有太
醫御醫之稱乃是在太醫院應差者
如有人請馬錢二千四百四千八百
不等到門首看病給錢一吊名曰門
脈

137. "This is a depiction from the practice of Chinese medicine. In the capital, there are Eminent Physicians and Imperial Physicians. They perform their activities in the Highest Bureau of Medicine. When someone asks them [to make a visit], a road fee of 2,400 to 4,800 [pieces of cash] is due. Then, when they arrive at the entrance [to the patient's house] and examine the patient there, they receive another string of cash. This is called '[to feel] the pulse [at the] door'." Gouache, second half of the nineteenth century. Museum für Völkerkunde, Berlin.

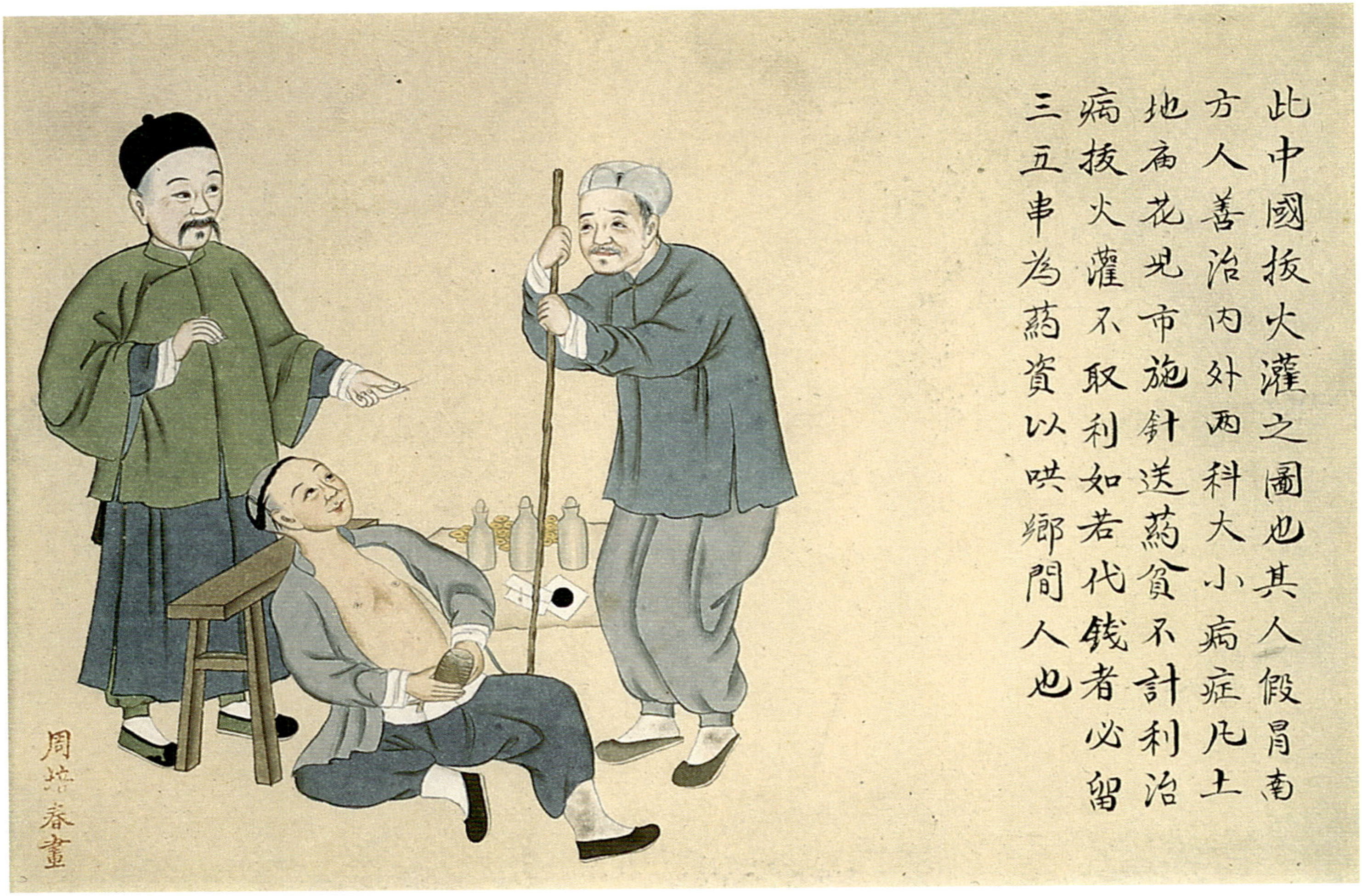

此中國拔火灌之圖也其人假冒南
方人善治內外兩科大小病症凡土
地庙兒市施針送葯資不計利治
病拔火灌不取利如若代錢者必留
三五串為葯資以哄鄉間人也

138. "This illustration depicts cupping by fire in China. The people are pretending to be from the South and to be capable of curing any major or minor illness from internal as well as external medicine. In local temples and markets, they use needles and dispense medicine. In the case of poor [patients], they do not look for a profit. When they treat an illness by way of fire cupping, they do not make a profit. When [the patients] carry money on them, however, they keep three or five coins as a fee for the medicine. In this way, they deceive the country people." Gouache, second half of the nineteenth century. Museum für Völkerkunde, Berlin.

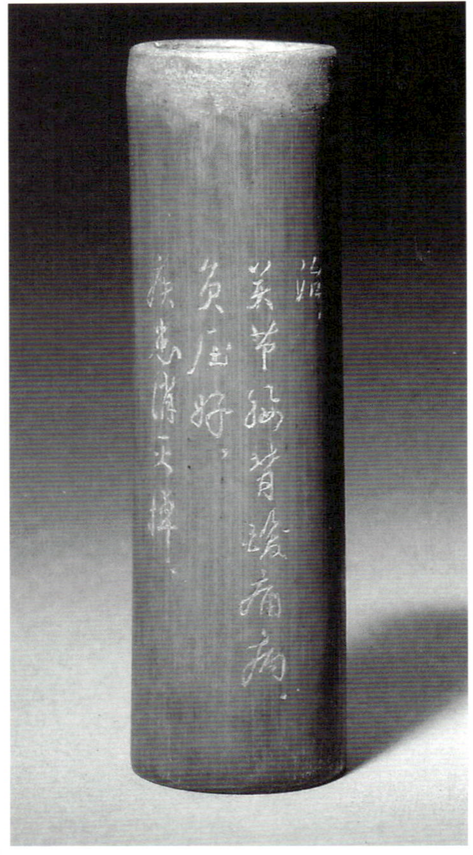

139. Cupping instrument with carved writing: "For the treatment of painful illnesses in the joints and lower back. Press firmly, and the problem will disappear completely." Bamboo, length 13.3 cm.

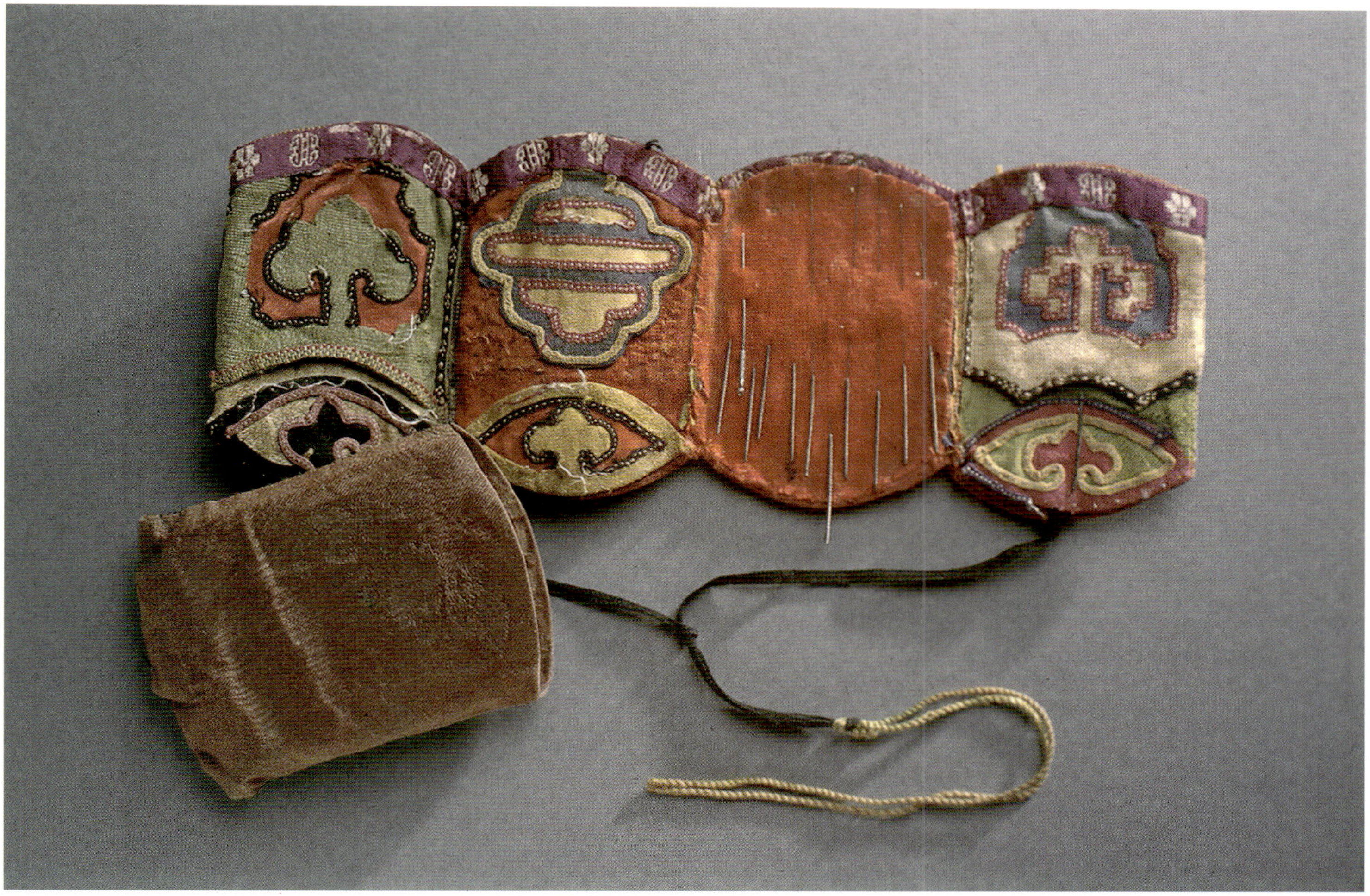

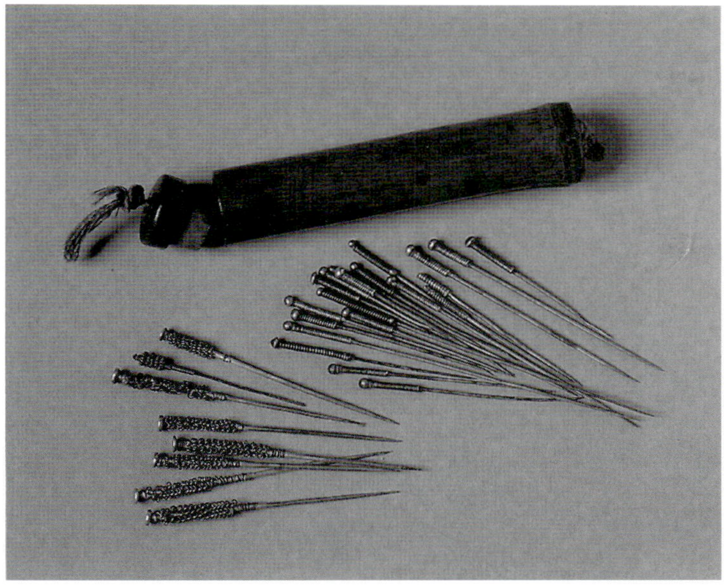

140. Acupuncture needles. Silver, on a pin-cushion with cloth embroidery and with a silk case woven with bat symbol, early twentieth century.

141. Acupuncture needles. Silver, bamboo container, length 9.5 cm, early twentieth century.

142. Acupuncture needles in embroidered case. Mid-twentieth century.

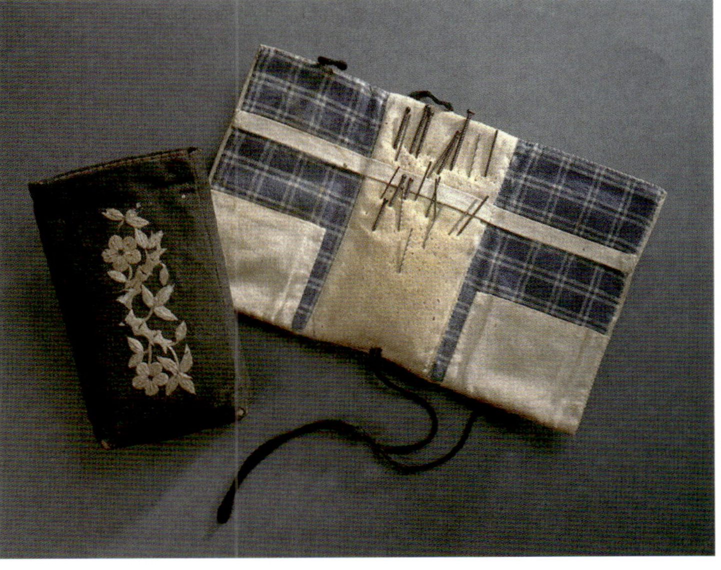

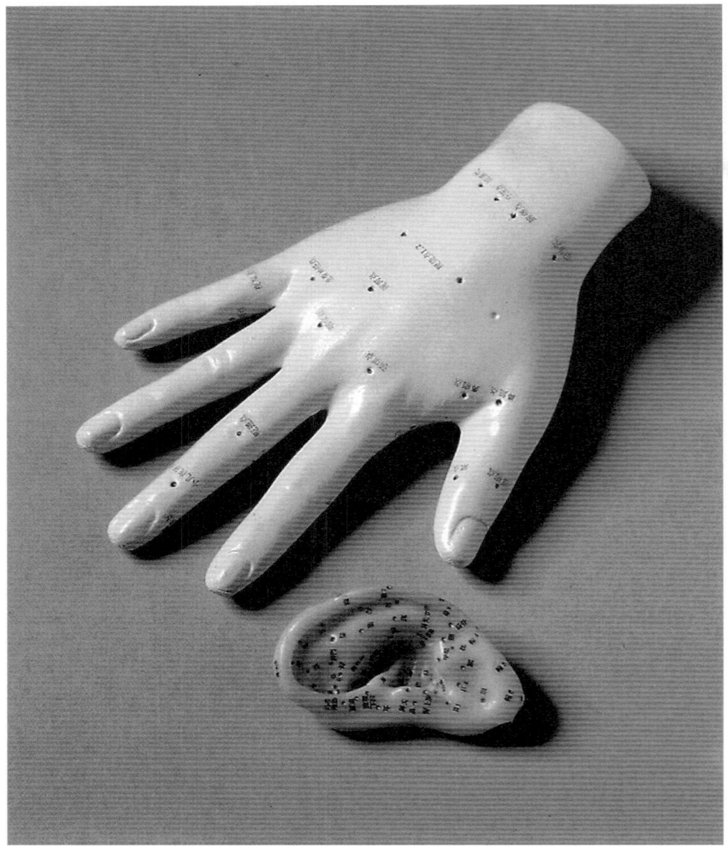

143. Acupuncture models made of plastic. (a) Ear model with locations and names of the insertion points. (b) Hand model with locations and names of the insertion points.

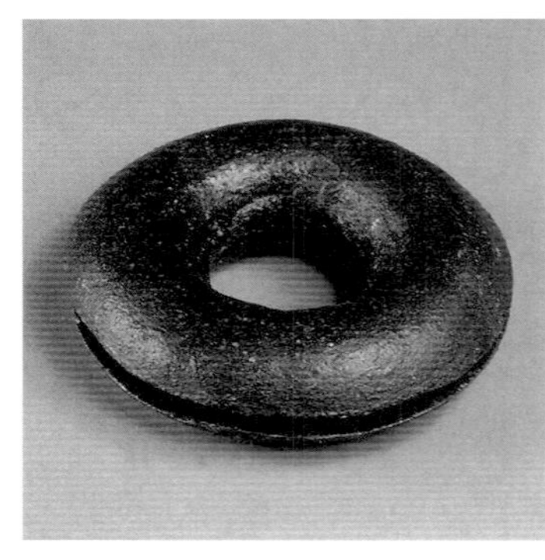

144. "Tiger sting," an itinerant doctor's rattle. Iron, circumference 10.5 cm.

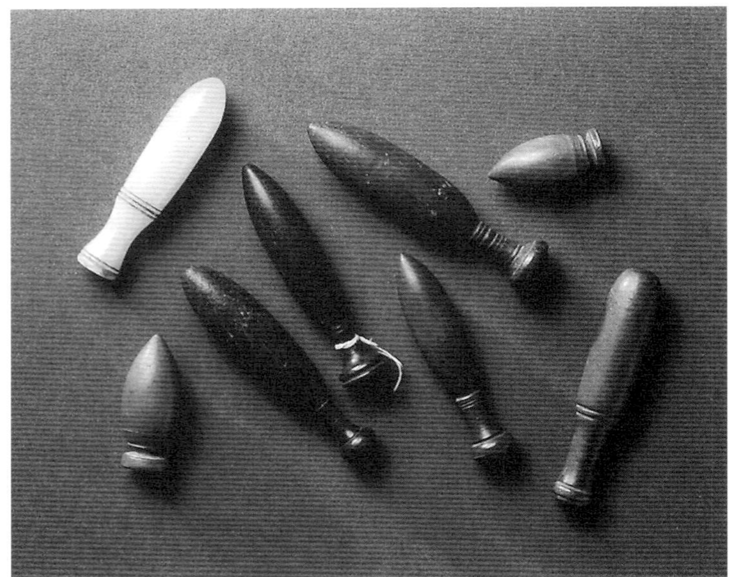

145

145. Eight acupressure sticks with partially detachable handle to be used as medicine container. Turned wood or soapstone, length 4.2–10.4 cm.

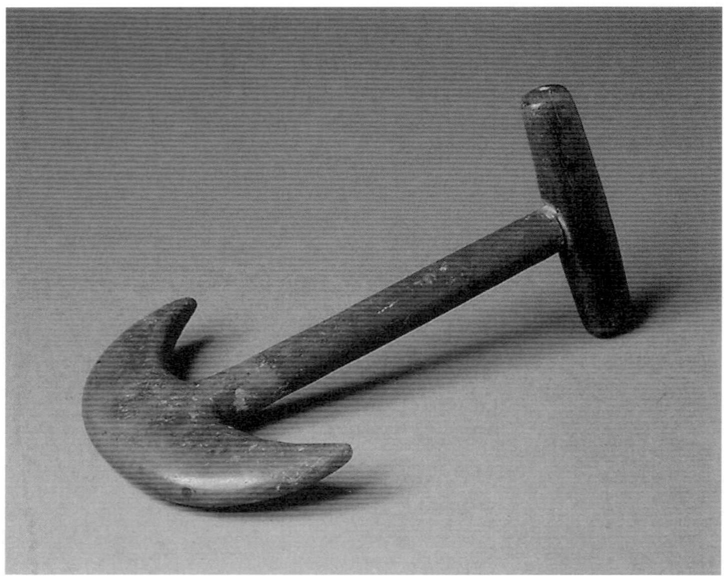

146

146. "Massage anchor." An instrument for abdominal massage. Wood, length 16 cm.

147. Different massage instruments. (a) Conical, jade, length 8.7 cm. (b) Cylindrical, jade, length 8.7 cm. (c) Turned, wood, length 17.8 cm. (d) Roller, wood, length 18 cm.

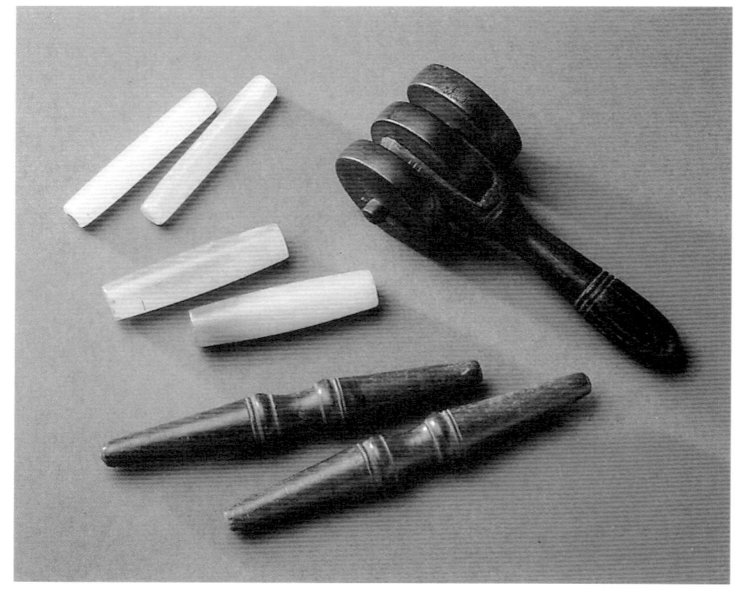

147

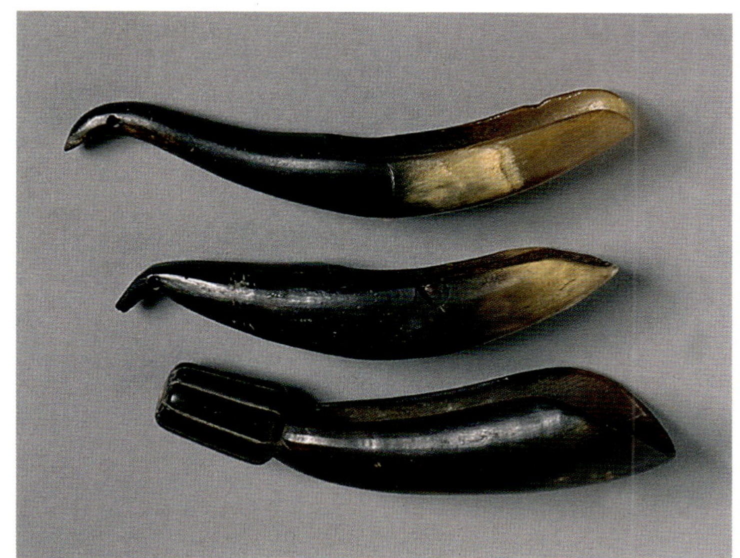

148. Three spoons for dispensing powder. Horn, length 13.2–13.9 cm.

149. Seven instruments for blowing in powder. Brass, length (including extended nozzle) 13–21.7 cm.

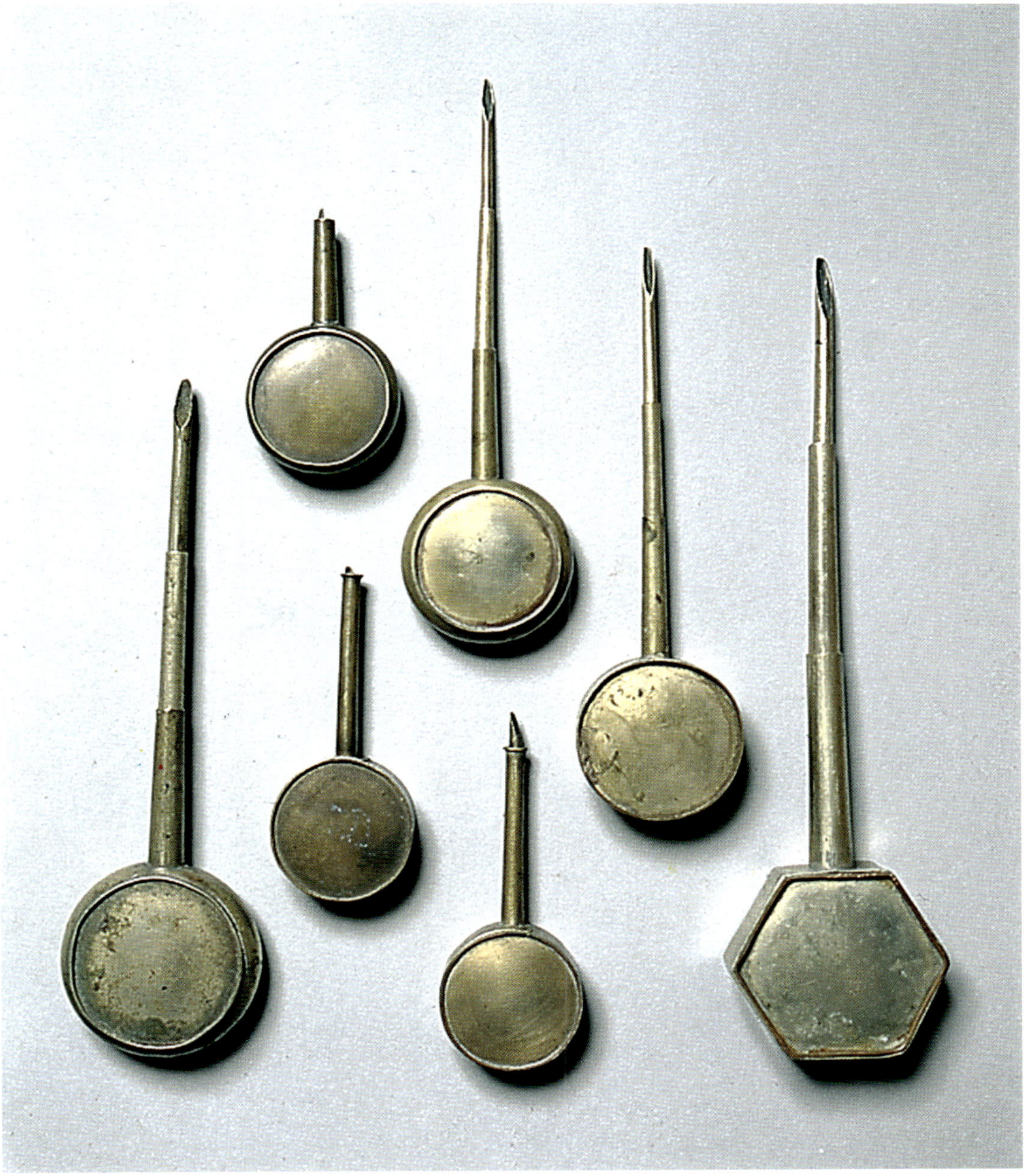

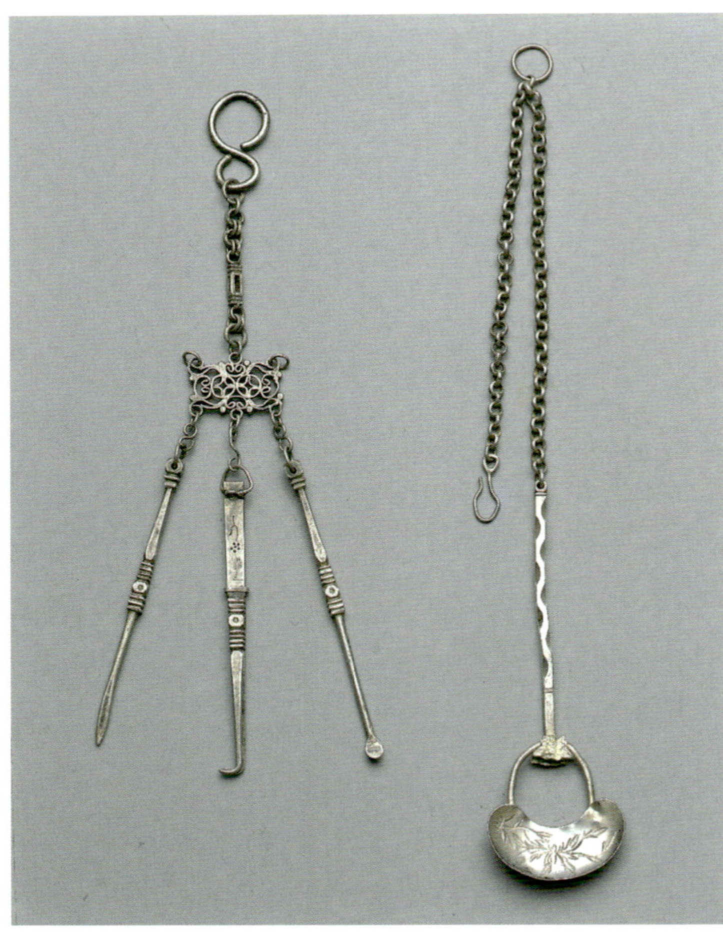



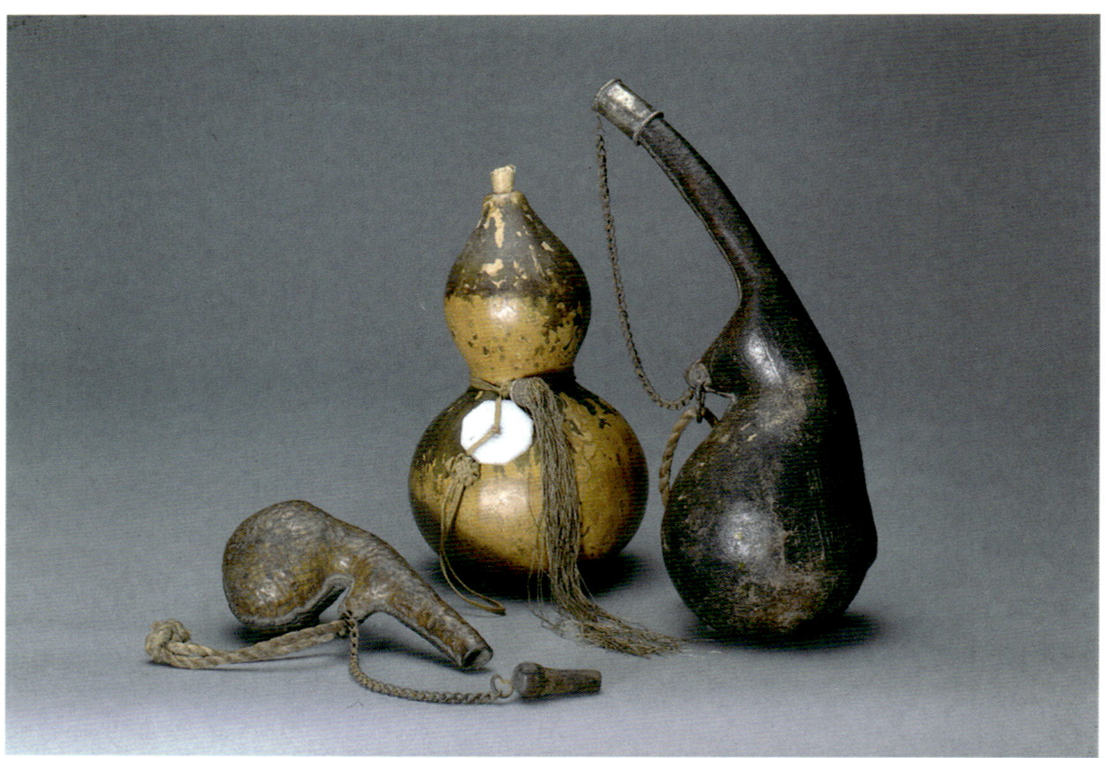

151. Left and right: leather medicine containers in the shapes of
gourds from the possessions of an
itinerant doctor. Left: Wooden
plug, length 17 cm. Right: Silver
stopper, length 28 cm. Center:
Dried squash bottle, residual
gold-plating, paper plug, frosted
glass pendant in trigram shape,
silk tassel, height 21.5 cm.

Beginning in the third century B.C.E., a form of medicine developed in China which attempted to influence human health and illness exclusively in the context of natural law. However, even now the older concept that there are magical and religious connections to illness and healing has not been completely refuted. Amulets and invocations that exorcise malevolent demons and prayers that seek the assistance of deities have been widespread at all times, and not only outside of the formally educated classes.

The Tang period physician Sun Simiao, in particular, has been worshipped as a medicine god since approximately the thirteenth century. In response to the favor of being brought back to the human world by believers as a wooden sculpture, he was expected to fulfill the requests of donors. Two other ancestors of Chinese medicine, Shennong, the legendary founder of Chinese pharmaceutics and Damo (Bodhidharma), the patron saint of chiropractics, have survived until the present only in the pantheon of Japanese religion.

Although the Buddha—similar to Christ—is referred to as the savior of all creatures and as the "physician" of humanity, in Chinese art he has never been used to address the tension between suffering and healing or to heighten it metaphorically. Thus, illustrations of this type, related to a medical content, are, in Chinese art, mostly coincidental appearances in non-medical contexts.

It is not known when portraits of eminent figures from the history of Chinese medicine and pharmaceutics first appeared, since older paintings and sculptures of this kind are not documented. It appears that the cultural need to artistically represent figures such as the great materia medica author Li Shizhen has arisen only in the recent past—heroic depiction of the distinguished representatives of past culture is supposed to increase pride and respect for China's own history in light of the prevalence of Western lifestyles.

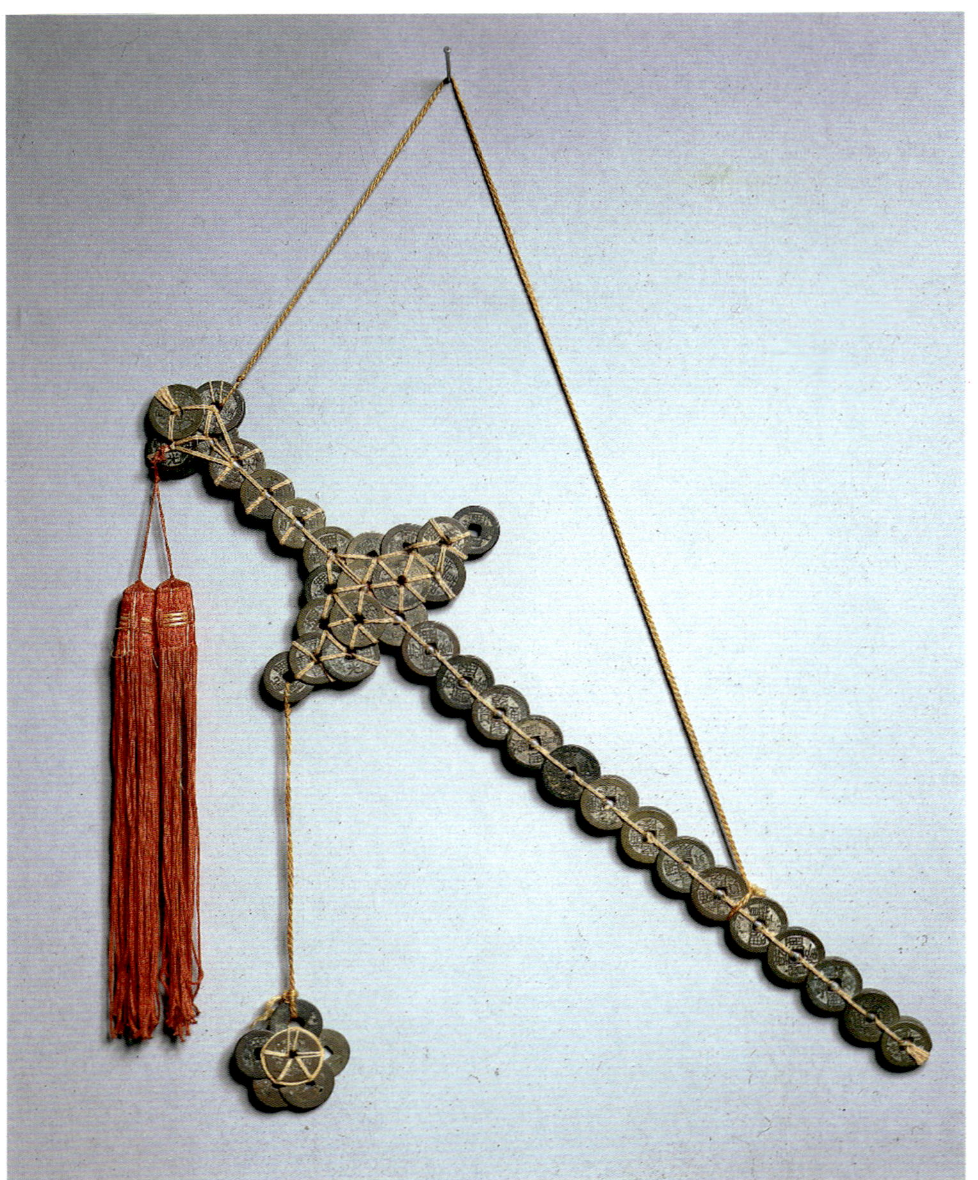



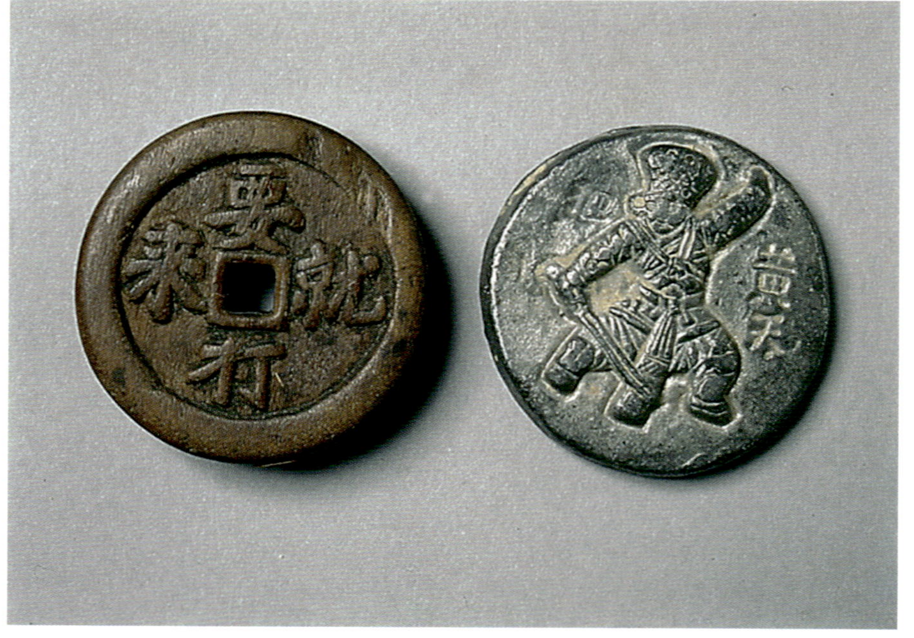

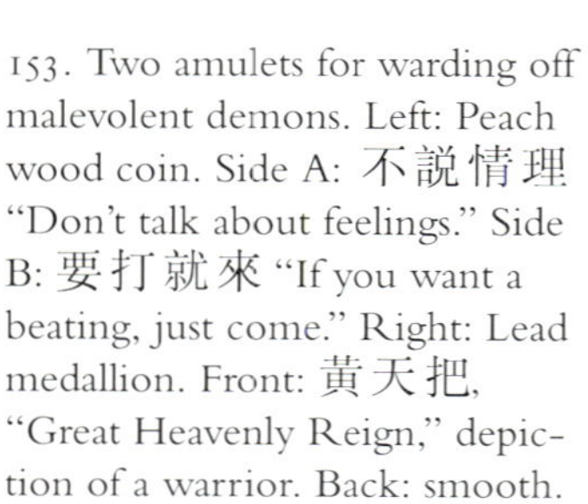

153. Two amulets for warding off
malevolent demons. Left: Peach
wood coin. Side A: 不説情理
"Don't talk about feelings." Side
B: 要打就來 "If you want a
beating, just come." Right: Lead
medallion. Front: 黄天把,
"Great Heavenly Reign," depiction of a warrior. Back: smooth.

200

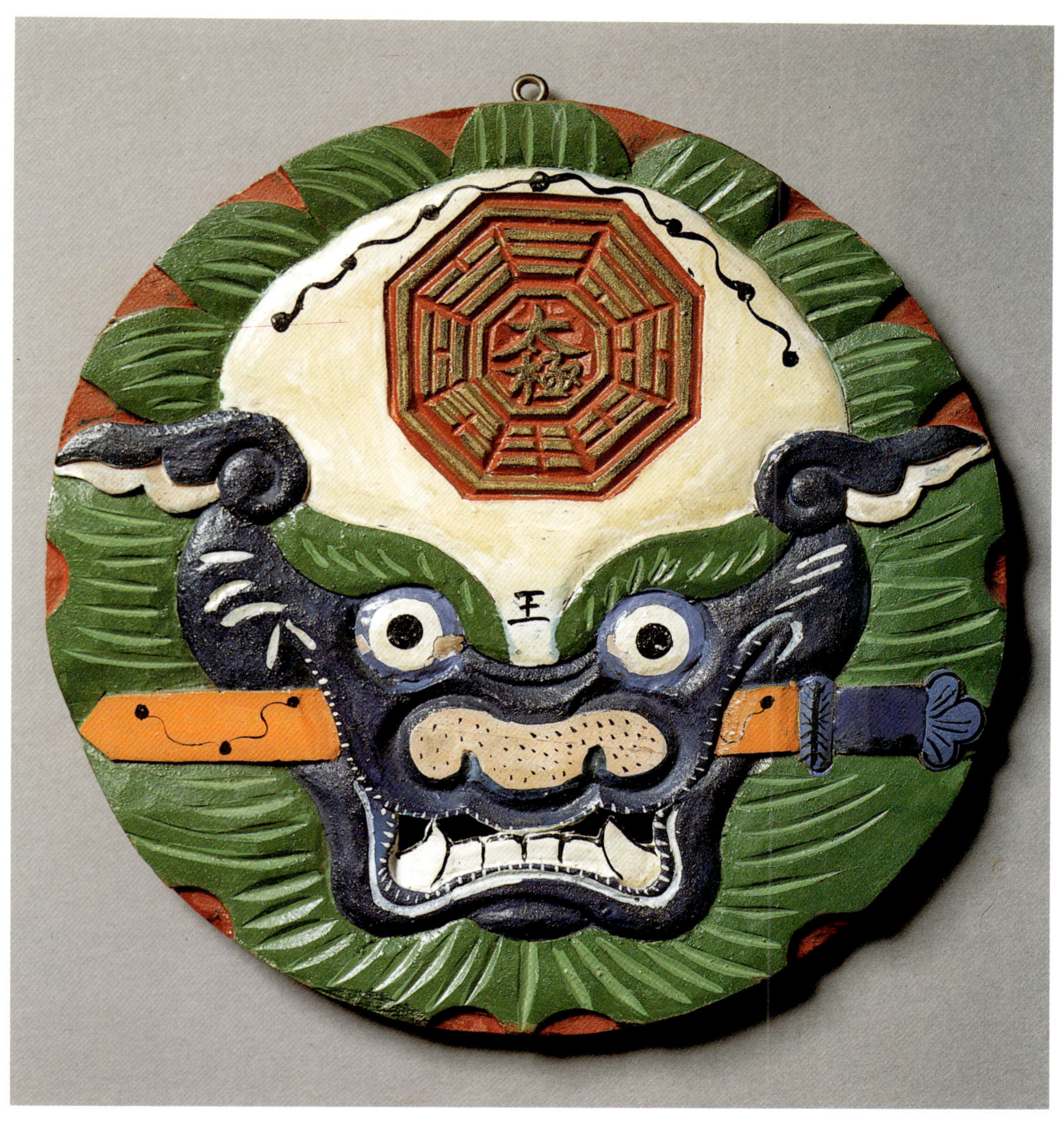

154. Traditional door amulet for
warding off malevolent demons in
the shape of a demon's head with
insignia of power: a sword, the
character "king" between the
eyes, the eight trigrams of the
*Yijing* with the Taiji characters on
the forehead, and the Seven Star
constellation on top of the head.
Multicolored wood relief,
diameter 21 cm, Hong Kong
1975.

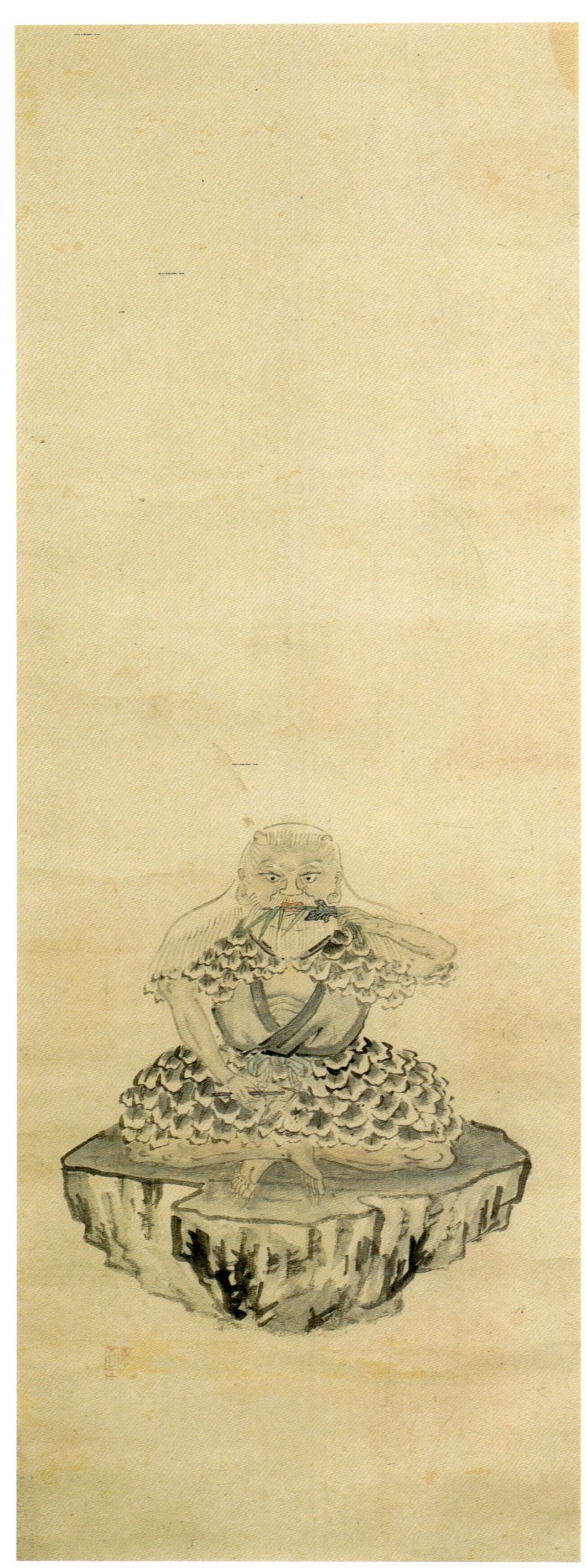

155. Shennong 神農, legendary
ancestor of Chinese pharmaceutics. Colored ink on paper,
163 x 50 cm, Japan.

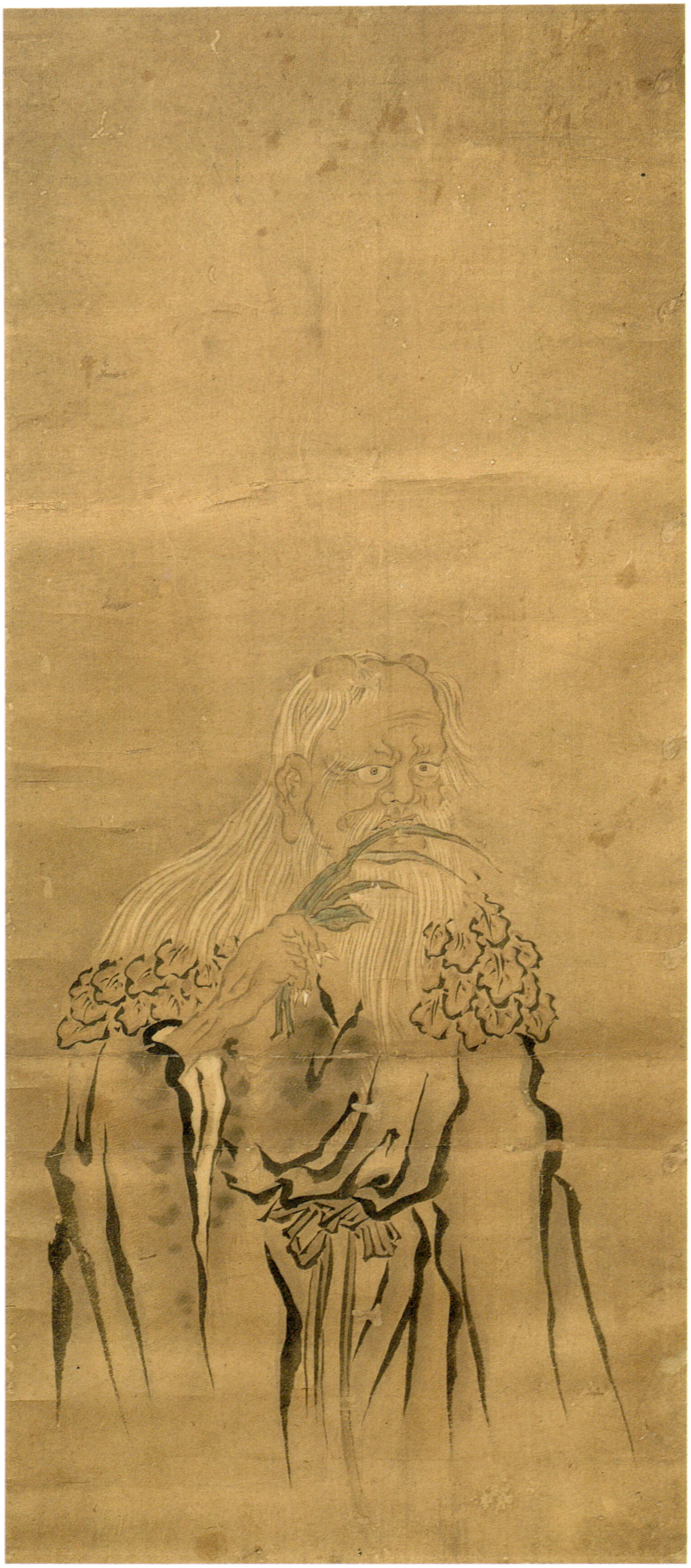

156. Shennong 神農, legendary
ancestor of Chinese pharmaceutics. Colored ink on paper,
60 x 25.5 cm, Japan.

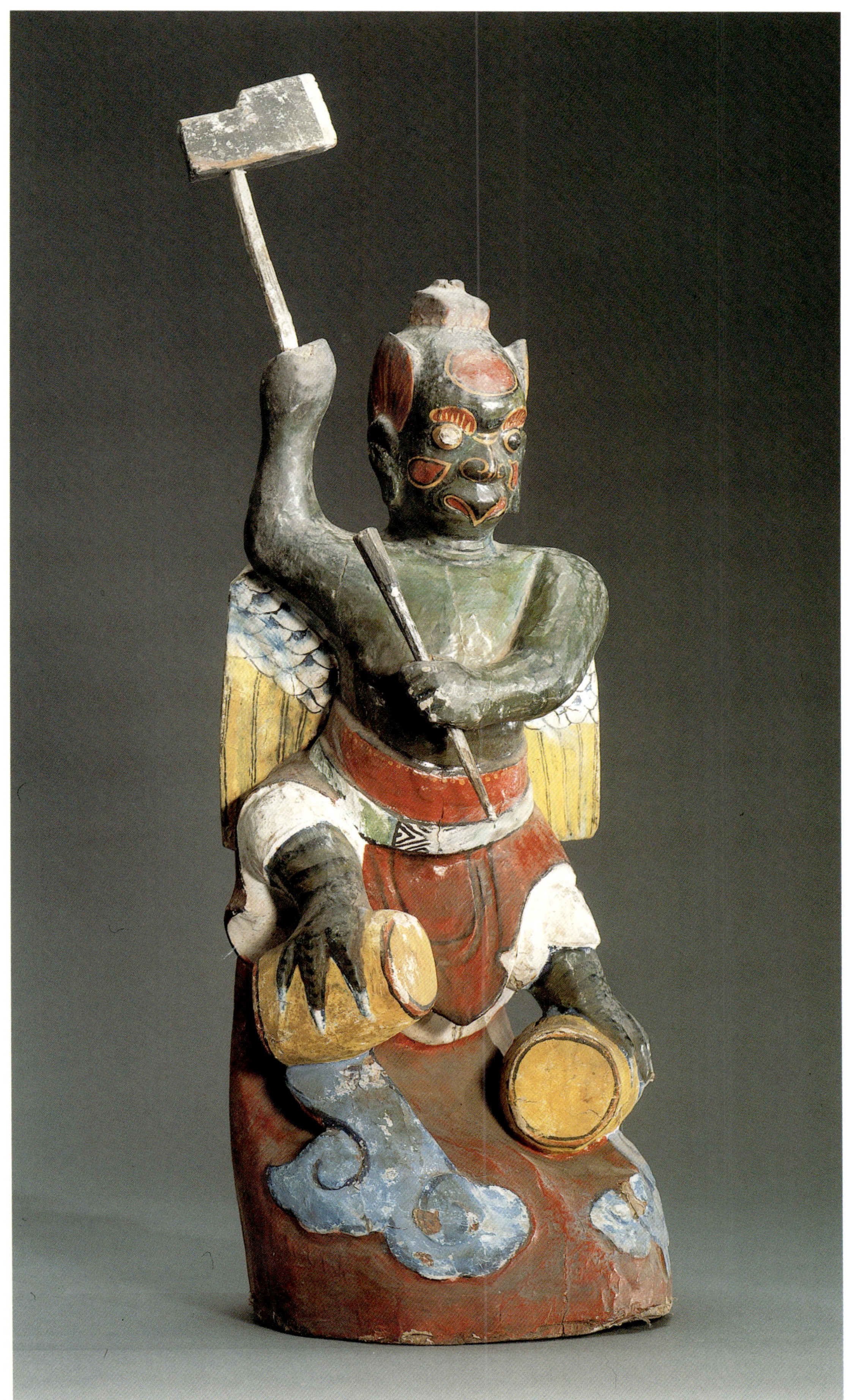

157. Leigong 雷公, "The Lord of Thunder." The thunder spirit of ancient Chinese mythology; a preferred ally in the protection from malevolent demons, and one of the dialogue partners of Huang Di in the medical classic *Huang Di Neijing.* Also the namesake of the standard text of pharmaceutical technology, the *Leigong paozhi lun* 雷公炮炙論 (*Leigong on the Preparation [of drugs] with Heat*), by Lei Xiao (fifth century) Wooden sculpture with applied color, height 64 cm, Hunan Province, China.

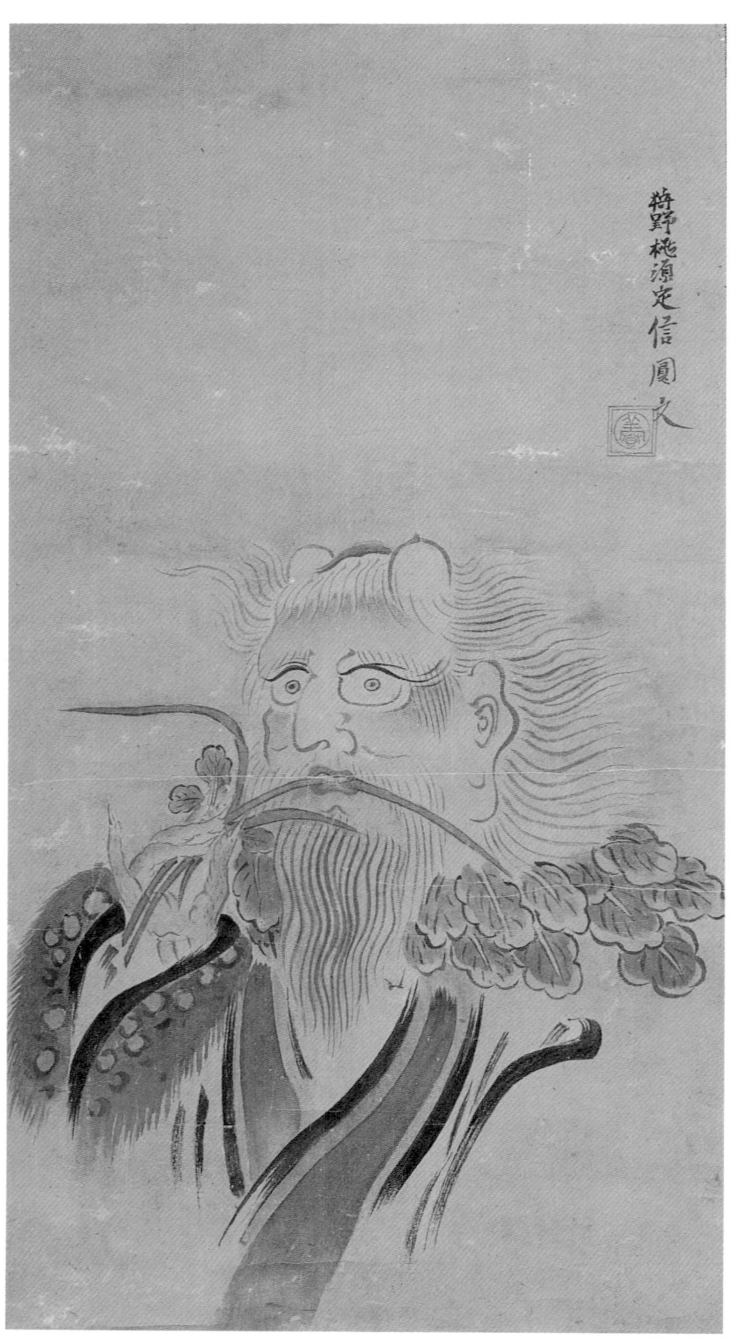

158. Shennong 神農, legendary ancestor of Chinese pharmaceutics. Signature: Kanoo Sadanobu 狩野定信 1722 (Ryuuhaku 1666–1722). Colored ink on paper, 164 x 59 cm, Japan, eighteenth century.

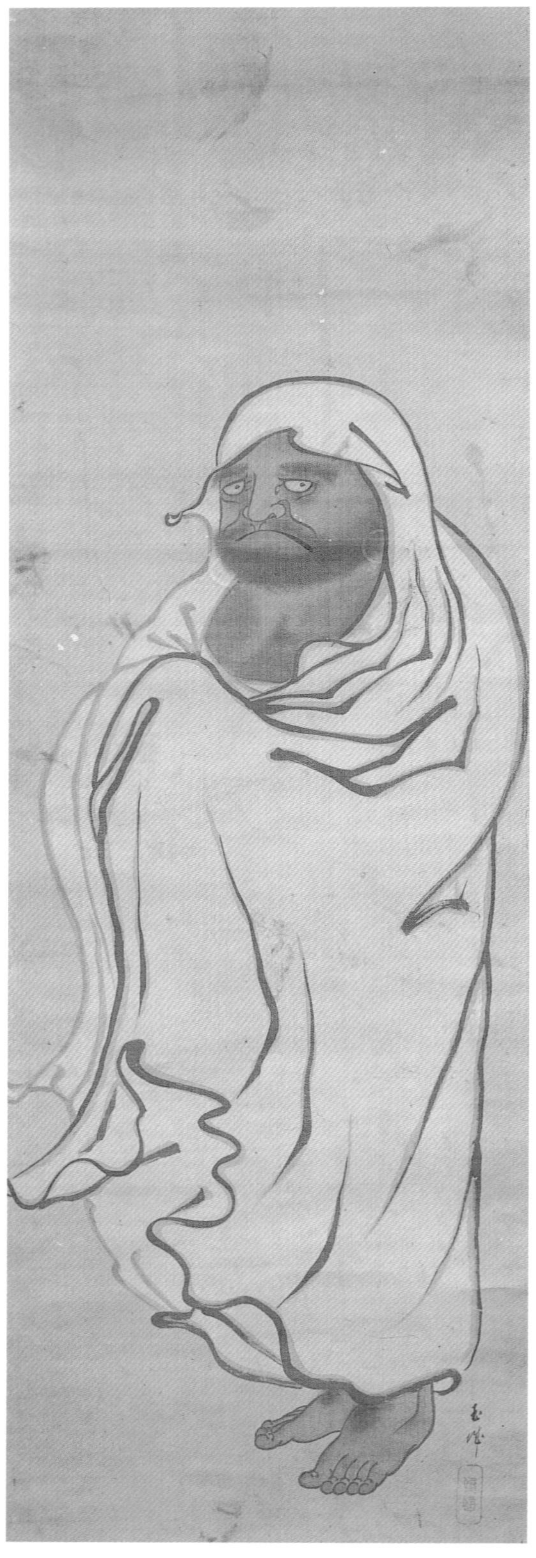

159. *Bodhidharma.* Damo 達摩 (ca. 535). Indian patriarch of Buddhism who arrived in China ca. 520. Founder of a tradition of fighting and movement techniques, and grandfather of Chinese chiropractics. Colored ink on silk, 110.5 x 34.5 cm, Japan.

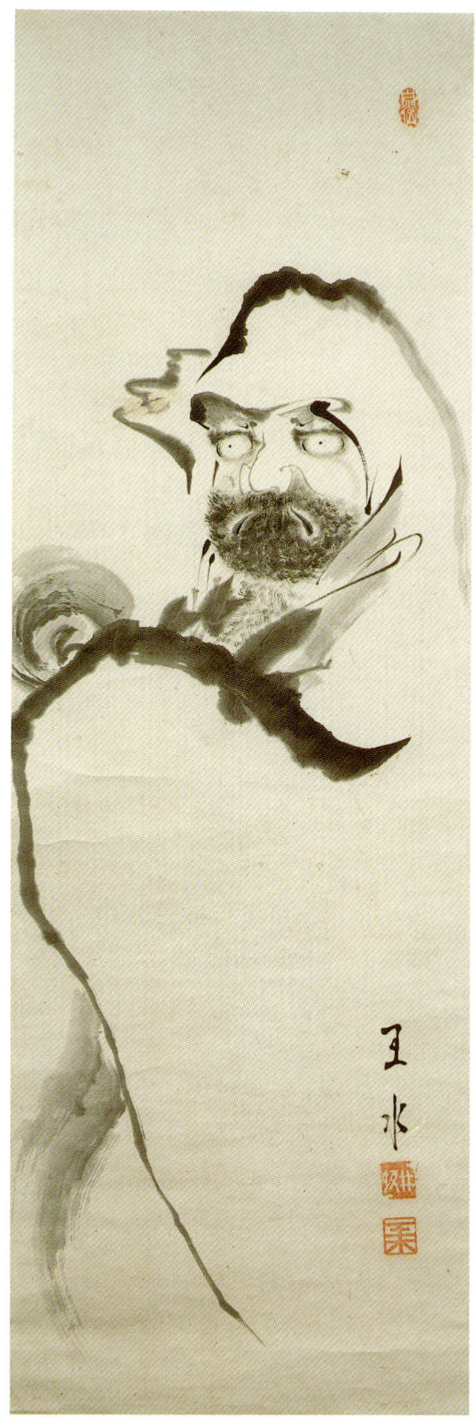

160. *Bodhidharma*. Ink on paper,
124 x 39.5 cm, Japan.

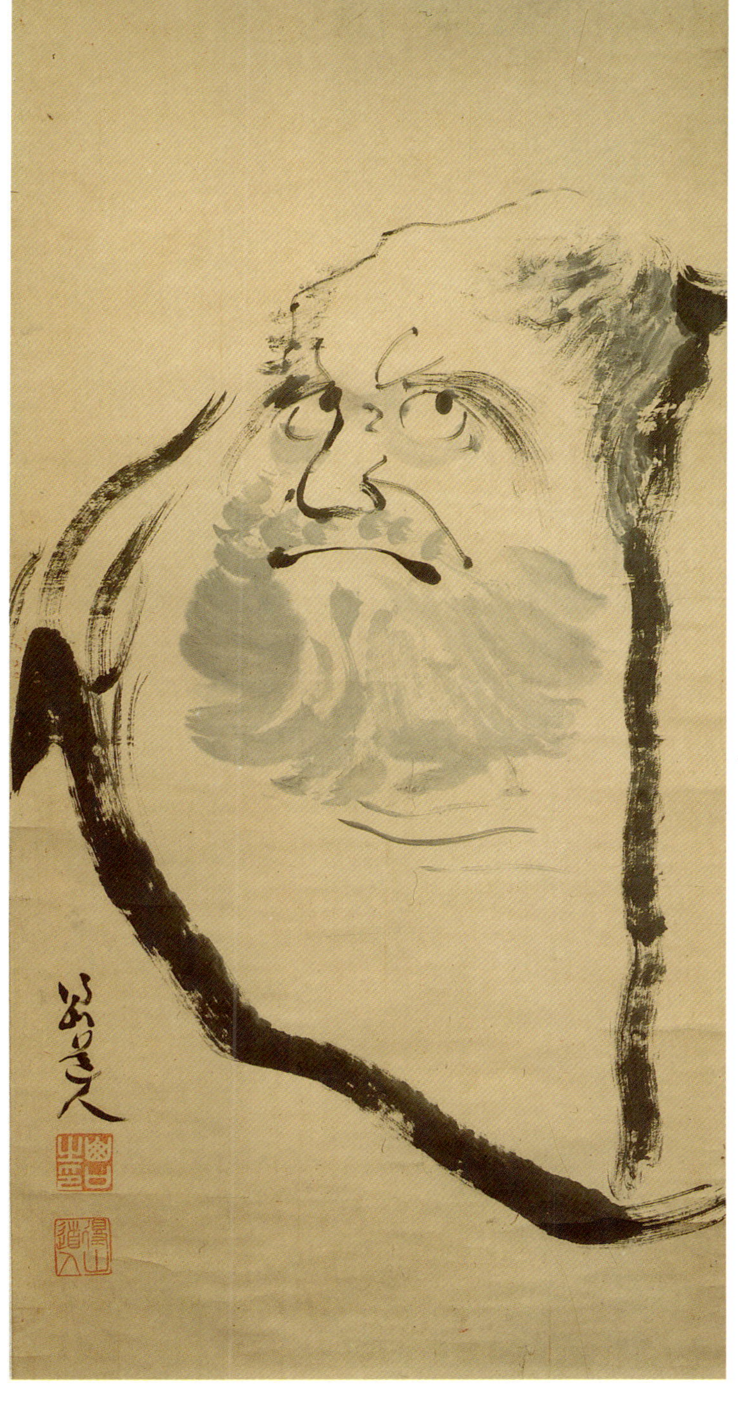

161. *Bodhidharma*. Ink on paper,
135 x 68.2 cm, Japan.

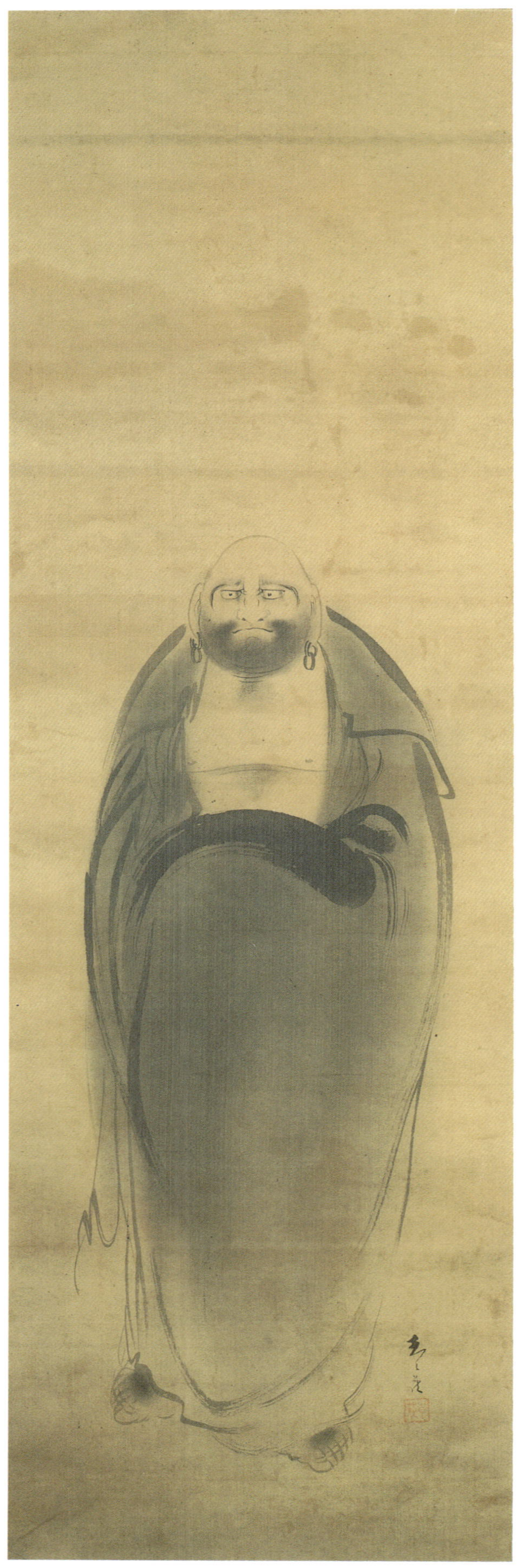

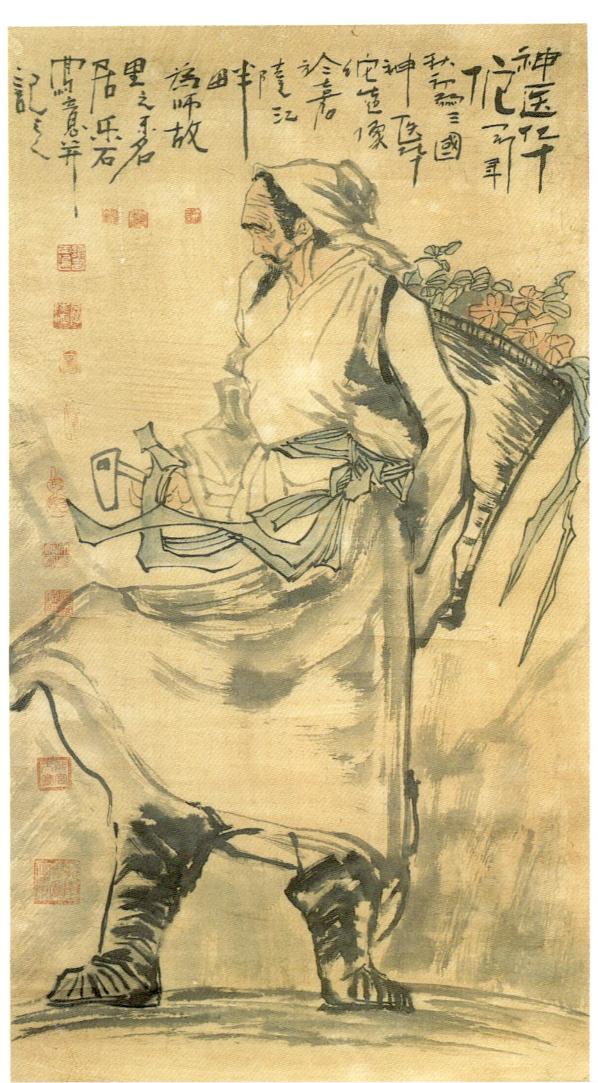

162. *Bodhidharma.* Colored ink
on silk, 102.5 x 34 cm, Japan.

163. Hua Tuo 華佗 (d. 208).
Chengdu, Sichuan. Heroic representation of the late-Han doctor
as an herb gatherer. Text: "The
divine doctor Hua Tuo. In the
year of [ ], in the first month of
fall, a likeness of the divine doctor
Hua Tuo from the time of the
Three Kingdoms was constructed
on the shores of the river Jialing,
so that he might serve as a teacher
for his homeland. By Ju Leshi,
[adult name] Zhile, roughly
drawn and provided with this
inscription." Original drawing,
95.5 x 50 cm, ca. 1980.

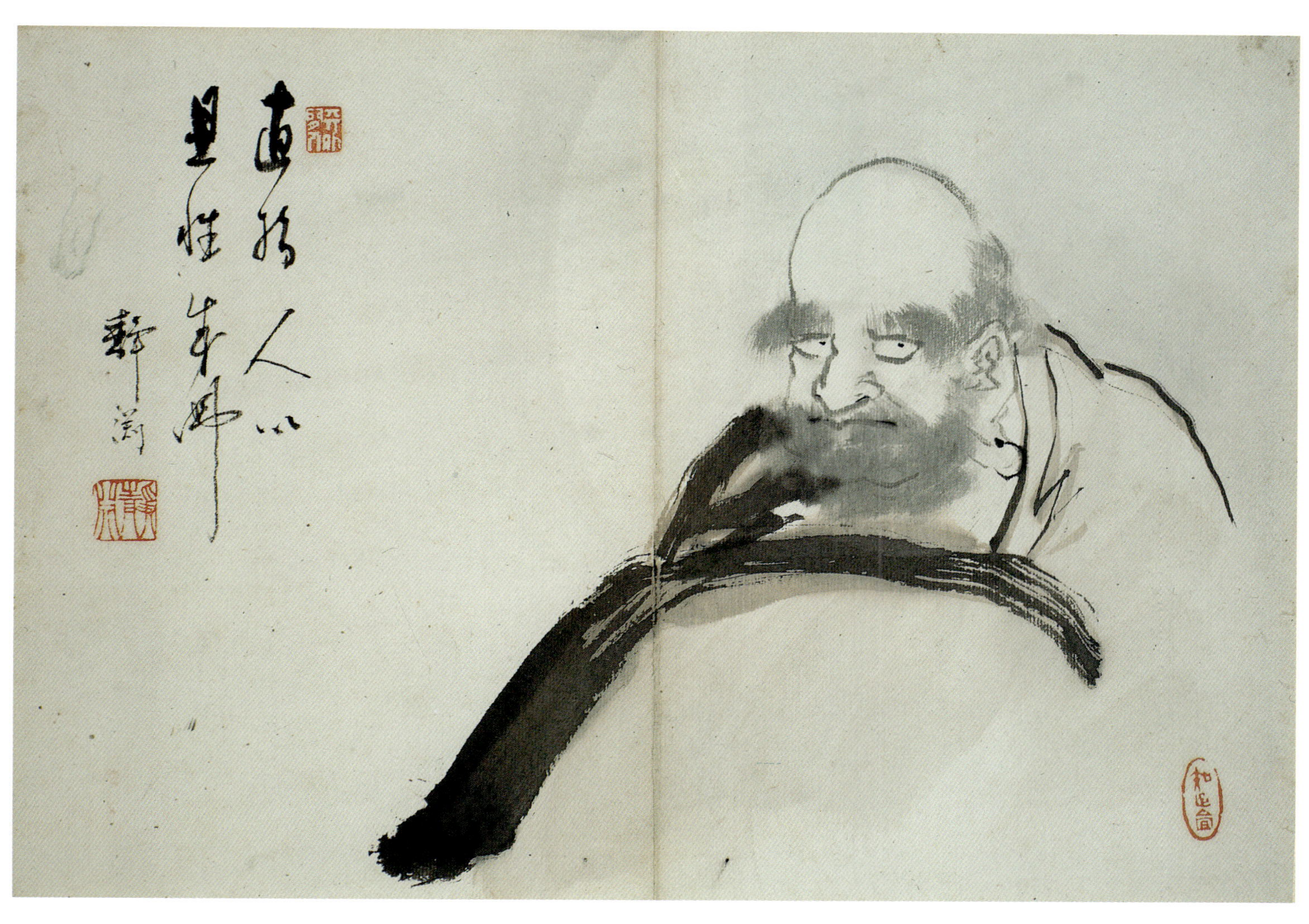

164. Shennong 神農,
*Bodhidharma*. Leporello with
guest signatures. Ink on paper,
21 x 29.5 cm, Japan.

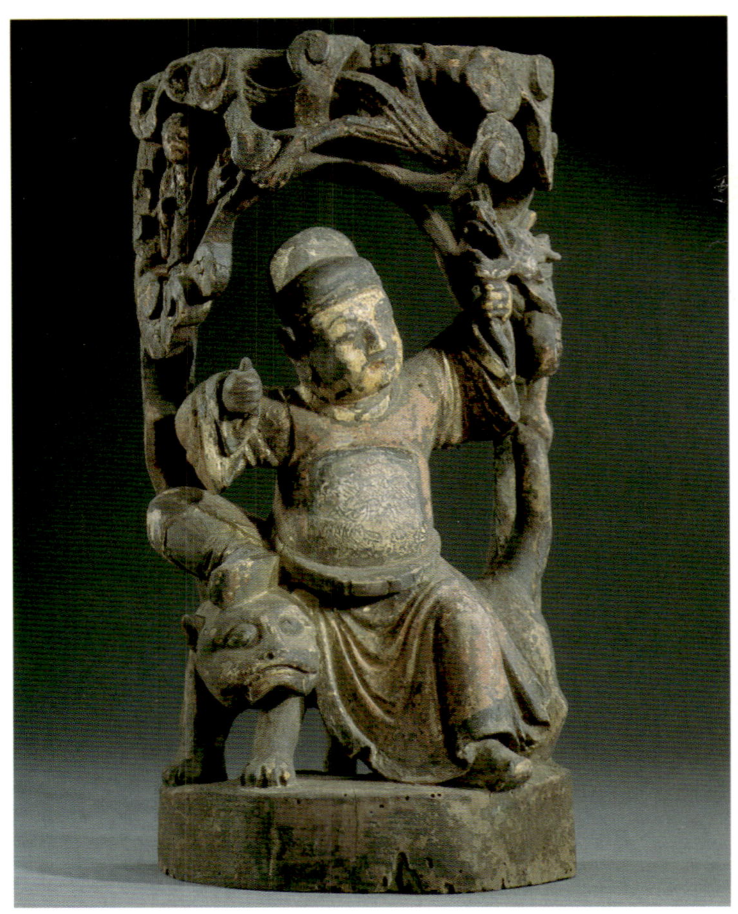

165

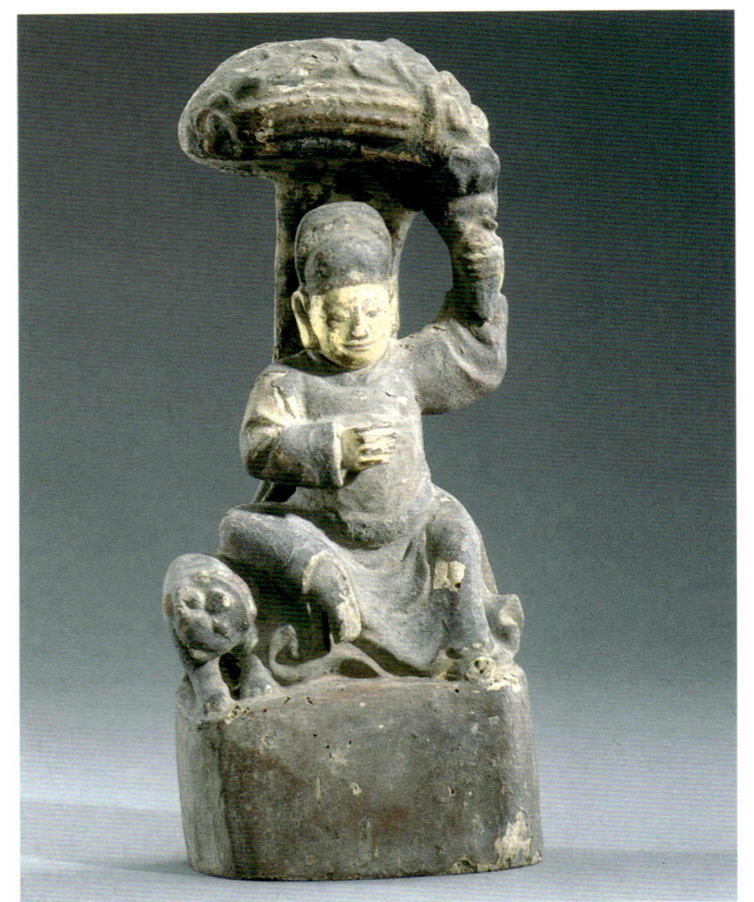

166

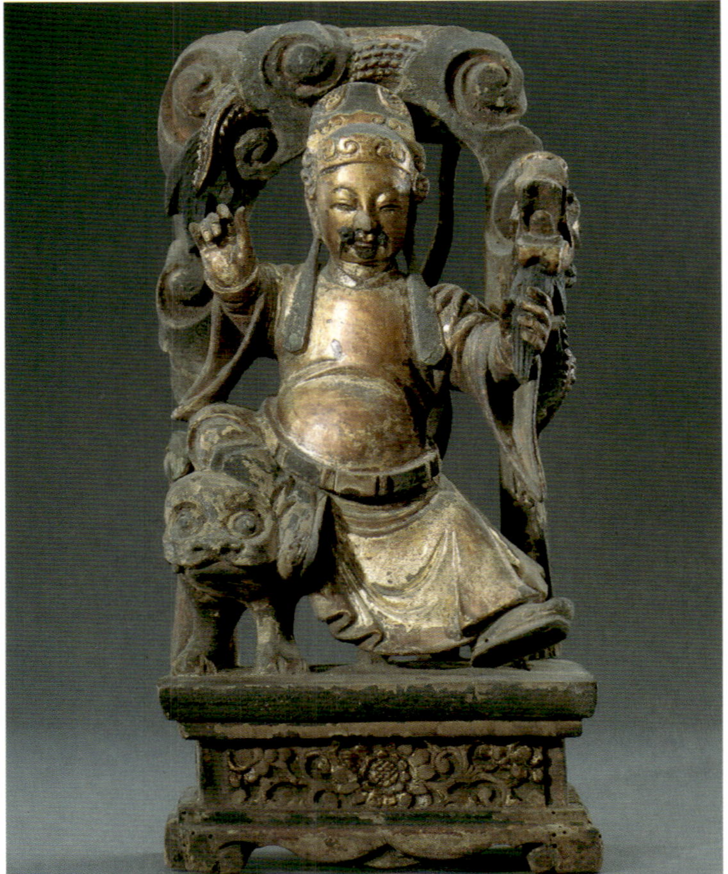

167

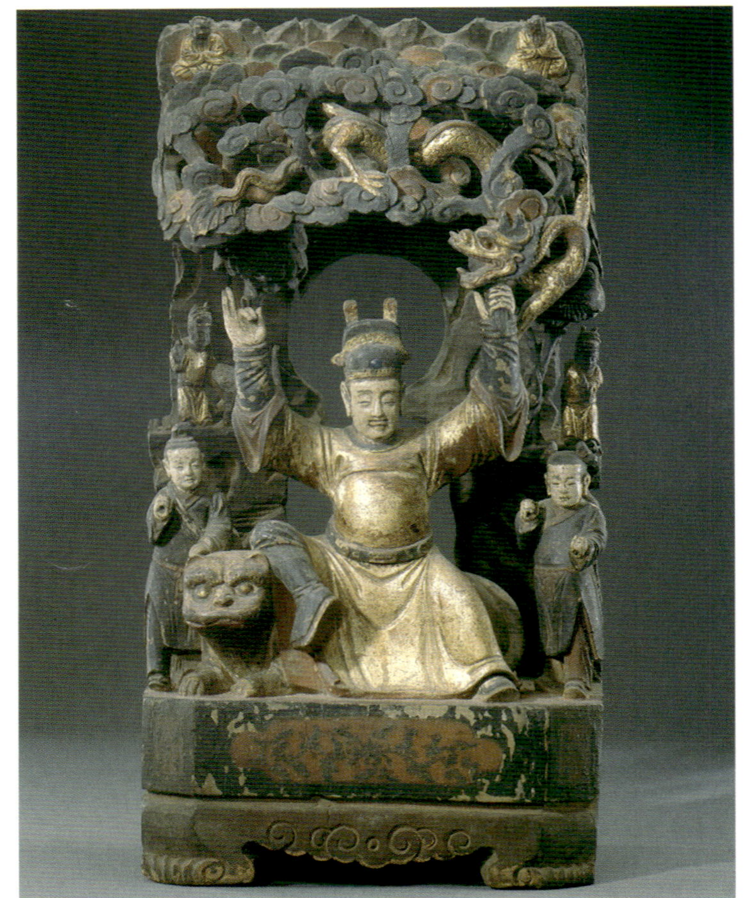

168

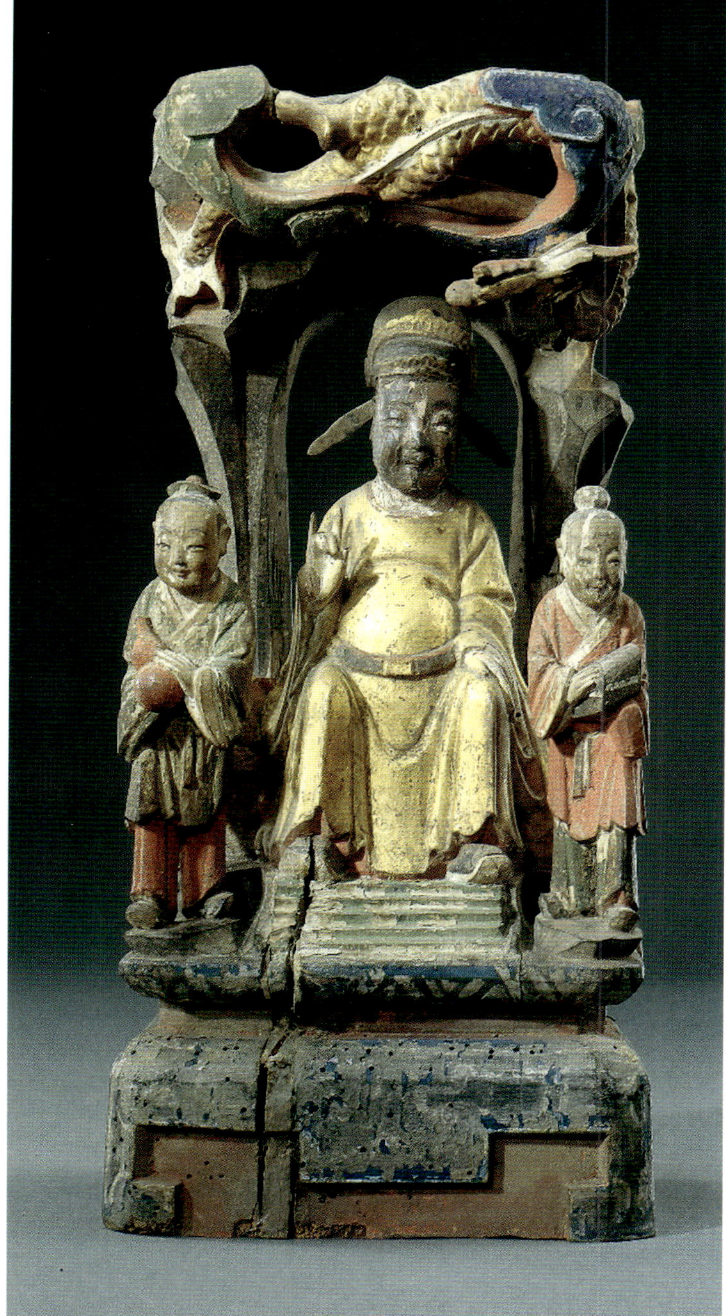

165. The Medicine God Sun Simiao seated on the tiger. He is holding the beard of the dragon in his left hand, and over his right shoulder is a small figure (in the interlaced ornament). Wooden figure with applied color, height 40 cm. Hunan, China, nineteenth century.

166. The Medicine God Sun Simiao with the tiger to his right and the stylized dragon as canopy. Wooden figure with applied color, height 30 cm, Hunan, China, nineteenth century.

167. The Medicine God Sun Simiao seated on the tiger. He is holding the beard of the dragon in his left hand. Wooden figure with applied gold-bronze and color, height 39 cm, Hunan, China, nineteenth century.

168. The Medicine God Sun Simiao seated on the tiger. He is holding the beard of the dragon in his left hand. There are assistants to his right and left sides. Above them, on the left: Sun Simiao's encounter with the tiger. On the right: Another figure of Sun Simiao. In the canopy: two small figures, possibly Huang Di (left) and Shennong (right). Wooden figure with applied gold-bronze and color, height 56 cm, Hunan, China, nineteenth century.

169. The Medicine God Sun Simiao with the tiger (behind the left figure) and the dragon as canopy. Two assistants with gourd (left), book (right). Wooden figure with applied color, height 39 cm, Hunan, China, nineteenth century.

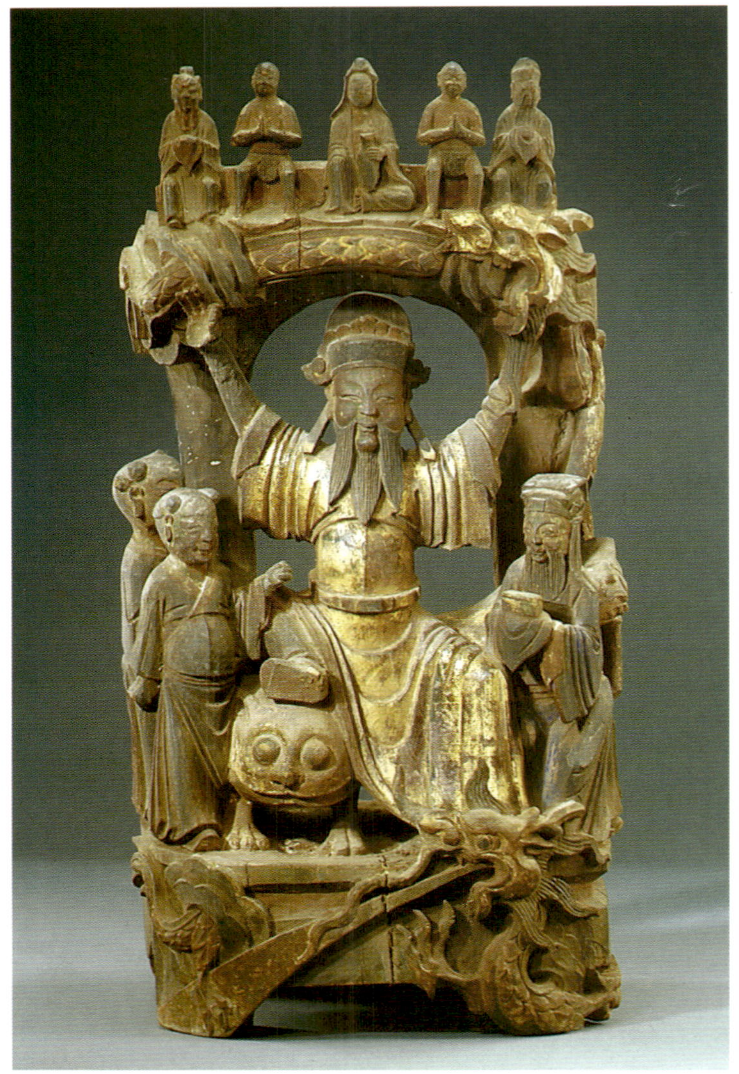

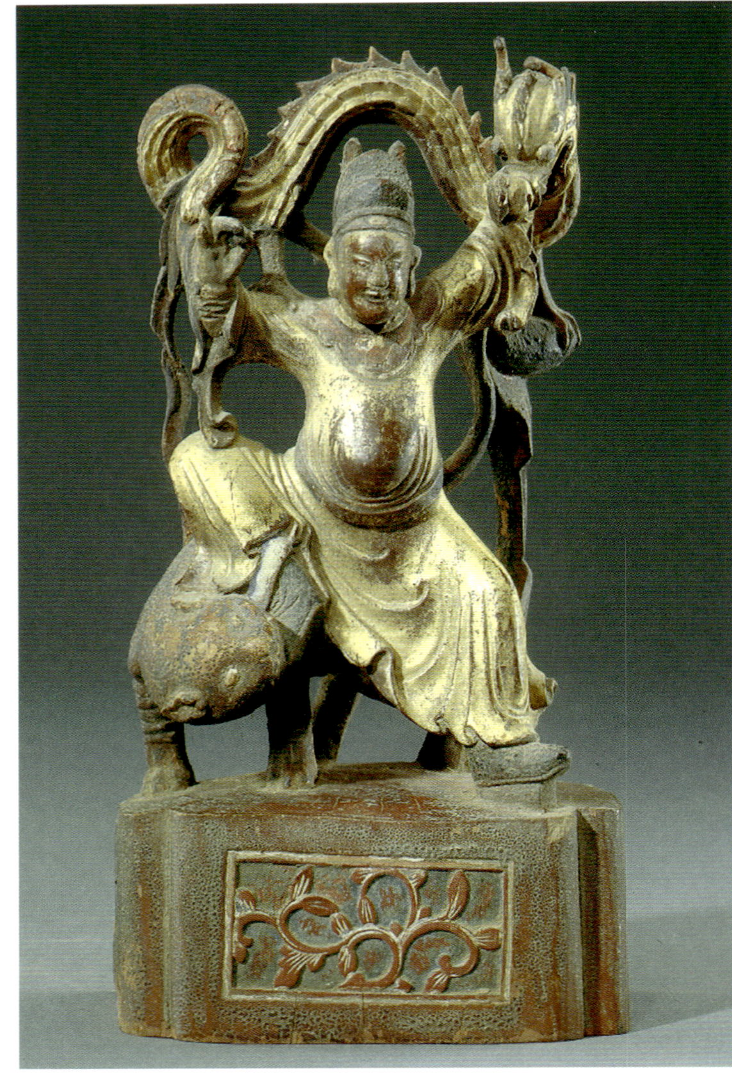

170. The Medicine God Sun Simiao seated on the tiger. He holds the dragon's beard in his left hand. Left: next to the tiger's head, two assistants. Right: the dragon god presenting his formulas to Sun Simiao. Behind: a sleeping Sun Simiao. Above center: Guanyin, the Goddess of Mercy, with a child on each side. Top left: Shennong. Top right: Huang Di. Wooden figure with applied gold-bronze and color, height 60 cm, Hunan, China, nineteenth century.

Detail of the sleeping Sun Simiao.

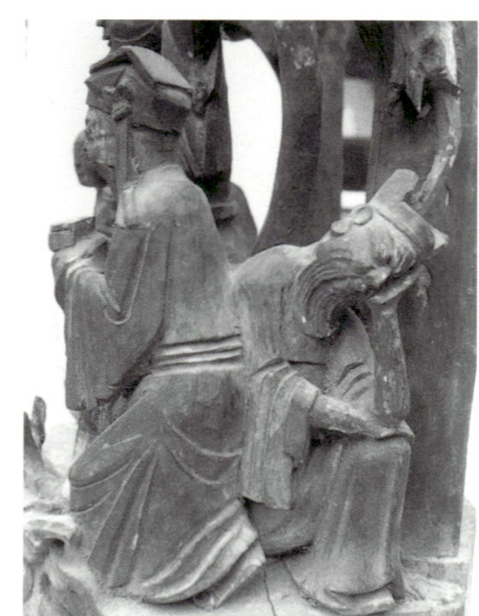

171. The Medicine God Sun Simiao seated on the tiger. He holds the dragon's head in his left hand. Wooden figure with applied gold-bronze and color, height 24 cm, Hunan, China, donor slip in the back dated to 1917.

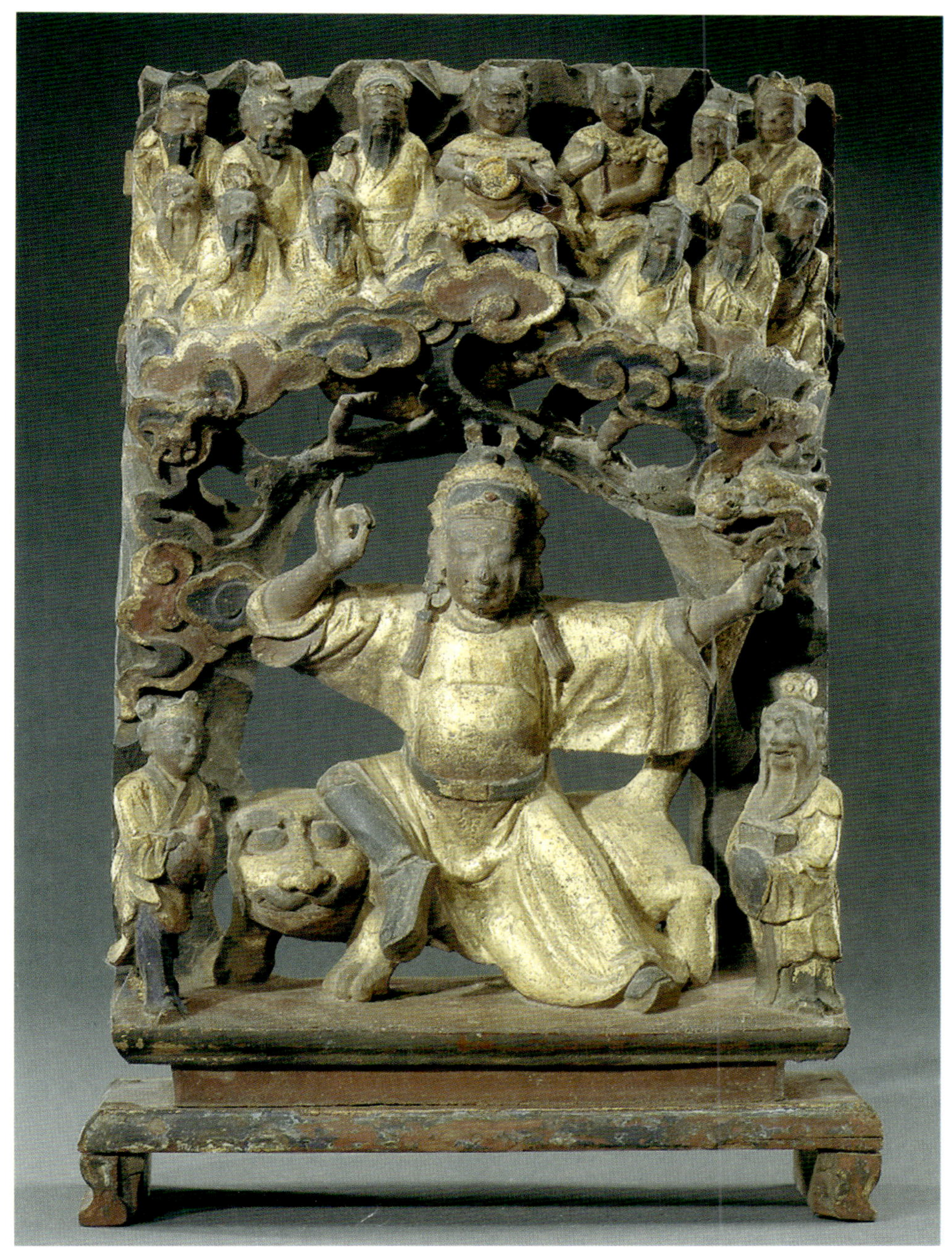

172. The Medicine God Sun
Simiao seated on the tiger. The
left hand is holding the dragon's
beard. Left: an assistant with
gourd. Right: the dragon god
presenting his formulas to Sun
Simiao. Above: thirteen figures.
Center: Fuxi, to his left Huang
Di, to his right Shennong.
Wooden figure with applied
gold-bronze and color, height
37.3 cm, Hunan, China, donor
slip in the back dated to 1758.

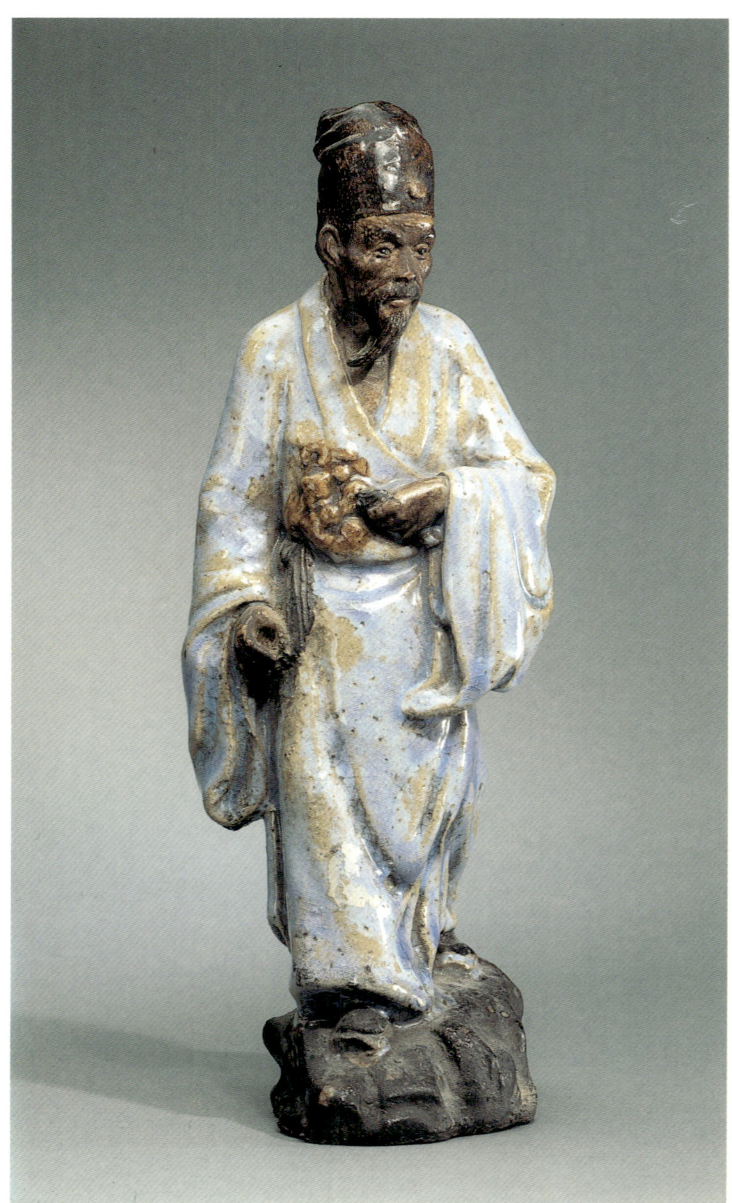

174. Barefoot doctor. Redwood, height 27 cm, South China, 1976.

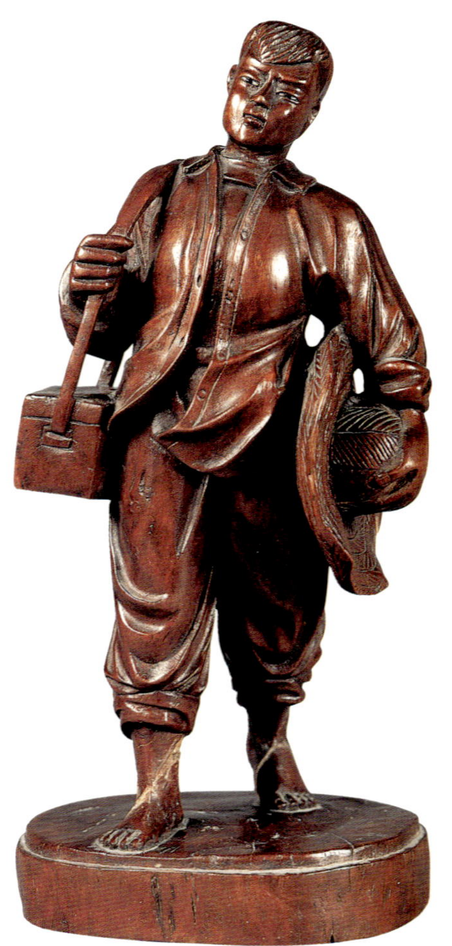

173. Li Shizhen 李時珍 (1518–1593), author of the encyclopedia of natural history and pharmaceutics *Bencao gang mu* 本草綱目. Stoneware, height 29.5 cm, South China.

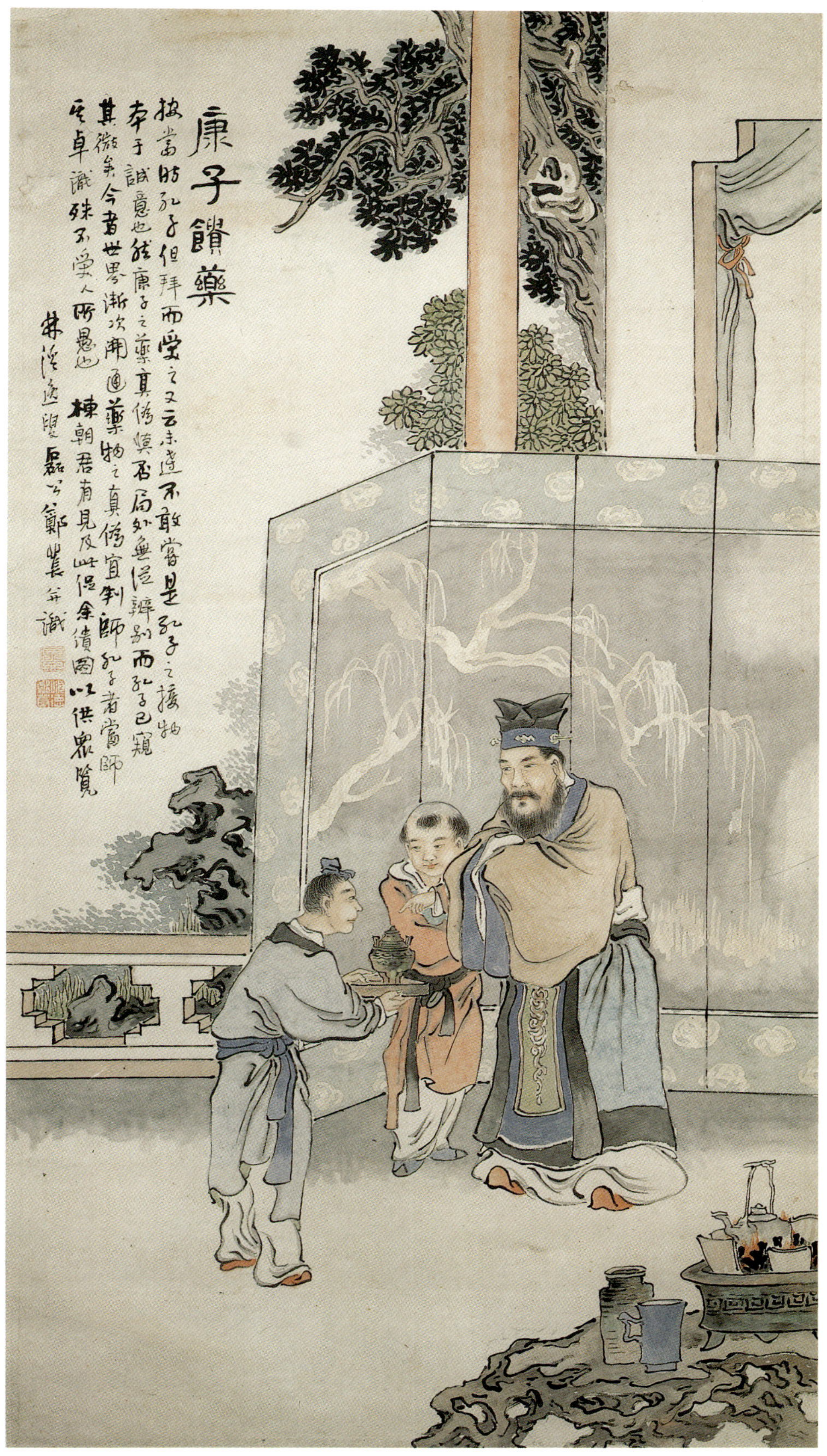

175. "Kangzi offers medicinal drugs [to Confucius]." Scroll drawing by Zheng Chang 鄭葨 from Canton, height 102 cm, width 55 cm, early twentieth century.

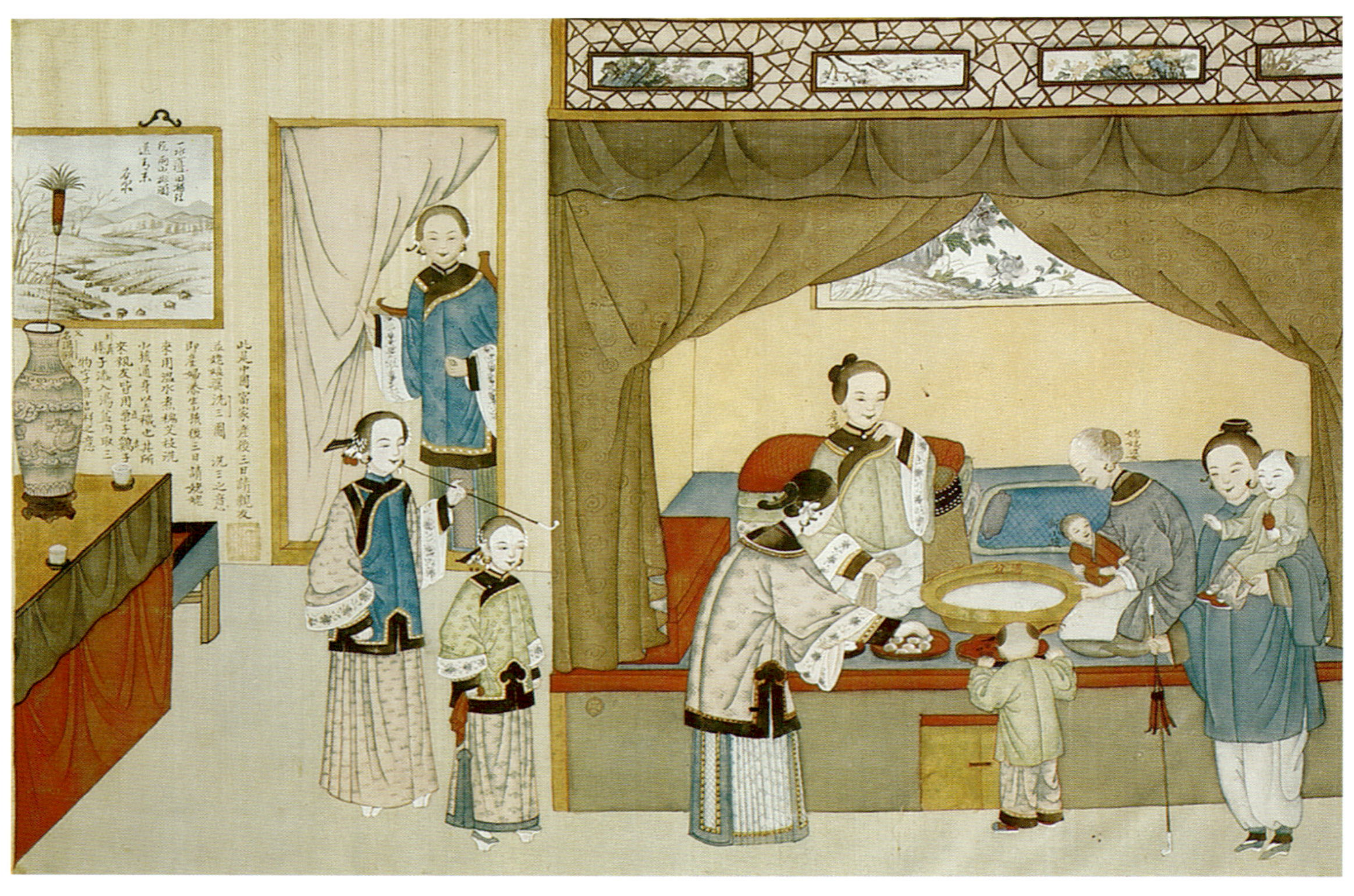

176. *Xi san* 洗三 "The bathing on the third day." Depiction of the bathing of a newborn on the third day after birth, common in well-off families of the late-Imperial period. For this, the oldest sister-in-law of the child's father was invited to wash the infant's entire body in warm water in which *hui* and *ai* branches had been boiled. This removed all impurities. Relatives and friends put *lizi* (chestnuts), *jizi* (chicken eggs), and *zhenzi* (hazelnuts) in the water, in order to attract good fortune [for the child], as it was implied by the pronunciation of these three substances: *li ji zhen*, "to provide with fortune and treasures." Museum für Völkerkunde, Berlin.

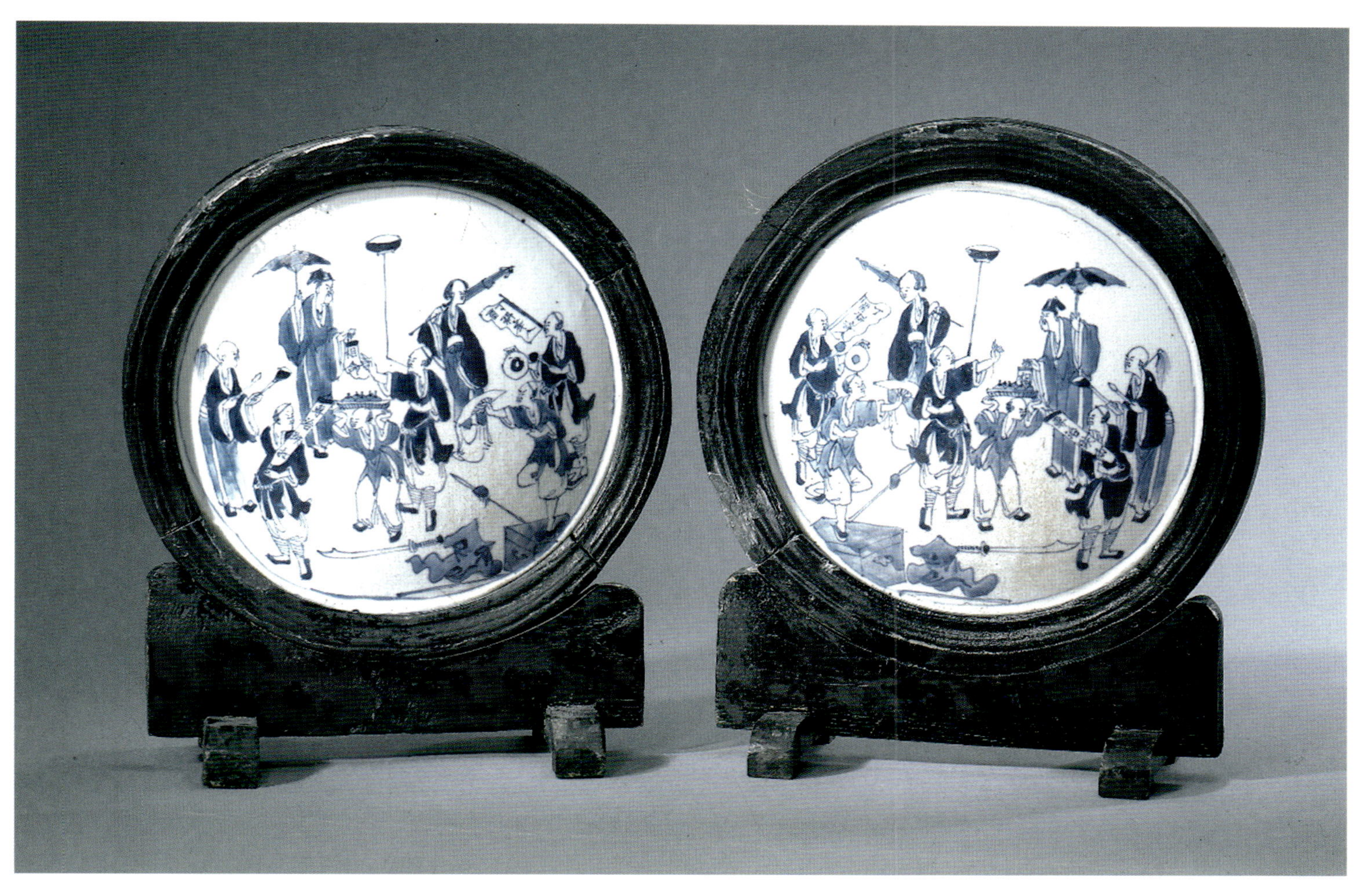

177. A market scene depicting an artist, a fortune teller, a fruit peddler, a messenger announcing the results of the examination for the official's career, and an itinerant doctor and medicine merchant. The four characters on the sign state: *zhuanzhi die da* "Curing especially [injuries from] falling or hitting." Two porcelain disks, mirror images, diameter 24 cm.

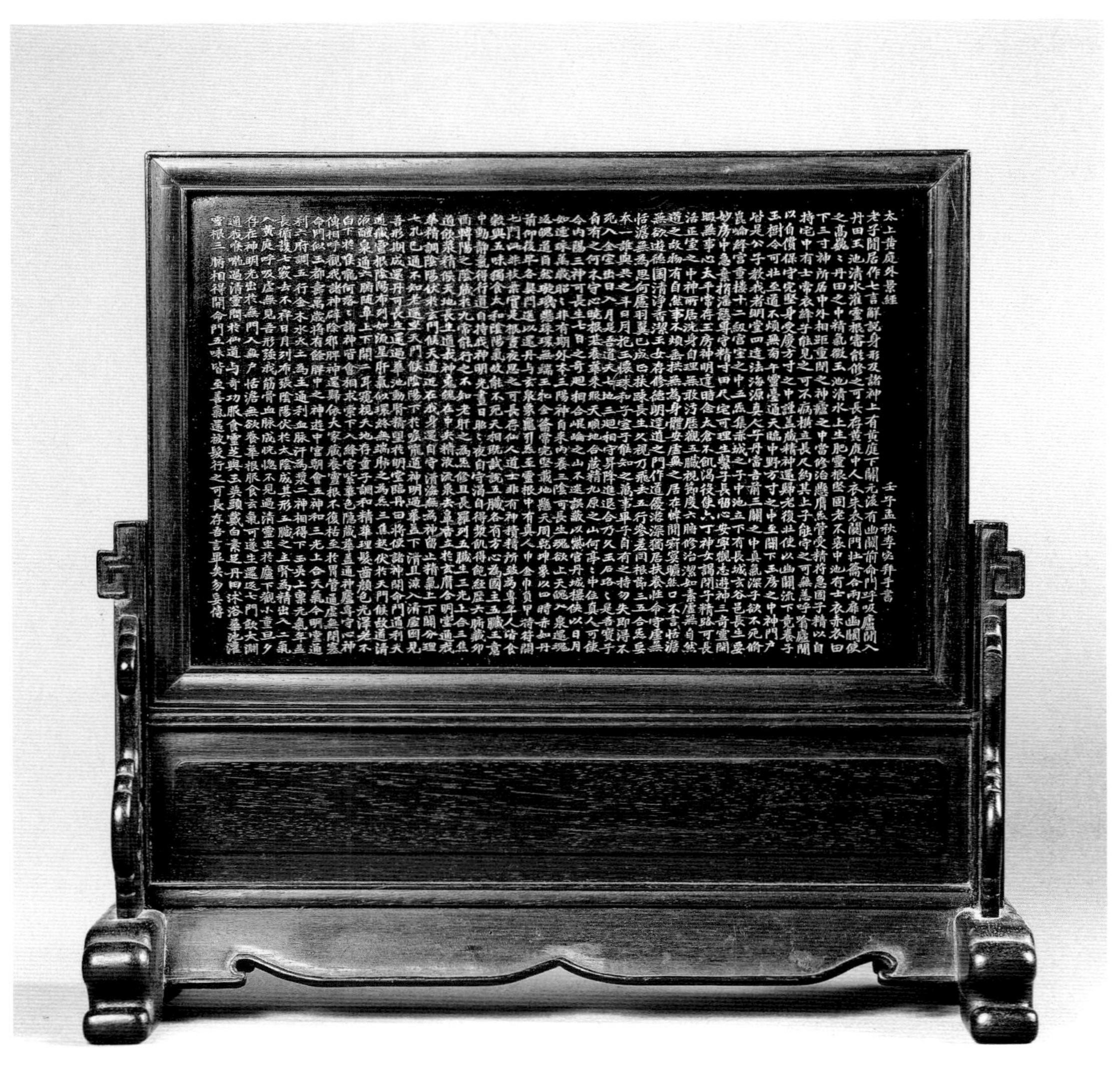

178. 太上黃庭外景經壬子
孟秋李宓拜手書 "Classic of
the External Appearance of the
Uppermost Yellow Pavilion. In
[the year of] *renzi*, in the first fall
month, handwritten respectfully
by Li Mi." Slate board, wooden
frame, wooden stand, engraving
of a medical text from the Daoist
canon *Daozang* 道藏 (Depository
of the Way), 1465 characters, gold
inlay, 25.5 x 18 cm.

# CHRONOLOGICAL CHART

| | |
|---|---|
| **Xia dynasty** | 21st–16th century B.C.E. |
| **Shang dynasty** | 16th–11th century B.C.E. |
| **Western Zhou dynasty** | 11th century–771 B.C.E. |
| **Eastern Zhou dynastie** | 770–256 B.C.E. |
| Spring and Autumn period | 722–481 B.C.E. |
| Warring States period | 481–222 B.C.E. |
| **Qin dynasty** | 221–206 B.C.E. |
| **Western Han dynasty** | 206 B.C.E.–C.E. 9 |
| **Xin dynasty** ( Wang Mang interregnum ) | C.E. 9–24 |
| **Eastern Han dynasty** | C.E. 25–220 |
| **Three Kingdoms period** | C.E. 220–265 |
| Wei dynasty | C.E. 220–266 |
| Shu Han dynasty | C.E. 221–263 |
| Wu dynasty | C.E. 222–280 |
| **Southern dynasties ( Six dynasties period )** | C.E. 221–589 |
| Western Jin dynasty | C.E. 266–313 |
| Eastern Jin dynasty | C.E. 317–420 |
| Liu Song dynasty | C.E. 420–479 |
| Southern Qi dynasty | C.E. 479–505 |
| Liang dynasty | C.E. 502–557 |
| Chen dynasty | C.E. 557–589 |
| **Sixteen Northern Kingdoms** | C.E. 304–439 |
| Wei dynasty | C.E. 385–557 |
| Northern Qi dynasty | C.E. 550–577 |
| Northern Zhou dynasty | C.E. 557–581 |
| **Sui dynasty** | C.E. 581–618 |
| **Tang dynasty** | C.E. 618–906 |
| **Five Dynasties period** | C.E. 907–960 |
| **Liao dynasty** | 907–1125 |
| **Song dynasty** | |
| Northern Song dynasty | 960–1127 |
| Southern Song dynasty | 1127–1279 |
| **Jin dynasty** | 1115–1234 |
| **Yuan dynasty** | 1279–1368 |
| **Ming dynasty** | 1368–1644 |
| **Qing dynasty** | 1644–1912 |
| **Republic/People's Republic** | since 1912/1949 |

# INDEX

acupressure 196

acupuncture 7, 11, 13, 19, 20, 22, 27, 31, 33, 35, 37, 42, 52, 57, 60, 63–66, 68, 83–85, 89, 92, 103, 104, 109, 127, 135–141, 191, 195, 196

advertisement, advertising 23, 56–61, 71, 72, 95, 142–149

alchemy, alchemists 27, 88, 89

amulet 54, 89, 96, 199–201

anatomy, anatomical knowledge 16, 33, 35, 39–41, 98, 103

ancestral healing 9, 10

aphrodisiacs 55, 56

aspirin 60

Ba Jin 107–109

bacteriology 14, 16, 35, 37

barefoot doctor 17, 99, 212

baths 11, 20

*Beijing minsu baitu* 75

*Bencao beiyao* 24

*Bencao gang mu* 24, 25, 43, 44, 98, 99

Berg, Daria 110

Bi Gongchen 39

Bian Que 22, 65–68, 97, 99

blood-letting 9, 11, 31, 83, 85, 104

Bodhidharma 204–207

breathing exercises 20, 37

Buddhism, Buddhist 15, 51, 69, 70, 72, 89, 90, 92, 95, 100, 128

*caozeyi* (country doctors) 73

Cao Yingfu 29

cauterization 11, 20, 27, 33, 80, 86, 104, 127

Chang E 104

Chao Yuanfang 33, 64

chemotherapy 16, 17

Cheng Yangqing 66

*Chuanya* 36–38, 73, 74, 79

Chunyu Yi 65–67

Cleyer, Andreas 7

coin swords, coins 96, 200

cold-related illnesses 26, 27, 66

Colledge, Dr. Thomas R. 16

compresses 11, 20, 37, 65

conduits 13, 30, 31, 40, 57, 66, 85

Confucianism 14, 26, 51, 62, 69, 71, 78, 95

Confucius 63, 101, 213

Cornaby, W.A. 61

cupping 20, 64, 86, 87, 194

Dai Sigong 64

*Danjing* 89

Daoism, Daoist 11, 14, 15, 26, 89, 216

*Daozang* 216

*De Humani Corporis Fabrica Libri Septem* 39

decoction, medicinal 7, 32, 44, 47

delivery containers 52, 54–56, 162–190

demonism, demonological 9, 10, 11, 14, 28, 36, 64, 89, 96, 100, 199–201, 203

dietetics 13, 15, 20, 22, 27

*Dongjing menghualu* 49

door gods 54

*Douzhen jingyan* 32

*douzhen niangniang* (Smallpox Empress) 96

Dragon King 90–92

"drug boat" 50, 109, 151

drugs 11, 17, 22, 30, 37, 46, 50, 63, 65, 68, 79, 89, 91

ear acupuncture 85

eight genies 55

ethical standards 38, 68–72, 89, 90

exorcistic, exorcism 9–11, 20, 28, 37, 63, 89, 134

*Falü yixue* 41

Five Phases 12, 31, 34

Fleck, Ludwik 34

folk medicine 27, 28, 36–38

formulary literature 11, 21, 24, 27–30, 32, 38, 42, 45, 49, 57, 66, 81, 88, 90

Fryer, John 41

*fu* (palaces or prefectures) 13, 30, 40, 77

fumigation 20, 37

functional centers 13, 27, 30

Gong Tingxian 65

Gong Xin 65

gourd, calabash 48, 100, 102, 198

Gray's *Anatomy* 41

grinding bowl 51, 155, 159

Guan Maocai 16, 40

Guanyin 92, 95, 96, 99

Guo Ziyi 182

gynecology 27, 33, 49, 65, 82, 106

Han Kang 53

Harper, Donald 20

*heihua* ("dark speach"), see secret language

He Xiangu 183

Hippocratic oath 68, 88, 90

Hobson, Benjamin 16, 40

*Hu bencao* 24

*Hu Qingyu tang* 51, 52

Hua Tuo 67, 99, 206

*Huainanzi* 15

Huang Di 70, 71, 92

*Huang Di hamajing* 103, 104

*Huang Di neijing* 19, 20, 30, 31, 39, 83, 203

*Huang Di neijing lingshu* 30, 83

*Huang Di neijing suwen* 11, 30, 31

*Huang Di neijing taisu* 31

Huangfu Mi 33

*hulu*, see gourd

Idema, Wilt 110

itinerant doctors 36–38, 62, 65, 66, 68, 73–82, 99, 100, 102, 111–113, 214

itinerant medicine peddlers 51, 62, 63, 65, 101, 111, 112

Jenner, Edward 16

*Jiang sangzhen Cai Shun fengmu* 108

*Jianghu neimu heihuakao* 79

*jianghuyi* (doctors [who pass] over rivers and lakes) 73

*Jingshi zhenglei daguan bencao* 24

*Jingui yaolüe fang lun* 26, 66

*Jinjing* 89

*Jinpingmei* 50, 69, 109, 110

*jiyi* (physicians for illnesses) 63

*Kaibao xin xiangding bencao* 23, 24

*kampo* (Chinese formula) 60

Kanban (advertising board) 148, 149

Kangzi 63, 213

*Kangzi kuiyao* 101

Kuhn, Thomas 34

*A Laborer's Love* 107, 108

Lao She 109

Le Fengming 51

Le Xianchang 51

Legalism 14

Leigong 52, 96, 203

*Leigong paozhi lun* 203

Li Cikou 74

Li Gao 34

Li Ji 23

Li Shizhen 24, 43, 98, 99, 199, 212

Li Yanwen 24

*Liaofengqi zhufang* 64

*lingyi* (bell doctors) 73, 110

Liu Fang 33

Liu Han 23

Liu Wansu 34

*Lü chanyan bencao* 22, 104, 105

Lu He 24

Lu Xun 107–109

*Lun taiyi jingcheng* 88

magic, magical 7, 9, 11, 20, 21, 36, 43, 89, 94, 96, 199

Mai Sun 74, 79

*Maijing* 33

*maiyaosuo* (Store for Selling Medicines) 49

malpractice legislation 67, 68

Mao Zedong 99

massage 9, 11, 20, 63, 64, 87, 191, 196

materia medica 9, 15, 22–24, 29, 42–45, 52, 92, 98, 104, 105

Mawangdui 10, 11, 13, 19, 20, 21, 23, 24, 36, 42, 48, 55, 86, 103

Medicine King, medicine god 88, 90–94, 99, 108, 143, 208–211

Medicine of Systematic Correspondences 12

Meiji 17, 60

Meng Yuanlao 49

mortar 50, 51, 153–155, 159

*moxa*, moxibustion 35, 37, 52, 57, 80, 86, 89, 109

Nagai 44
*Nanjing* 31, 39
*Neijingtu* 14

ophthalmology 33, 39, 41, 60, 90, 105, 106, 125
opium 16, 43, 44, 56
opium containers 56, 172
oracle bones 8

Pang Anshi 24
Paracelsus 36
Parker, Dr. Peter 16, 18
peach wood 54, 96, 200
Pearson, Dr. 16
pediatrics 27, 33, 49, 64, 65, 87
pharmaceutical literature 22, 23, 29, 30, 43
pharmeceutics 10, 14, 23, 40, 42–48, 81, 100, 142, 150, 203
pharmacies, pharmacist 27, 29, 42–61, 63, 68, 82, 98, 100, 101, 111, 142, 145, 148, 150–190
physical exercises 11, 20, 21, 89
point ointment , see topical ointment
processing of medicinal drugs 45–48, 49
psychological methods 38, 75–81
public health measures 27, 28, 29
public welfare pharmacies 29
pulse 7, 20, 31, 33, 66, 81, 82, 83, 84, 191
pulse pillow 83, 84, 85, 191, 192

qi 13, 20, 22, 31, 32, 37, 44, 45, 51, 57, 77, 81, 84–87, 125, 132, 145
Qi Bo 70, 71
Qian Yi 64
*Qianjin fang* 89
*Qianjin yifang* 22, 89
Qin Chengzu 67
Qin Linbing 56
*Qingming shanghetu* 29, 49, 50, 111
*Qingrentang yaomu* 53
*Quanti xuzhi* 41
*Quantu niumatuojing* 33

rattle 51, 73, 74, 75
religious, religion 9, 11, 20, 88–92, 95, 96, 199
*Renzhen zhuan* 24
*ruyi* (scholar physicians) 65, 67, 68

Schreck, Johann 39, 40
secret language 79–81
*Shanghan lun* 24, 26, 66
*Shanghan zabing lun* 24, 66
*shangyaojian* (Director of Palace Medications) 48
*shangyaoju* (Palace Office of Pharmaceutics) 48, 49, 63
*Shengji zonglu* 28
Shennong 15, 23, 92, 202, 204
*Shennong bencaojing* 23
*Shennong bencaojing jizhu* 14
*Shenshi yaohan yanke daquan* 125
*Shiji* 11, 65
*Shiwu bencao* 24
*Shiwubencao huizuan* 26
*shiyi* (dietary physicians) 63
*shouyi* (veterinarians) 63
*shuiluhui* (Water-and-Land Ritual) 99–102
*shuyaosuo* (Pharmacies for Processed Medicines) 49
Sima Qian 11, 65
Sivin, Nathan 88
Song Ci 33
*Songfentang* 51
*Specimen Medicinae Sinicae sive Opuscula Medica ad mentem Sinensium* 7
Stein, Sir Aurel 11
Stove God 9
Su Jing 23
Sudhoff, Karl 103
Sun Simiao 22, 27, 33, 68, 69, 72, 88–95, 99, 108, 109, 208–211
Sun Yatsen 107
surgery 11, 20, 98

*Taiping huimin hejiju fang* 28
*Taiping shenghui fang* 27
*taipinghuiminju* (Office for the Provision of the Population in Great Peace) 49
*Taixi renshen shuogai* 39, 40
*taiyi* (palace physicians, eminent or outstanding physician) 48, 63–66, 69, 108–110
*taiyiju* (Imperial Office of Medicine) 64, 65
*Taiyiju fang* 27
*taiyiling* (Office of the Palace Physician) 63
*taiyishu* (Imperial Department of Medicine) 64, 67
*taiyiyuan* (Imperial Academy of Medicine) 64

talisman 10, 36, 55, 56
Tang Shenwei 24
Tang Zonghai 41
Tao Hongjing 14, 15
"tiger sting," see rattle
*Tongren shuxue zhenjiu tujing* 85
*Tongrentang* 51
topical ointments 56, 57, 58, 59, 60, 143
trigrams 34, 55, 74, 171
Triple Burner 13
*tuina* (pushing and pulling) 34, 87, 133
*Tuxiang bencao mengquan* 66, 67
*Tuzhu nanjing maijue* 31, 126

Vesalius 36, 103
vessels 13, 20, 30, 66
veterinary medicine 25, 33, 128
von Kalkar, Stefan 103
von Wesel, Andreas, see Vesalius

*Waitai biyao* 27
*Wanbing huichun* 65
Wang An 24
Wang Anshi 49
Wang Bing 31
Wang Dao 27
Wang Huaiyin 27
Wang Jie 104
Wang Qingren 35, 40
Wang Shuhe 24, 33
Wang Weiyi 85
Western medicine 8, 16, 17, 29, 39, 40, 41, 60, 61, 70, 81, 82, 97, 105, 108, 109
*Wushier bingfang* 10, 11, 20, 23, 24, 42, 43

*Xi xuan jilu* 33
Xia Liangxin 24
*Xianchun Lin'an zhi* 48
*Xiao'er tuina guangyi* 34
*Xiaoeryaozheng zhijue* 64
*Xingshi yinyuan zhuan* 109, 110
*Xinxiu bencao* 23, 43
*Xinyixue tushuo* 39
*xiuheyaosuo* 49
*Xiuzhi yao fa* 24
*Xiyi luelun* 16, 40
Xu Dachun 15, 16, 62, 72
Xu Mai 53
Xu Yanzuo 69
Xue Mo 79

*Yanfang xinbian* 32
Yang Shangshan 31
*yangyi* (physicians for ulcers) 63
*Yangyi daquan* 125, 128
*Yanke daquan* 41
*Yijing* 34, 55
*Yilin gaicuo* 35, 40
*Yinhai jingwei* 33, 90
yin-yang 12, 26, 55, 66, 170
yin-yang and Five Phases theories 15, 21, 26, 30, 35, 36, 37, 45
*yixue tijusi* (Bureau for the Supervision of Medical Schools) 64
*Yixue Yuanliu lun* 15
*yiyaohejiju* (Office for the Composition of Medicinal Drugs) 49
*yiyaohuiminju* (Office for the Provision of the Population with Medicinal Drugs) 49
*yongyi* (common physicians) 67
*Youyou xinshu* 33
*Yuan Heng liaomaji* 33, 103, 128
*Yucuan yizongjinjian* 33, 124, 127, 129, 130
*yuyaofang, yuyaoju, or yuyaoyuan* (imperial pharmacy) 49
*Yuzhi bencao pinghui jingyao* 42, 43, 105, 121–123

*zang* (depots) 13, 30, 40
Zhang Bozu 66
Zhang Congzheng 34
Zhang Ji 22, 24, 26, 27, 66, 67
Zhang Shicuang 107, 108
Zhang Wenzhong 64
Zhang Zeduan 50
Zhang Zhongjing, see Zhang Ji
Zhao Xuemin 36, 38, 73, 79
Zheng Chang 63, 101
Zheng Qian 24
*Zhengbuhuitu zhenjiudacheng* 35
Zhenghe 28
*Zhengzhi yaojue* 65
*Zhenjiu jiayijing* 33
*Zhiwu mingshitu kao* 105
*Zhongxi huitong yijing jingyi* 41
Zhu Xi 98
Zhu Zhenheng 28
Zhuangzi 15
*Zhubing yuanhou lun* 33, 64
Zong Boyun 36, 38
*zou fang yi* (wandering doctors) 73